Nuclear Medicine
A Case-Based Approach

Nuclear Medicine
A Case-Based Approach

Editor-in-Chief

Munir Ghesani MD FACNM
Assistant Professor of Radiology
Director of PET/CT Fellowship
NYU Langone Medical Center
New York City, New York, USA

Section Editors

Nasrin Ghesani MD
Associate Professor of Radiology
Rutgers New Jersey Medical School
Newark, New Jersey, USA

E Gordon DePuey MD
Professor of Radiology
Director of Nuclear Medicine
Mount Sinai, St Luke's-Mount Sinai
Roosevelt Hospitals
New York, NY, USA

Amir Kashefi MD
Board Certified in Nuclear Medicine
Abdominal Imaging and Interventional Radiology Fellow
Massachusetts General Hospital
Harvard Medical School
Boston, Massachusetts, USA

Yi Chen Zhang MD
Radiology Resident
Mount Sinai, St Luke's-Mount Sinai
Roosevelt Hospital
New York, NY, USA

Foreword

Satoshi Minoshima MD PhD

JAYPEE *The Health Sciences Publisher*
Philadelphia | New Delhi | London | Panama

Jaypee Brothers Medical Publishers (P) Ltd

Headquarters
Jaypee Brothers Medical Publishers (P) Ltd.
4838/24, Ansari Road, Daryaganj
New Delhi 110 002, India
Phone: +91-11-43574357
Fax: +91-11-43574314
E-mail: jaypee@jaypeebrothers.com

Overseas Offices
J.P. Medical Ltd.
83, Victoria Street, London
SW1H 0HW (UK)
Phone: +44-20 3170 8910
Fax: +44(0)20 3008 6180
E-mail: info@jpmedpub.com

Jaypee-Highlights Medical Publishers Inc.
City of Knowledge, Bld. 237, Clayton
Panama City, Panama
Phone: +1 507-301-0496
Fax: +1 507-301-0499
E-mail: cservice@jphmedical.com

Jaypee Medical Inc.
325 Chestnut Street
Suite 412
Philadelphia, PA 19106, USA
Phone: +1 267-519-9789
E-mail: support@jpmedus.com

Jaypee Brothers Medical Publishers (P) Ltd.
17/1-B, Babar Road, Block-B, Shaymali
Mohammadpur, Dhaka-1207
Bangladesh
Mobile: +08801912003485
E-mail: jaypeedhaka@gmail.com

Jaypee Brothers Medical Publishers (P) Ltd.
Bhotahity, Kathmandu, Nepal
Phone: +977-9741283608
E-mail: kathmandu@jaypeebrothers.com

Website: www.jaypeebrothers.com
Website: www.jaypeedigital.com

Inquiries for bulk sales may be solicited at: jaypee@jaypeebrothers.com

Nuclear Medicine: A Case-Based Approach

First Edition: **2016,** Reprint: 2024

ISBN: 978-93-5152-965-1

Printed in India

Dedicated to

My parents, my wife, my children and my sister for their selfless love, inspiration and support and in loving memory of my mother...

Munir Ghesani MD FACNM

My mother...

Nasrin Ghesani MD

My wife, Golnaz and my daughter, Keemia for their kindness, devotion and endless support. My mother, for her unconditional love and in loving memory of my dad...

Amir Kashefi MD

Contributors

Ramsey D Badawi PhD
Associate Professor of Radiology
and Biomedical Engineering
Director of Nuclear
Medicine Research
Molecular Imaging
Chair in Radiology
Sacramento, California, USA

Mohsen Beheshti MD FEBNM FASNC
Associate Professor in
Nuclear Medicine
Deputy Director PET/CT
Center Linz
Department of Nuclear Medicine
and Endocrinology
St Vincent's Hospital
Seilerstaette 4, Linz, Austria

Abhijit J Chaudhari PhD
Assistant Professor of
Radiology UC Davis
School of Medicine
Sacramento, California, USA

E Gordon DePuey MD
Professor of Radiology
Director of Nuclear Medicine
Mount Sinai
St Luke's-Mount Sinai
Roosevelt Hospitals
New York, NY, USA

Munir Ghesani MD FACNM
Assistant Professor of Radiology
Director of PET/CT Fellowship
NYU Langone Medical Center
New York City, New York, USA

Nasrin Ghesani MD
Associate Professor of Radiology
Rutgers New Jersey Medical School
Newark, New Jersey, USA

Amir Kashefi MD
Board Certified in Nuclear Medicine
Abdominal Imaging and Interventional
Radiology Fellow
Massachusetts General Hospital
Harvard Medical School
Boston, Masschusetts, USA

Jonathan Kuo MD
Nuclear Medicine Chief Resident
Department of Nuclear Medicine
UC Davis Medical Center
Sacramento, California, USA

Werner Langsteger MD FACE
Professor in Internal and Nuclear Medicine
Head of PET/CT Center Linz
Department of Nuclear Medicine
and Endocrinology
St Vincent's Hospital
Seilerstaette 4, Linz, Austria

Johan Löfgren MD Ian Law MD DMSc PhD
Department of Clinical Physiology
Nuclear Medicine and PET
Rigshospitalet, Copenhagen, Denmark

Stephen Malutich MD
Nuclear Medicine Resident
Department of Nuclear Medicine
UC Davis Medical Center
Sacramento, California, USA

Christian Pirich MD
Professor in Internal
and Nuclear Medicine
Head of Department
of Nuclear Medicine and
Endocrinology
Paracelsus Private
Medical University
Strubergasse 21, Salzburg, Austria

Yi Chen Zhang MD
Radiology Resident
Mount Sinai
St Luke's-Mount Sinai
Roosevelt Hospital
New York, NY, USA

Foreword

I am very happy to see Dr Ghesani's first edition of *Nuclear Medicine: A Case-Based Approach*. This book presents excellent case-based nuclear medicine studies that should be useful for trainees, practicing physicians, and technologists. Dr Ghesani was able to assemble a team of Section Editors and contributing authors across the world. Not only general nuclear medicine studies, but also nuclear cardiology and PET/CT studies are well-represented in this book. This is a clear reflection of Dr Ghesani's well-regarded expertise in clinical nuclear medicine and also his enthusiasm for nuclear medicine education. I hope this book will be read by many and serve as an indispensable case reference. Congratulations for the publication.

Satoshi Minoshima MD PhD
Professor and Chair
Department of Radiology
University of Utah
Salt Lake City, Utah, USA

Preface

Throughout my training and years in practice the concept of case-based learning has appealed me tremendously. While preparing for nuclear medicine and radiology board examinations, I relied heavily on the case-based teaching material, and have supplemented it considerably with my own teaching file cases created over the years. In order to communicate key learning principles, I have published a few of these cases in the form of case reports and have included several others in various sections of this book. It is my sincere hope that the potpourri of cases covering broad areas of nuclear medicine and molecular imaging will enrich and enhance the knowledge of the reader without making the learning process unwieldy.

Munir Ghesani

Acknowledgments

First and foremost, I acknowledge unconditional support and understanding of my wife and my children in making this book a reality. I acknowledge the contribution of several mentors who have motivated me during my training and my two decades of practice to aim higher. I truly value my interactions with medical students, radiology residents and fellows. In the process of preparing for the conferences and contributing to review sessions, I myself continue to learn tremendously from them.

I am very thankful to Mr Jitendar P Vij (Group Chairman), Mr Ankit Vij (Group President), Ms Chetna Malhotra Vohra (Associate Director), Ms Sheetal Arora Kapoor (Development Editor) and production team of Jaypee Brothers Medical Publishers (P) Ltd., New Delhi, India for providing me with the exciting opportunity to write this book, for their patience through this journey and for providing kind words of encouragement and support.

Munir Ghesani

I would like to thank Stephen Malutich MD, and Jonathan Kuo MD, for their help and contribution to chest and abdomen PET/CT cases; and Mohsen Beheshti MD, Werner Langsteger MD, Ramsey Badawi PhD, Abhijit Chaudhari PhD, Christian Pirich MD, Johan Löfgren MD, Ian Law MD PhD, and Andrea Ferrerod for their help and contribution to Non-FDG PET cases. I would also like to thank faculty and technologists at UC Davis Medical Center for all that they taught me. I would like to acknowledge their efforts, without whom this book would not be possible.

Amir Kashefi

Contents

Section 1: General Nuclear Medicine

Nasrin Ghesani, Yi Chen Zhang, Munir Ghesani

Section 2: Nuclear Cardiology

E Gordon DePuey, Munir Ghesani

Section 3: PET/CT

Amir Kashefi, Munir Ghesani

Section 1

General Nuclear Medicine

Nasrin Ghesani, Yi Chen Zhang, Munir Ghesani

Cases

CASE 1: ASSESSMENT OF OSSEOUS METASTATIC DISEASE IN THYROID CANCER

Brief History

A 63-year-old female with left leg pain. Plain radiographs showed a lytic bony lesion in the proximal left femur associated with intertrochanteric hip fracture and a soft tissue mass. A whole body bone scan was performed for evaluation of osseous metastatic disease.

Findings

Whole body bone scan demonstrates increased tracer uptake corresponding to the pathologic fracture. Uptake on the bone scan in this case may be due to metastatic disease itself, post-traumatic remodeling or a combination thereof. In contrast, significant increased uptake in the left hip on whole body iodine scan is more likely to represent metastatic thyroid carcinoma. Follicular carcinoma is more likely than papillary carcinoma to metastasize to skeleton. Foci of uptake in the neck on the iodine scan may be due to residual thyroid gland after thyroidectomy, local/marginal recurrence of thyroid malignancy or due to regional nodal metastatic disease.

Main Teaching Points

- With regards to skeletal metastatic disease from thyroid carcinoma uptake of radioiodine corresponding to the suspected lesion is more specific for metastatic disease than any uptake on bone scan. Follicular carcinoma is

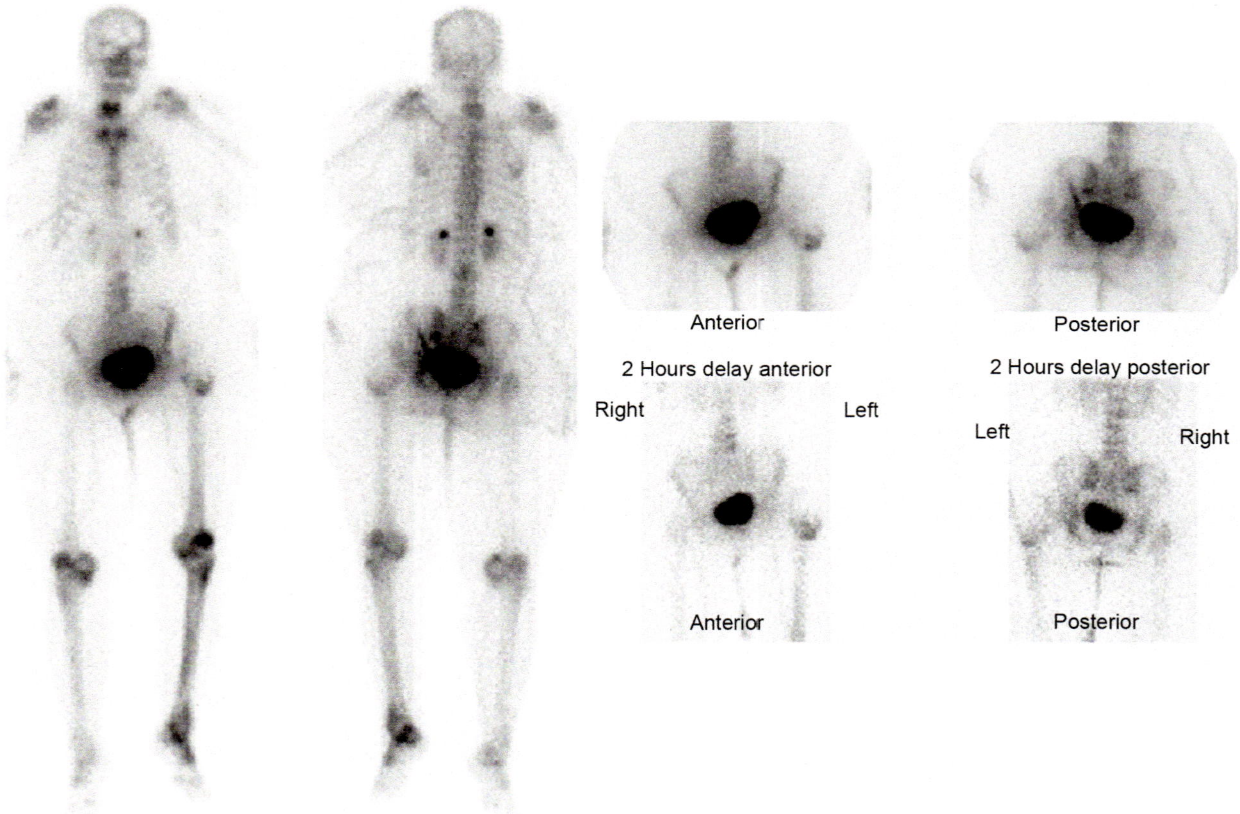

Fig. 1: Whole Body Tc-99m methylene diphosphonate (MDP) Bone Scan demonstrated increased radiotracer uptake in the left proximal femur, at the site of known pathological fracture through the known soft tissue mass.

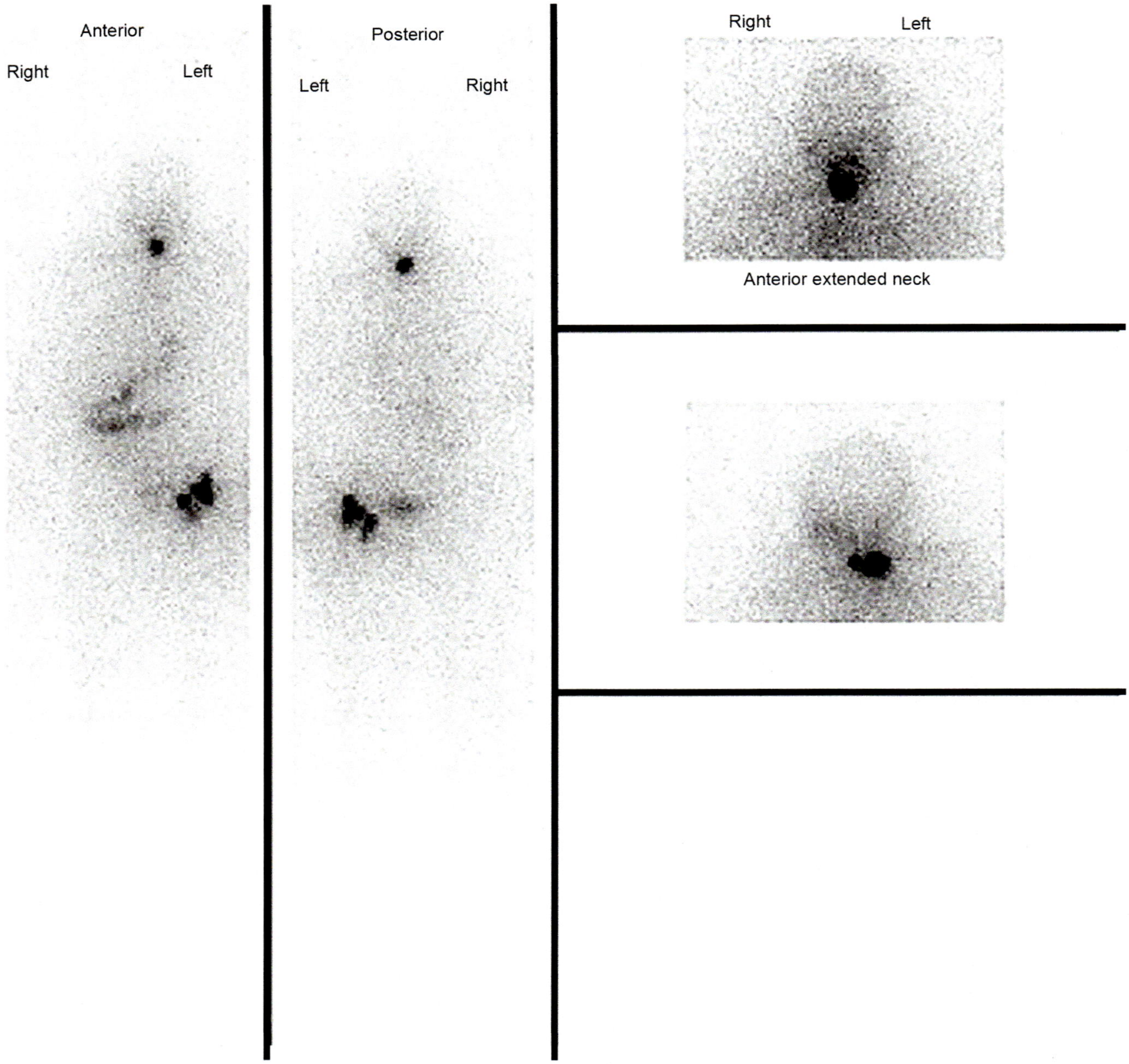

Fig. 2: Whole body ^{131}I scan performed after total thyroidectomy demonstrated increased radiotracer uptake in the thyroidectomy bed, compatible with residual thyroid tissue/residual neoplasm. Markedly abnormal uptake was noted in the left him metastatic lesion.

more likely to metastasize to skeleton whereas papillary carcinoma more commonly spreads to regional lymph nodes in the neck, in the mediastinum and in the lungs.

- If papillary/follicular tumor dedifferentiates and is no longer ioxdine-avid, but the patient has a rising serum thyroglobulin (Tg), ^{18}F Fluorodeoxyglucose-positron emission tomography/computed tomography (FDG-PET/CT) may identify metabolically active tumor.

REFERENCE

1. Coleman RE. Skeletal complications of malignancy. Cancer. 1997;80(8 Suppl):1588-94.

CASE 2: EVALUATION OF HYDRONEPHROSIS

Brief History

A 36-year-old woman is incidentally diagnosed with right-sided hydronephrosis.

Findings

Diuretic Furosemide was administered at the time of tracer injection (F0). Dynamic phase of Tc-99m mercaptoacetyltriglycin (MAG3) scan shows normal activity in the abdominal aorta with prompt and normal flow to the left kidney. However, there is moderate impairment of flow to the right kidney. In function phase images, there is normal cortical transit and prompt excretion of radiotracer from the left kidney. There is persistent retention of radiotracer in the enlarged right kidney with no evidence of radiotracer excretion. The T1/2 Lasix washout time of the left kidney is 4.9 minutes and the right kidney is >20 minutes. The findings are compatible with high grade ureteropelvic junction obstruction.

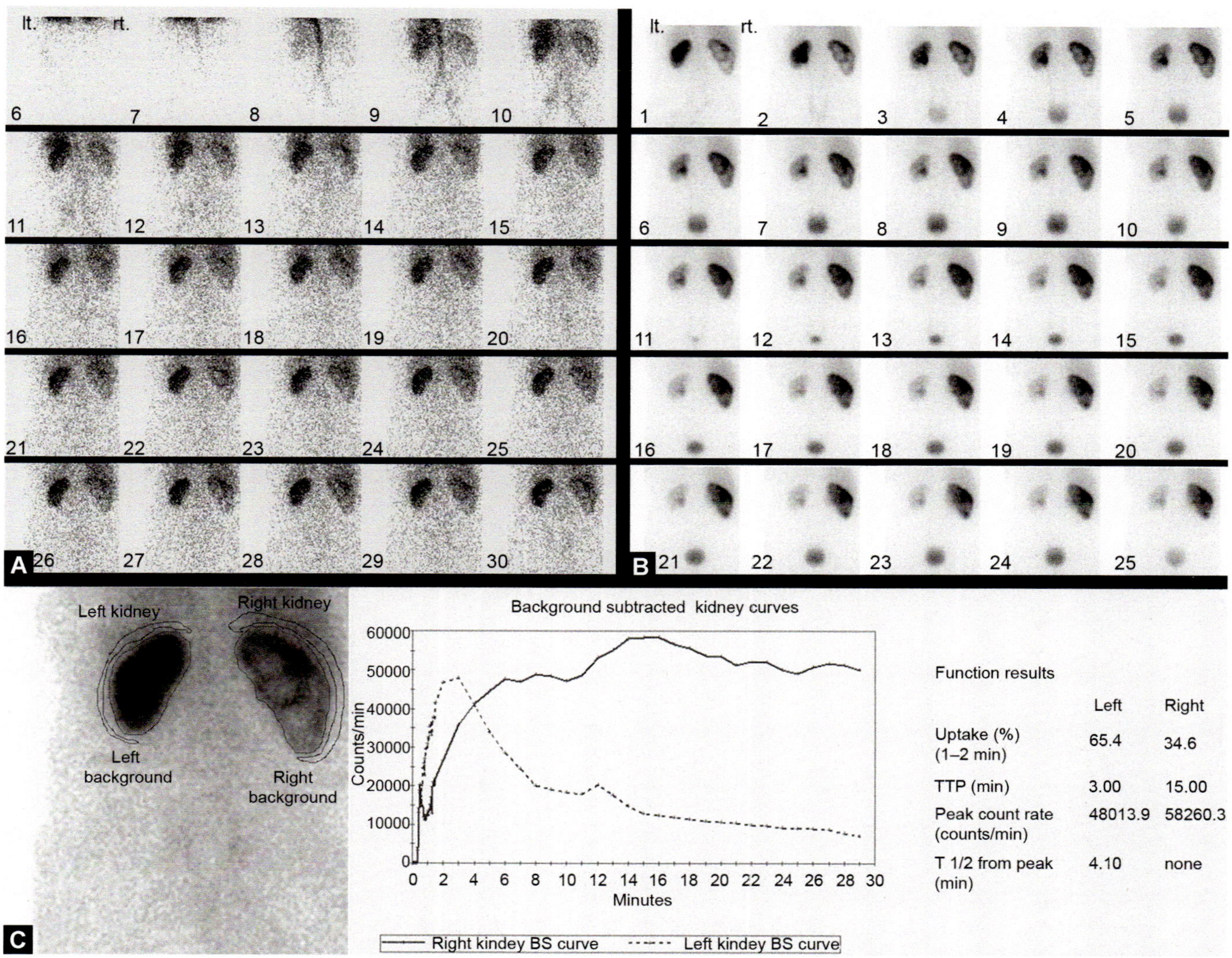

Figs. 1A to C: F-0 Diuretic renography with Tc-99m MAG-3 in posterior projection. Radionuclide angiographic images (A) demonstrate prompt blood flow to the left kidney and delayed and diminished blood flow to the enlarged right kidney. Function phase images (B) demonstrate normal cortical transit and prompt excretion of radiotracer from the left kidney and persistent retention of radiotracer with no evidence of radiotracer excretion in the right kidney. The findings are compatible with right UPJ obstruction. Renogram (C) confirms the findings.

Main Teaching Points

- Urinary obstruction can lead to forniceal rupture and urine leak in the acute setting and can cause parenchymal atrophy and renal failure on a chronic basis. A finding of dilated collecting system on CT or ultrasound is not specific for obstruction as a similar pattern can on seen on these imaging modalities irrespective of presence or absence of dynamic obstruction. Diuretic renography is an excellent and more specific method for evaluating patients with suspected urinary obstruction. In general, an emptying half-life (T1/2) of less than 10–15 minutes supports lack of obstruction, greater than 20 minutes is considered obstructive, and values in between are indeterminate. Irrespective of presence or absence of dynamic obstruction the Lasix administration cannot facilitate washout from the cortical into collecting system.
- Serial diuretic renography can be performed to determine the significance of a partial obstruction and to assess effectiveness of stenting or surgical correction. Pyeloplasty is performed with a high success rate, although residual obstruction on diuretic renography may persist.

REFERENCE

1. Sarhan O, Helmy T, Abou-El Ghar M, et al. Long-term functional and morphological outcome after pyeloplasty for huge renal pelvis. BJU Int. 2011;107(5):829-33.

CASE 3: ASSESSMENT OF GASTROINTESTINAL (GI) BLEEDING SITE

Brief History

A 62-year-old woman presents with acute bright red bleeding per rectum. A tagged red blood cell (RBC) scan was performed to localize the bleeding site.

Findings

Sequential images of a Tc-99m tagged RBC scan show abnormal accumulation of tracer activity at the hepatic flexure representing GI hemorrhage into the large bowel lumen. Over time, the hemorrhage traveled with peristalsis in an antegrade direction through the bowel. Small bowel bleeding, in contrast to large bowel, may show serpiginous activity, which changes rapidly over time.

Main Teaching Points

- Etiologies for lower GI hemorrhage include angiodysplasia, diverticula, polyps and neoplasm. A bleeding site is identified as a focal area of increased activity in the abdomen, within the right upper quadrant, which progresses distally in to the transverse colon. Criteria for a positive GI bleed study include a focal accumulation of abnormal activity, which moves over time.
- Gastrointestinal bleeding study with in vitro Tc-99m tagged RBC can detect bleeding rates as low as 0.3–0.5 mL/min when performed during an active bleed compared to a threshold of 1 mL/min by catheter angiography. Delayed images may show tracer accumulation at a site distant from the location of bleed due to peristalsis that transports Tc-99m tagged RBC in an antegrade or retrograde direction through the bowel. Tc-99m tagged RBC method is more sensitive than Tc-99m sulfur colloid imaging and has largely replaced the latter as a preferred method of imaging in an effort to localize the site of GI bleeding.
- Methods of Tc-99m RBC labeling include in vivo method (labeling efficiency: 75–80%), modified in vivo method (labeling efficiency: 85–90%), and in vitro commercial kit (ULTRATAG) (labeling efficiency: >97%).

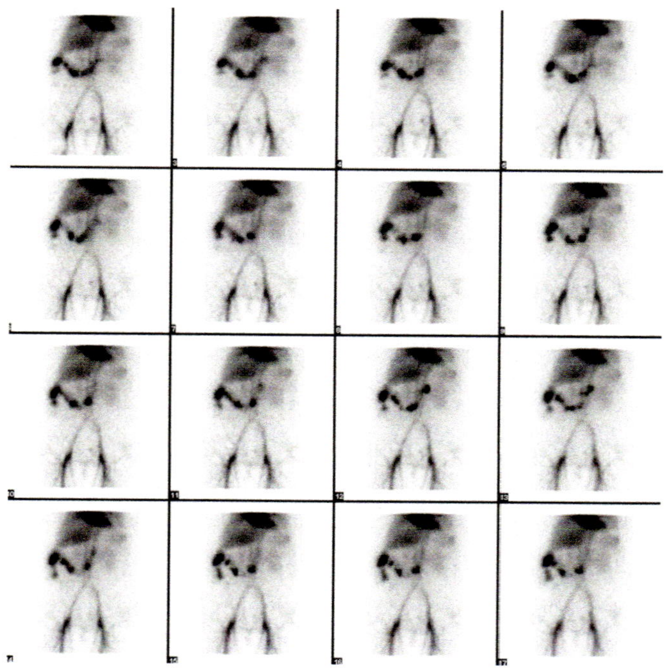

Fig. 1: Dynamic images of gastrointestinal bleeding scan performed with Tc-99m labeled red blood cells demonstrate prompt radiotracer uptake in the hepatic flexure of the colon and antegrade migration of activity in the transverse colon. In subsequent images, retrograde migration of radiotracer activity is seen in the ascending colon. The findings are compatible with active gastrointestinal bleeding in the hepatic flexure of the colon. The peripheral location and large-caliber configuration of the active bleeding site are characteristics of large colon bleed.

REFERENCE

1. Howarth DM. The role of nuclear medicine in the detection of acute gastrointestinal bleeding. Semin Nucl Med. 2006;36(2):133-46.

CASE 4: ASSESSMENT OF POSTRENAL TRANSPLANT COMPLICATIONS

Brief History

A 45-year-old patient with history of end-stage renal disease is referred for renal scintigraphy 4 days after cadaveric renal transplant to evaluate decrease urine output.

Findings

Arterial phase of a Tc-99m mercaptoacetyltriglycin (MAG3) scan demonstrates normal blood flow to the transplanted kidney in the right iliac fossa. Review of the time activity curves is also consistent with normal flow to the transplanted kidney. However, the nephrogram images show delayed excretion/increased renal transit time.

Main Teaching Points

- One-year allograft survival rates are 90–94% for living related donor kidneys and 88–90% for cadaveric transplants. Vasomotor nephropathy is most common in cadaveric kidneys, occurring up to 50% of the time. However, it can be seen in grafts from living donors (5%). Scintigraphy can assess many complications including acute rejection, acute tubular necrosis (or vasomotor nephropathy), vascular problems and obstruction.
- The pattern of normal blood flow but poor function during the first week after transplantation is typical of acute tubular necrosis (ATN). Acute tubular necrosis results from sloughing of tubular epithelial cells as a result of ischemic or toxic injury. Scintigraphic imaging demonstrates a relative preservation of arterial flow compared to renal function. Tc-99m MAG3 scan differentiates ATN from other causes of acute renal failure (such as acute rejection or renal artery stenosis) following renal transplant.

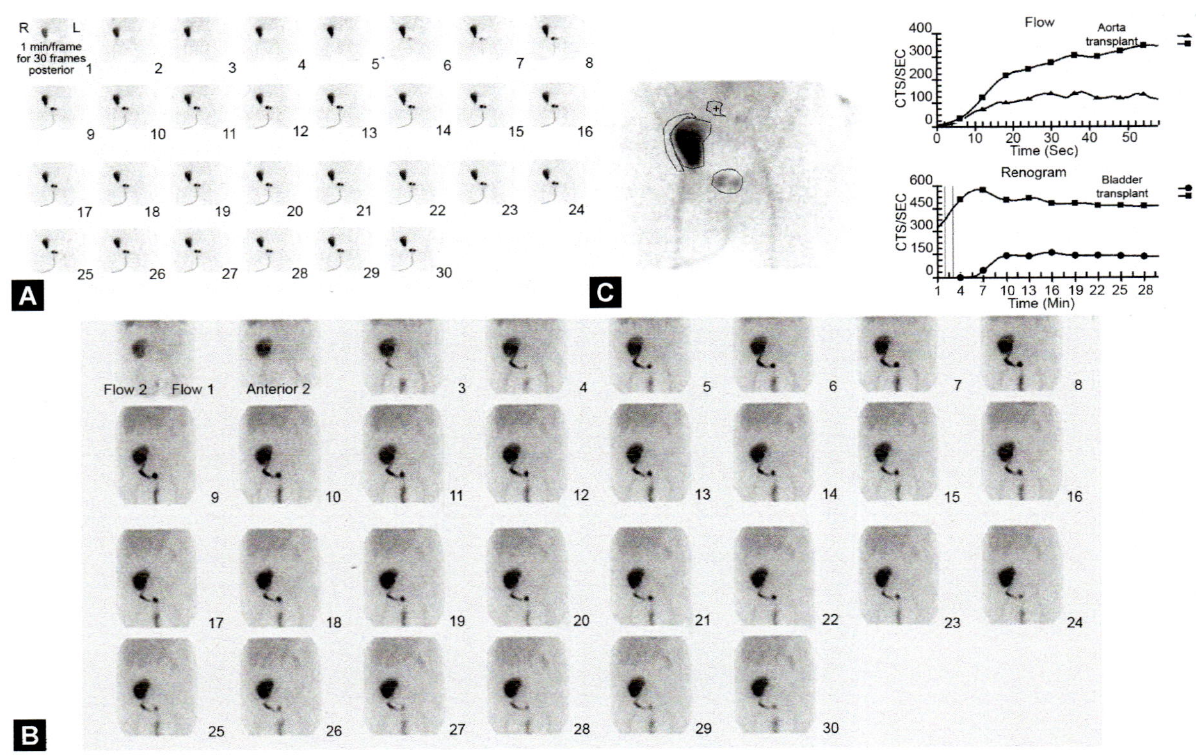

Figs. 1A to C: Tc-99m Mag 3 Renal scan. (A) Radionuclide angiographic images demonstrating prompt flow to the transplant in right iliac fossa. (B) Dynamic functional images demonstrating prompt and uniform uptake, normal cortical transit but impaired excretion and prolonged retention of radiotracer. The findings are compatible with acute tubular necrosis. (C) Renogram demonstrating similar findings.

REFERENCE

1. Sfakianaki E, Sfakianakis GN, Georgiou M, et al. Renal scintigraphy in the acute care setting. Semin Nucl Med. 2013;43(2):114-28.

CASE 5: ASSESSMENT OF BILATERAL BREAST UPTAKE IN GALLIUM SCAN

Brief History

A 36-year-old lactating woman with uveitis is referred for a whole body Gallium scan to evaluate for sarcoidosis.

Findings

Whole body Gallium scan with focal spot views of the thorax demonstrates symmetric bilateral breast uptake due to lactation. Otherwise, there is normal distribution of Gallium-67 (Ga-67) throughout the body with no evidence of active sarcoidosis.

Main Teaching Points

- The radiopharmaceutical Ga-67 citrate circulates in plasma bound to the protein transferrin. The Ga-67 transferrin complex is transported to the inflammatory site because of locally increased blood flow and vascular permeability. Sites of inflammation contain iron-binding compounds (e.g. lactoferrin released by leukocytes). After migration to an inflammatory site, neutrophils release large amounts of lactoferrin. Ga-67, with a higher binding affinity for lactoferrin than transferrin, localizes at the site of inflammation by dissociating from transferrin and binding to lactoferrin.
- Uptake is normal in the bone marrow and bone, and to a more variable extent in the spleen, salivary and

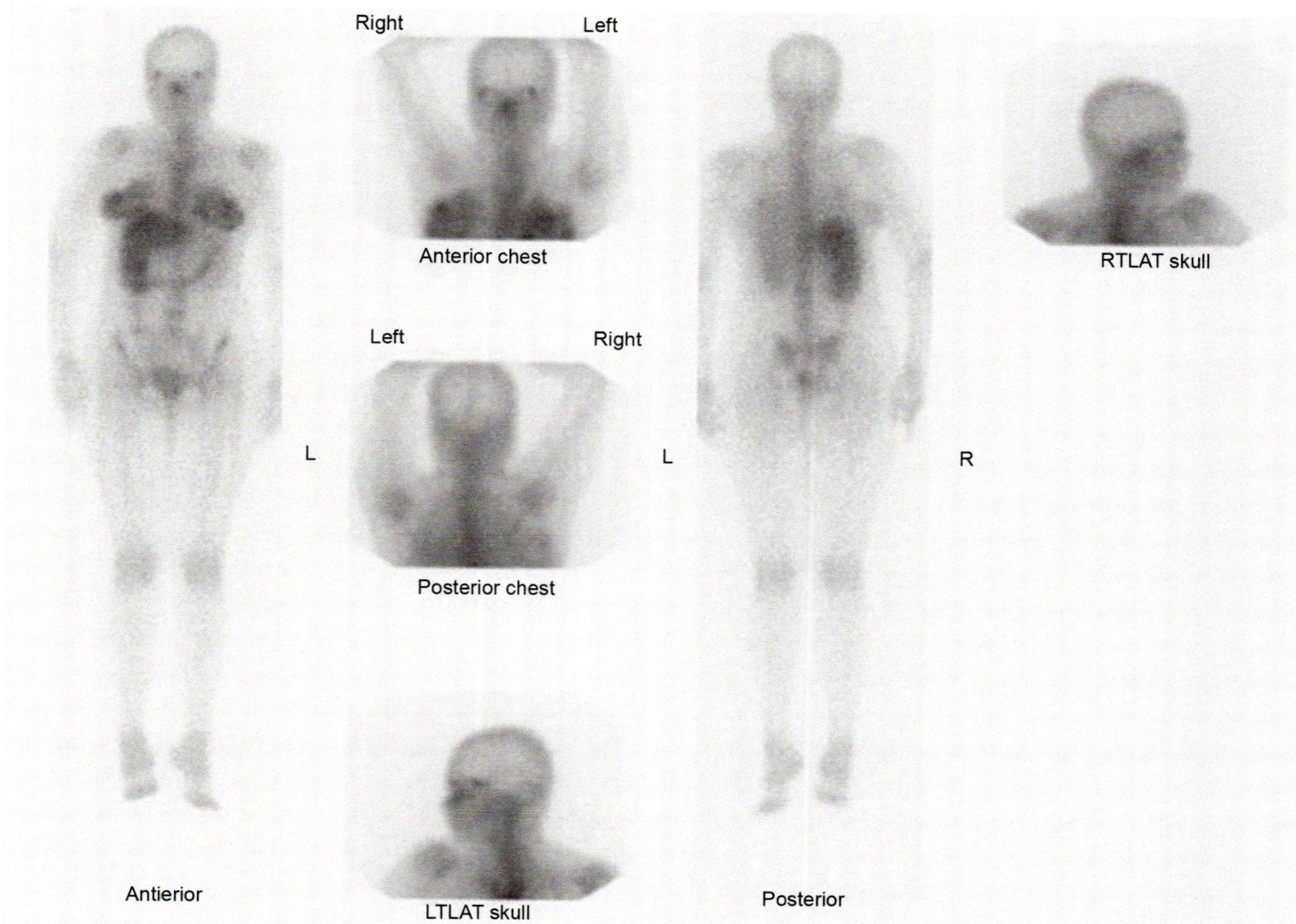

Fig. 1: Whole body and spot images of the 67Ga Citrate scan demonstrating diffuse radiotracer uptake in the right and left breasts.

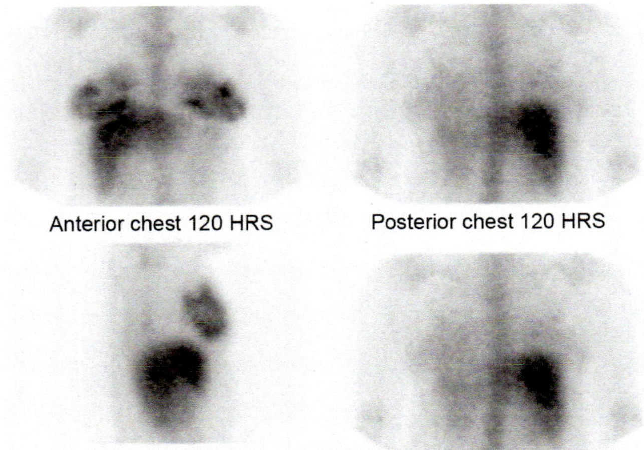

Fig. 2: Delayed 120-hour spot images of the 67Ga Citrate scan demonstrating similar findings of diffuse radiotracer uptake in the right and left breasts.

lacrimal glands. Lacrimal glands, salivary glands, and the breasts all produce lactoferrin. Inflammatory or stimulatory processes in these organs increase production and result in increased Ga-67 uptake (e.g. increased uptake is seen in the salivary glands in Sjögren's syndrome, the lacrimal glands in sarcoidosis, and the breast during lactation).

- Lactating women undergoing Gallium scans should discontinue breast-feeding for approximately 2 weeks to reduce the effective dose equivalent to the infant below 1 mSv.

REFERENCE

1. Rubow S, Klopper J, Scholtz P. Excretion of Gallium 67 in human breast milk and its inadvertent ingestion by a 9-month-old child. Eur J Nucl Med. 1991;18(10):829-33.

CASE 6: ASSESSMENT OF NEUROENDOCRINE MALIGNANCIES

Brief History

A 28-year-old male with uncontrolled hypertension and abnormal findings on abdominal computed tomography (CT) scan (two aortocaval soft tissue masses) is referred for metaiodobenzylguanidine (MIBG) scan to evaluate for pheochromocytoma.

Findings

Axial contrast-enhanced CT images demonstrate an enhancing midline retroperitoneal mass. Whole body MIGB scan demonstrates increased uptake in the midline abdomen. In the given clinical context, this is consistent with an extra-adrenal pheochromocytoma. Lugol's iodine or SSKI is given prior to MIBG injection as a thyroid protective measure by decreasing accumulation of radioiodine within the thyroid gland.

Main Teaching Points

- Extra-adrenal pheochromocytomas, which account for 10% of all pheochromocytomas, originate from paraganglionic chromaffin cells of the sympathetic nervous system. As such, they are considered as paragangliomas and can occur anywhere from the skull base to the urinary bladder, commonly in the retroperitoneum, bladder wall, heart, mediastinum and carotid bodies.
- Metaiodobenzylguanidine is a guanethidine analogue that accumulates in catecholamine-producing neuroendocrine tumors, commonly neuroblastoma in children and primary adrenal or extra-adrenal pheochromocytoma in adults. MIBG is particularly helpful in surveying the entire body for extra-adrenal tumors and metastatic disease. In addition, for some, the MIBG is a preferable alternative to octreotide for assessment of adrenal neuroendocrine tumors, given the normally intense adjacent renal cortical uptake of the latter.

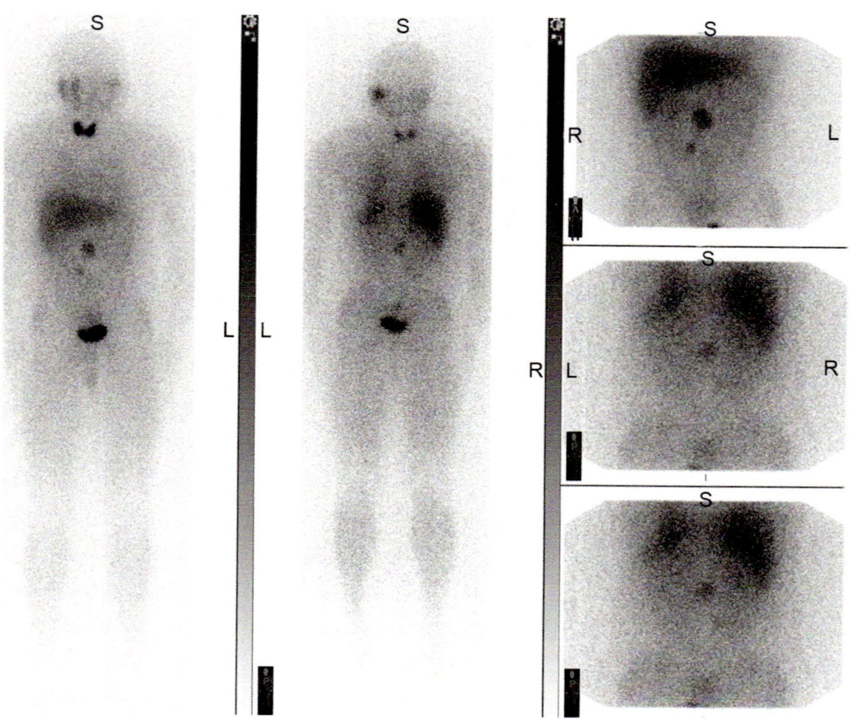

Fig. 1: Whole body and spot images of ^{123}I MIBG scan demonstrating abnormal radiotracer uptake in the mid-abdomen and a second smaller focus, right of the midline, inferior to the larger focus.

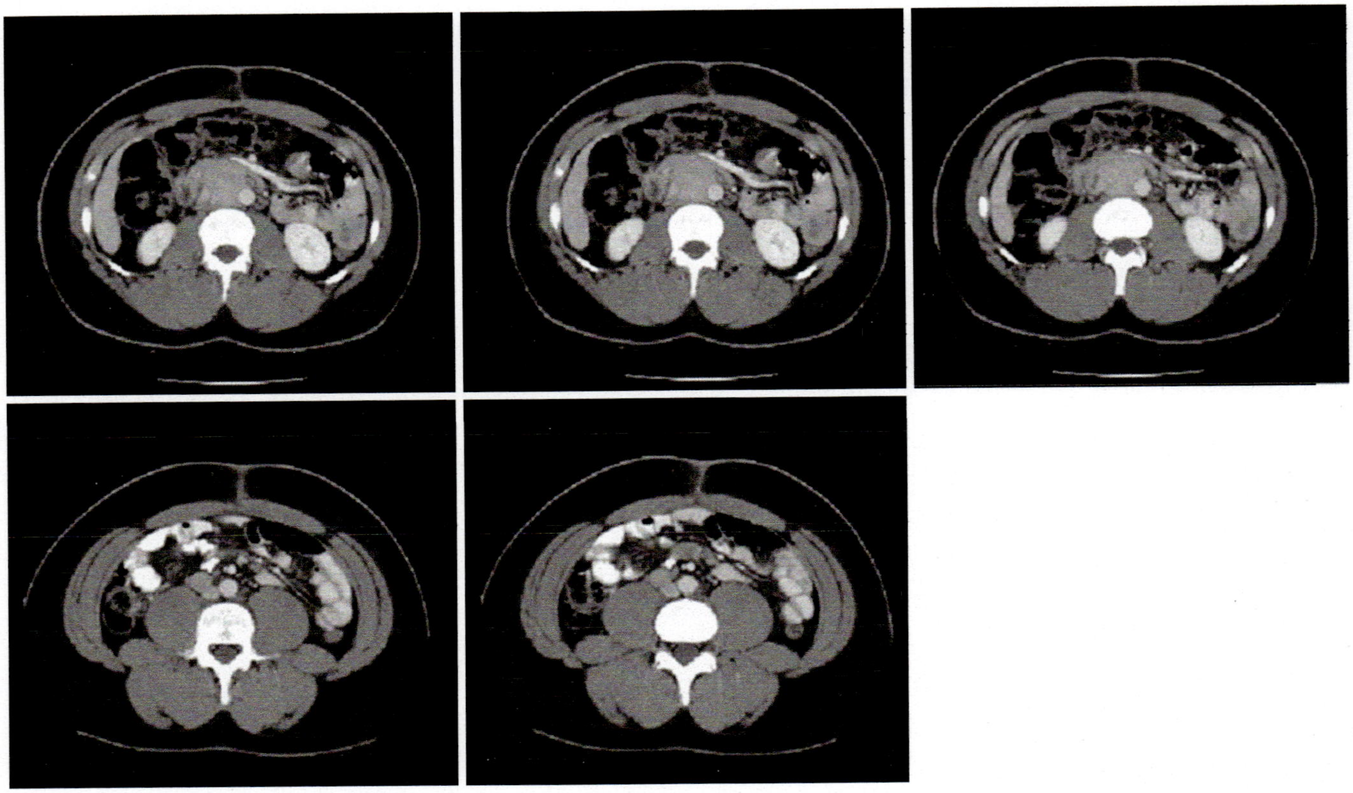

Fig. 2: Contrast enhanced CT scan of the abdomen demonstrating two soft tissue densities aortocaval region, corresponding to the increased radiotracer uptake seen on MIBG scan.

- Scintigraphy with MIBG is not recommended as a screening procedure for pheochromocytoma, and should only be performed after biochemical and CT assessment suggest the presence of a pheochromocytoma.

REFERENCE

1. Blake MA, Kalra MK, Maher MM, et al. Pheochromocytoma: an imaging chameleon. Radiographics. 2004;24 Suppl 1:S87-99.

CASE 7: ASSESSMENT OF LIVER AND SPLEEN USING TC-99M SULFUR COLLOID

Brief History

A 35-year-old female with history of idiopathic thrombocytopenic purpura (ITP) status post splenic artery embolism presents with persistent abdominal pain and is referred for a liver spleen scan to evaluate the efficiency of the treatment.

Findings

Sulfur colloid images demonstrate abnormal increased uptake in the spleen despite prior splenic artery embolization.

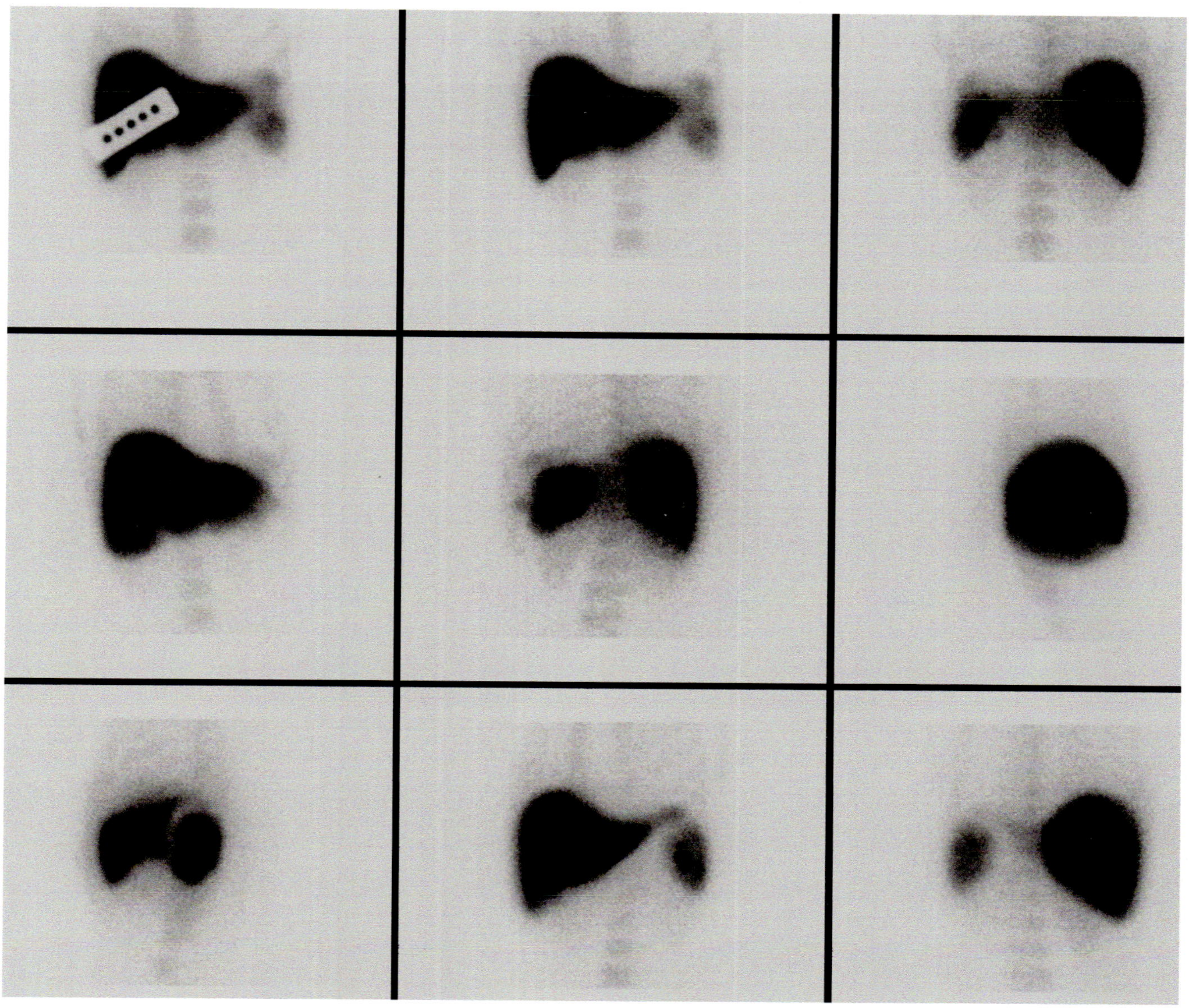

Fig. 1: Images of the Tc-99m Sulfur Colloid liver spleen scan in multiple projections demonstrating expected radiotracer uptake in the liver and the bone marrow. Unexpected radiotracer uptake in the spleen after splenic artery embolization.

Main Teaching Points

- Splenectomy is a surgical option for patients with clinically significant ITP in order to prevent platelet destruction within the spleen. Splenic artery embolism may be performed in high-risk nonsurgical candidates to treat hypersplenism or as an adjuvant procedure prior to elective splenectomy.
- A liver spleen scan can be performed to assess effectiveness of splenic artery embolization. After intravenous (IV) injection, Tc-99m sulfur colloid particles are extracted from the blood by reticuloendothelial cells of the liver (85%), macrophages of the spleen (10%), and bone marrow (5%). Tc-99m sulfur colloid has a single-pass liver extraction efficiency of 95% and a blood clearance half-life of 2–3 minutes. Uptake by liver, spleen and bone marrow is complete by 15 minutes. Visualization of the spleen post splenic artery embolization is consistent with nonoptimal embolization or regrowth of splenic tissue.

REFERENCE

1. Takahashi T, Arima Y, Yokomuro S, et al. Splenic artery embolization before laparoscopic splenectomy in children. Surg Endosc. 2005;19(10):1345-8.

CASE 8: ASSESSMENT OF PERCUTANEOUS TRANSHEPATIC CHOLANGIOGRAPHY COMPLICATIONS

Brief History

A 55-year-old man status post-percutaneous transhepatic cholangiography (PTC) presents with shortness of breath and right-sided pleural effusion. Patient is referred for a hepatobiliary iminodiacetic acid (HIDA) scan to evaluate for bile leak.

Findings

Hepatobiliary iminodiacetic acid (HIDA) scan demonstrates focal abnormal accumulation lateral to the right lobe of the liver which communicates to the right pleural cavity, consistent with biliary-pleural fistula along the surgical needle track.

Fig. 1: Dynamic Images of the Tc-99m DISIDA scan demonstrating extra-intestinal radiotracer extravasation in gallbladder fossa, along the track of PTC needle and upward tracking of radiotracer activity in the costophrenic recess and in the right pleural cavity.

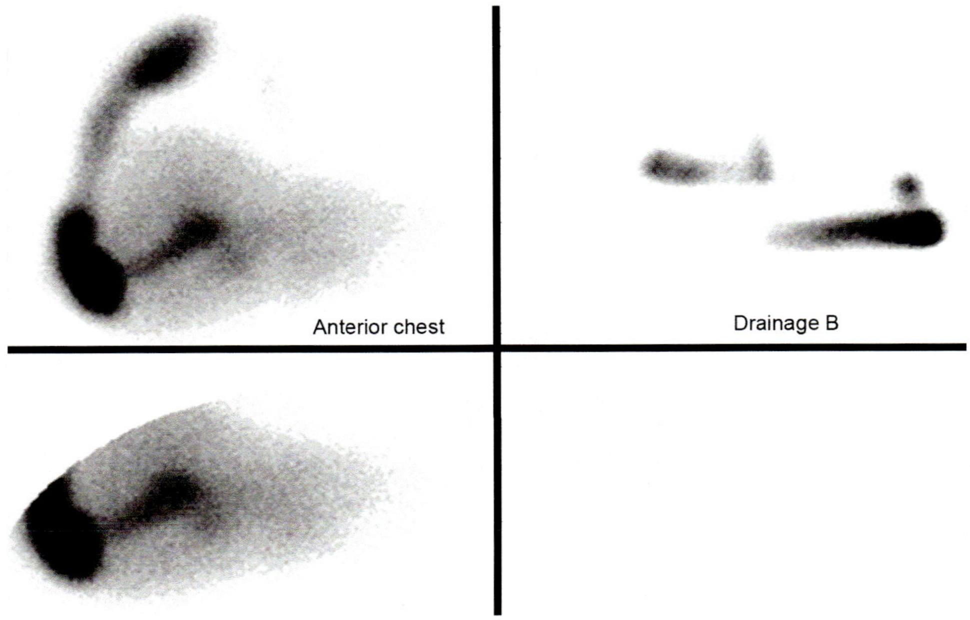

Fig. 2: Delayed spot images of the hepatobiliary study demonstrating similar findings of extravasation of radiotracer into the pleural recess and the right pleural cavity.

Main Teaching Points

- Although ultrasonography and computed tomography (CT) can detect fluid collections, the type and origin of the collection is often uncertain. Cholescintigraphy can determine whether the fluid collection is of biliary origin rather than due to ascites, hypoproteinemia, or other causes.
- Biliary-pleural fistula is a rare complication of PTC characterized by drainage of dark pleural fluid with high bilirubin content. When imaging for a possible bile leak, it is important to image the right paracolic gutter and to obtain pelvic images to look for subtle leaks, which may accumulate in the pelvis. Initial management of small leaks with thoracostomy drainage and antibiotics may lead to spontaneous fistula healing. Failure of response to conservative therapy may necessitate video-assisted thoracoscopic intervention.

REFERENCE

1. Lee MT, Hsi SC, Hu P, et al. Biliopleural fistula: a rare complication of percutaneous transhepatic gallbladder drainage. World J Gastroenterol. 2007;13(23):3268-70.

CASE 9: ASSESSMENT OF TRAUMATIC BILIARY INJURY

Brief History

A 35-year-old man status post-gunshot wound presents with left upper quadrant pain.

Findings

Hepatobiliary iminodiacetic acid (HIDA) scan demonstrates increased tracer uptake in the left upper quadrant consistent with a biliary leak. The photopenic defect along the right liver border represents the lodged bullet fragment.

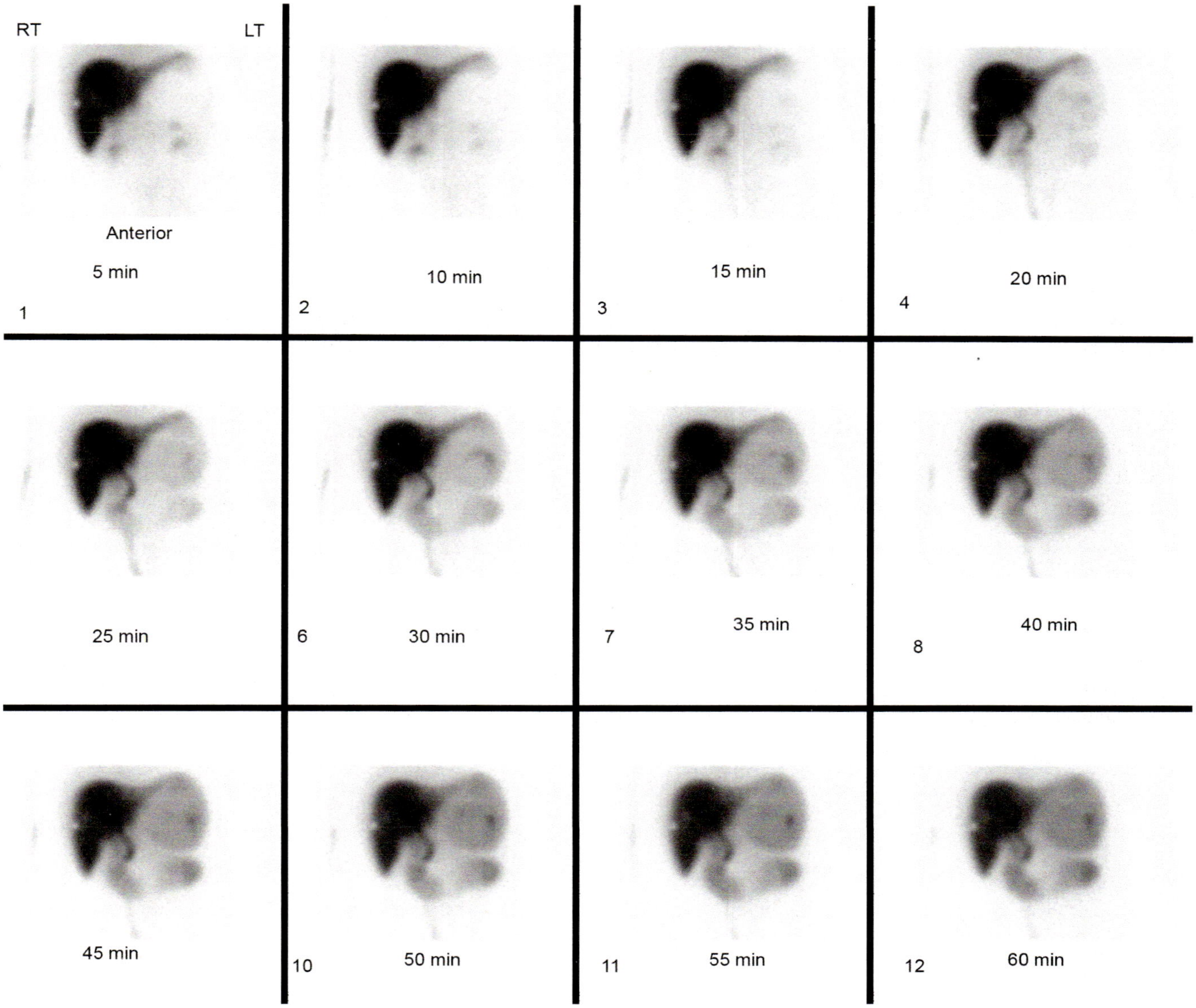

Fig. 1: Dynamic images of the Tc-99m Mebrofenin hepatobiliary scan demonstrating a photopenic defect, caused by bullet fragment in the right lobe of the liver and extra-intestinal extravasation of the radiotracer in the left subdiaphragmatic region and in the abdomen, compatible with the bile leak secondary to liver laceration caused by bullet fragment.

Main Teaching Point

- Nonoperative management of severe blunt liver injury is associated with lower mortality but subsequent clinical course is complicated by factors such as biliary leak. Scintigraphically, a bile leak often initially manifests as a progressively increasing collection of radiotracer in the region of the gallbladder fossa or hepatic hilum. The activity may progressively spread into the subdiaphragmatic space, over the dome of the liver, into the colonic gutters, or manifest as free bile in the abdomen. Delayed imaging may be required to detect a small or slow leak.

REFERENCE

1. Wahl WL, Brandt MM, Hemmila MR, et al. Diagnosis and management of bile leaks after blunt liver injury. Surgery. 2005;138(4):742-7; discussion 747-8.

CASE 10: ASSESSMENT OF PERIPROSTHETIC INFECTION

Brief History

A 40-year-old woman with a Harrington rod in the thoracolumbar spine presents with back pain and is referred for bone scan and Gallium scan for possible implant infection.

Findings

Whole body bone scan shows expected decrease of radiotracer uptake at the site of Harrington rod. However, there is greater intensity of Gallium uptake in the thoracic (left side of T8 and right side of T9) and lumbar spine (right side of L1) compared to methylene diphosphonate (MDP) uptake which strongly indicates the presence of infection/inflammation superimposed upon periprosthetic reactive changes.

Main Teaching Points

- Radionucleotide imaging is the modality of choice in evaluating periprosthetic infection because it is not limited by hardware artifacts seen on computed tomography (CT) and magnetic resonance (MR). Bone scintigraphy is used as a screening tool for prosthetic failure, but it cannot differentiate among different causes of failure. Since indium white blood cell (WBC) is known to have lower sensitivity for detection of infection in the spine, Ga-67 scans are often performed in conjunction with bone scans to assess for infectious etiologies of prosthetic failure in the thoracolumbar spine.
- Gallium-67 is a bone-seeking radiopharmaceutical also used as a tumor-imaging and infection/inflammation-imaging radiotracer. Ga-67 is cyclotron-produced and decays by electron capture with emission of a gamma ray spectrum (93, 185, 288, 394 keV).

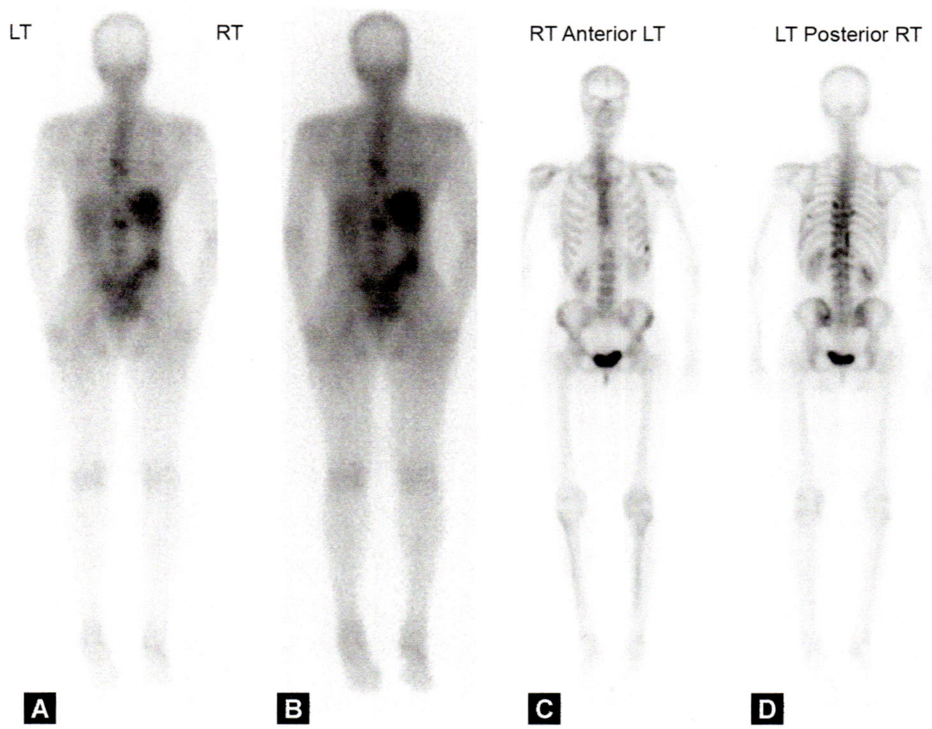

Figs. 1A to D: Whole body images of 67Ga Citrate scan (A and B) in posterior projection demonstrating abnormal uptake in the mid thoracic and mid lumbar spine. Whole body images of Tc 99m MDP bone scan in anterior (C) and posterior (D) projection demonstrating diffuse uptake in the lower mid and lower thoracic and upper lumbar spine from presence of Harrington Rod.

REFERENCE

1. Love C, Marwin SE, Palestro CJ. Nuclear medicine and the infected joint replacement. Semin Nucl Med. 2009;39(1):66-78.

CASE 11: ASSESSMENT OF HYPERTHYROIDISM

Brief History

A 36-year-old female with weight loss and palpitations referred for further evaluation of hyperthyroidism.

Findings

Iodine-123 (I-123) scan demonstrates a solitary toxic nodule with 40% uptake over 24 hours suppressing uptake in the remainder of the thyroid gland.

Main Teaching Point

- Thyroid scintigraphy is used to assess the functioning state of the thyroid in patients exhibiting signs of thyrotoxicosis. Hyperfunctioning thyroid adenomas characteristically suppress function in the remainder of the gland. Central photopenia in the functioning nodule in the right lobe is likely due to central necrosis within the rapidly growing nodule.

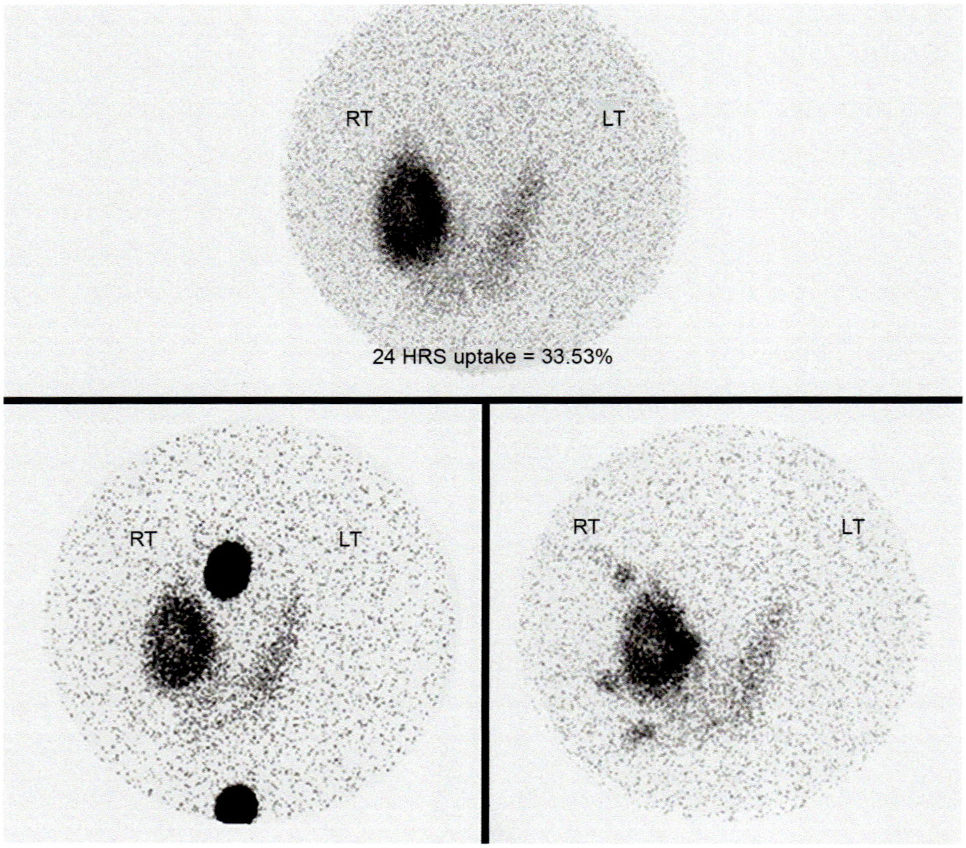

Fig. 1: Pinhole images of ^{123}I Na thyroid scan demonstrating intense radiotracer uptake in the right lobe of the thyroid compatible with "hot" nodule. Suppressed radiotracer uptake in the remainder of the thyroid gland.

REFERENCE

1. Intenzo CM, Dam HQ, Manzone TA, et al. Imaging of the thyroid in benign and malignant disease. Semin Nucl Med. 2012;42(1):49-61.

CASE 12: ASSESSMENT OF NEW HEARING LOSS

Brief History

A 64-year-old male with history of glomus jugulare tumor status post resection 5 years ago now presents with new hearing loss.

Findings

Whole body octreotide scan demonstrates uptake at the left skull base in the region of the left jugular canal consistent with recurrence.

Main Teaching Point

- Octreotide scintigraphy offers advantages over conventional MR or computed tomography (CT) in the evaluation of recurrent paragangliomas due to its intrinsic binding of somatostatin receptors (SSTRs) independent of radiotherapy or surgical changes. Octreotide scintigraphy, as compared to CT/MRI, provides more specific assessment of suspected recurrence although sometimes octreotide uptake can be seen in post therapy changes, decreasing the specificity of positive finding. In the skull base, differential diagnosis for an octreotide-positive tumor includes meningioma, lymphoma and low grade astrocytoma.

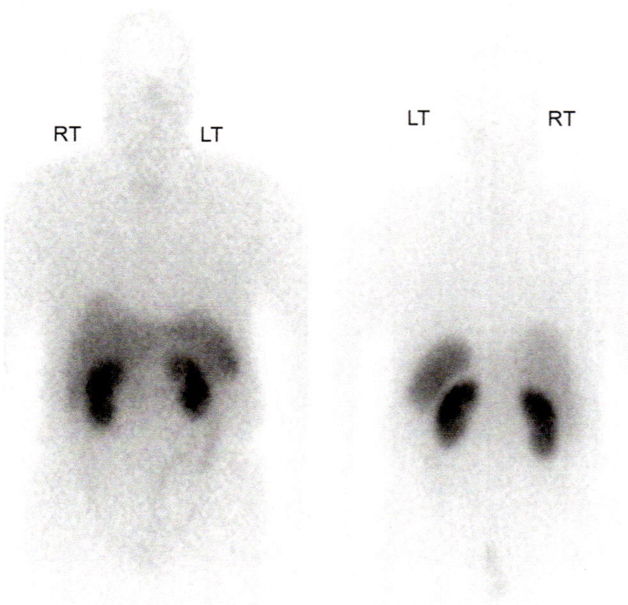

A

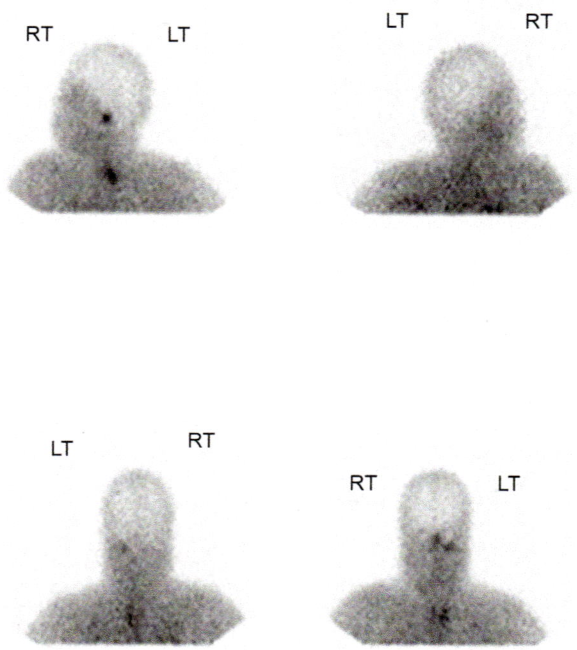

B

Figs. 1A and B: Whole body ^{111}In Octreotide scan (A) demonstrate expected radiotracer uptake in the liver, spleen and kidneys with physiologic excretion of radiotracer in the kidneys. The spot images of the skull (B) demonstrate increased radiotracer uptake in the posterior cranial fossa, left of the midline. The radiotracer uptake was in the recurrent glomus jugulare.

REFERENCE

1. Bustillo A, Telischi FF. Octreotide scintigraphy in the detection of recurrent paragangliomas. Otolaryngol Head Neck Surg. 2004;130(4):479-82.

CASE 13: ASSESSMENT OF OSSEOUS METASTASIS

Brief History

A 16-year-old male presents with bone pain.

Findings

Whole body bone scan demonstrates uptake in the left distal femur with synchronous regional bone metastasis (skip-lesions) to left acetabulum, lower thoracic spine, and left proximal tibia. Pathology results were positive for osteosarcoma.

Main Teaching Point

- Local resectability and sensitivity to chemotherapy are major determinants of osteosarcoma prognosis. Synchronous regional bone metastases (skip lesions) of osteosarcoma represents a major challenge in surgical management, as occult lesions beyond the local surgical resection margin will necessitate a more radical procedure or preclude curative resection.

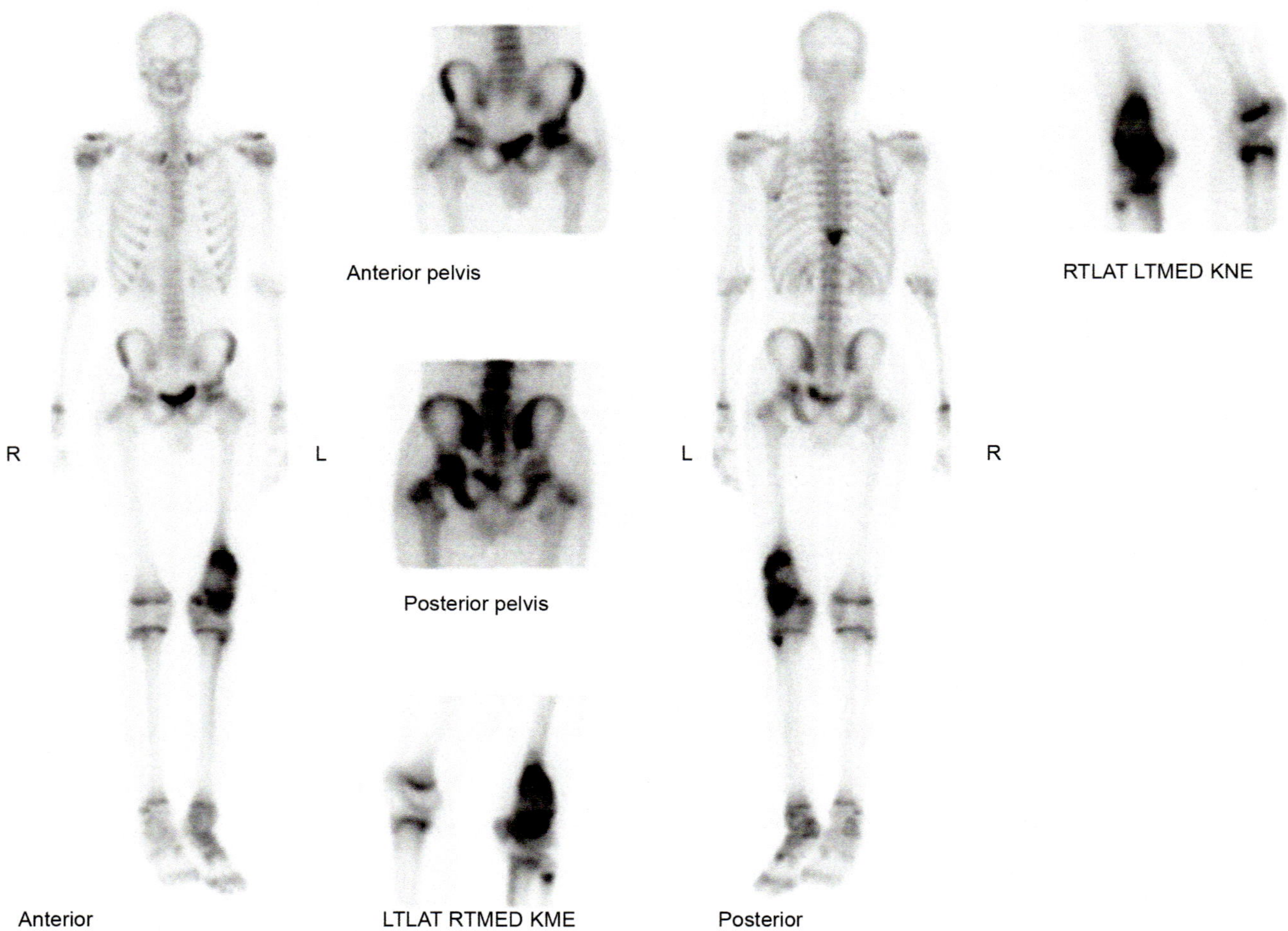

Fig. 1: Whole body 99mTc-Methyl diphosphonate (MDP) images demonstrate increased radiotracer uptake in the known osteosarcoma in the left distal femur. Skip metastatic lesion is seen in the left proximal fibula. Distant metastasis is seen in the 11th thoracic vertebra and in the left acetabulum.

REFERENCE

1. Kager L, Zoubek A, Kastner U, et al. Skip metastases in osteosarcoma: experience of the Cooperative Osteosarcoma Study Group. J Clin Oncol. 2006;24(10):1535-41.

CASE 14: ASSESSMENT OF PAROTID GLAND SWELLING

Brief History

A 45-year-old woman presents with bilateral parotid gland swelling.

Findings

Whole body Gallium scan demonstrates focal uptake in the lacrimal and salivary glands producing a "panda sign". There is also faint lung uptake.

Main Teaching Point

- The "panda sign" refers to the accumulation of Gallium citrate in the parotid glands in both acute and chronic inflammation secondary to sarcoidosis. Differential diagnosis of Gallium citrate uptake in this region includes lymphoma, bronchogenic carcinoma, Sjögren's syndrome and melanoma.

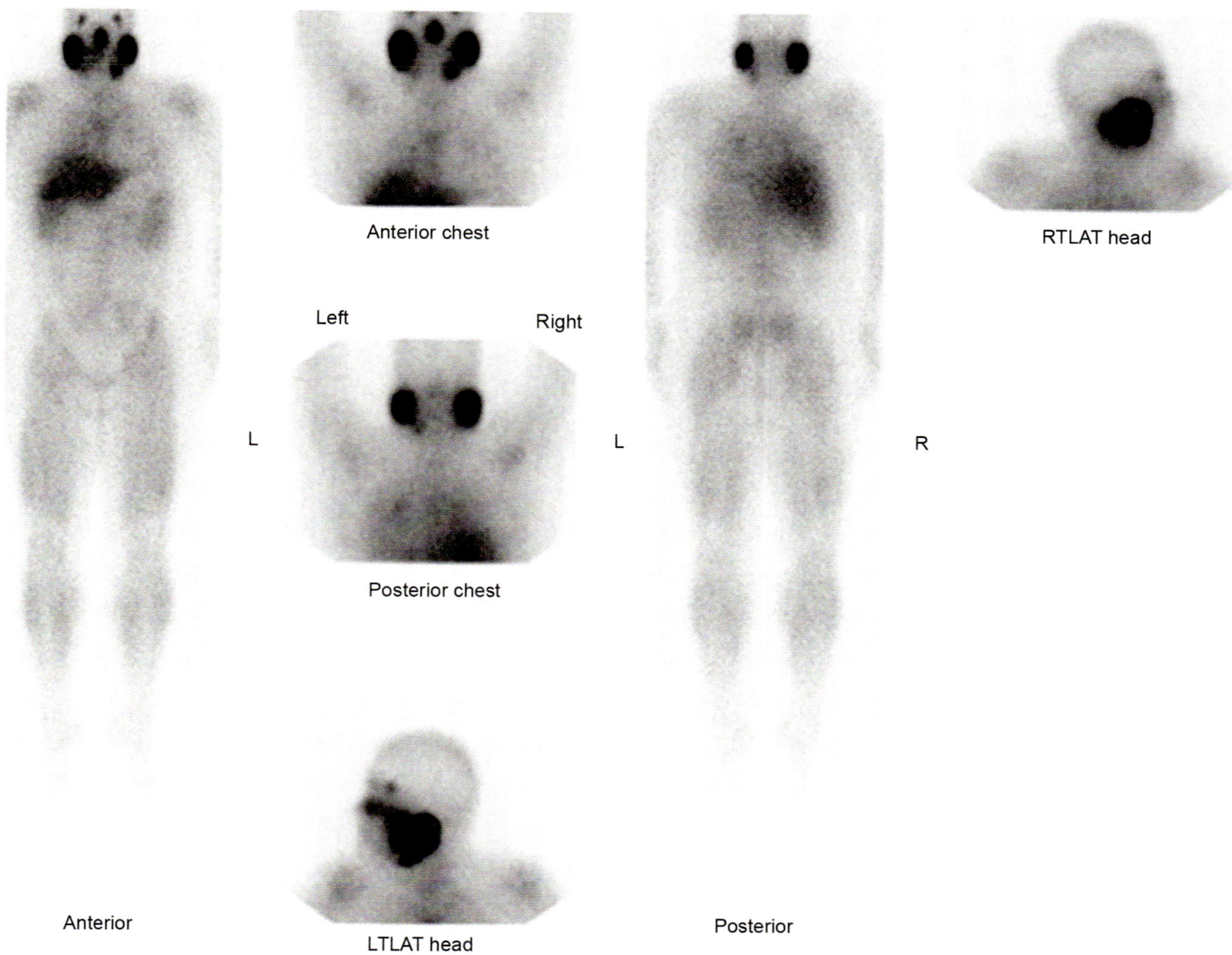

Fig. 1: Whole body 67Ga Citrate images demonstrate expected radiotracer uptake in the liver, spleen and bone marrow. Abnormal radiotracer uptake is seen in the parotid and submandibular salivary glands and in the lacrimal glands, in the typical pattern that is commonly seen in patients with sarcoidosis and is described as Panda's sign.

REFERENCE

1. Kurdziel KA. The panda sign. Radiology. 2000;215(3):884-5.

CASE 15: ASSESSMENT OF HEPATOPULMONARY SYNDROME

Brief History

A 65-year-old with end-stage liver disease undergoes evaluation for hepatopulmonary syndrome using Tc-99m Macroaggregated Albumin (MAA) scan.

Findings

Tc-99m MAA scan demonstrates uptake in the brain, kidneys and thyroid which can not be due to free pertechnetate and therefore confirms the diagnosis of hepatopulmonary syndrome (free pertechnetate can be taken up by thyroid and kidneys and not by brain parenchyma).

Main Teaching Point

- Hepatopulmonary syndrome is a characterized by shortness of breath and hypoxemia secondary to vasodilation in the lungs of patients with liver disease. The hepatopulmonary syndrome results from the formation of microscopic intrapulmonary arteriovenous dilatations in these patients which result in a right-to-left shunt.
- Whole-body nuclear imaging following IV injection of Tc-99m MAA is useful to document and quantify right-to-left shunt.

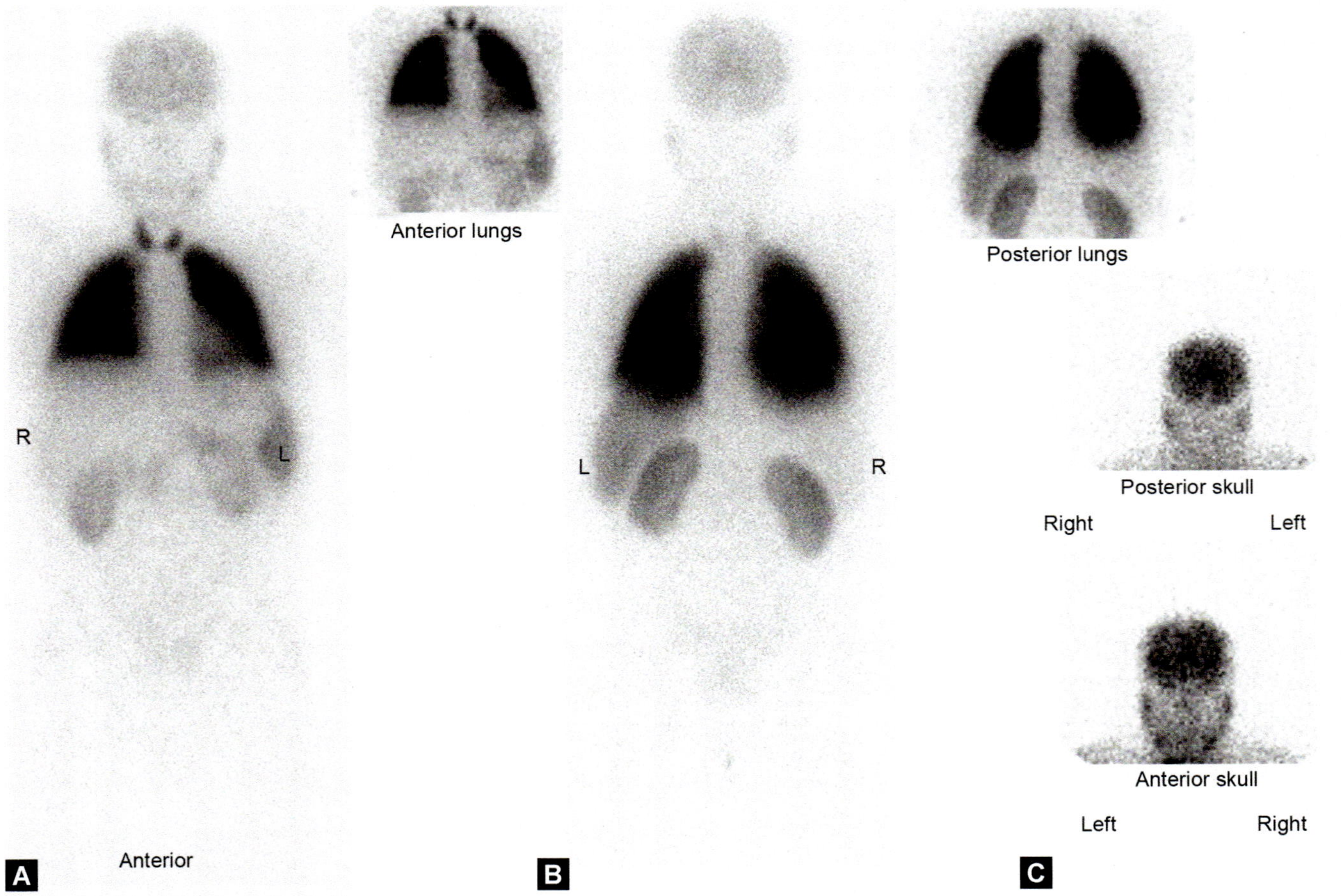

Figs. 1A to C: Whole body (A-Anterior, B-Posterior) images demonstrate expected radiotracer uptake in the lungs. Abnormal radiotracer uptake seen in the brain parenchyma (C) is indicative of right-to-left shunt. Radiotracer uptake seen in the kidneys and thyroid gland can be seen with right-to-left shunt or free pertechnetate. The brain radiotracer uptake confirms right-to-left shunt.

REFERENCE

1. Gandhi SJ, Babu S, Subramanyam P, et al. Tc-99m macro aggregated albumin scintigraphy—indications other than pulmonary embolism: A pictorial essay. Indian J Nucl Med. 2013;28(3):152-62.

CASE 16: ASSESSMENT OF OSSEOUS METASTATIC DISEASE

Brief History

A 60-year-old male with right tibial fracture and a large lung mass on chest X-ray.

Findings

Whole body bone scan demonstrates a focus of increase radiotracer in the distal right tibia consistent with a fracture. There is also periosteal uptake in the long bones consistent with hypertrophic osteoarthropathy. There is no definite scintigraphic evidence to suggest skeletal metastatic disease. Focal uptake in the left anterior

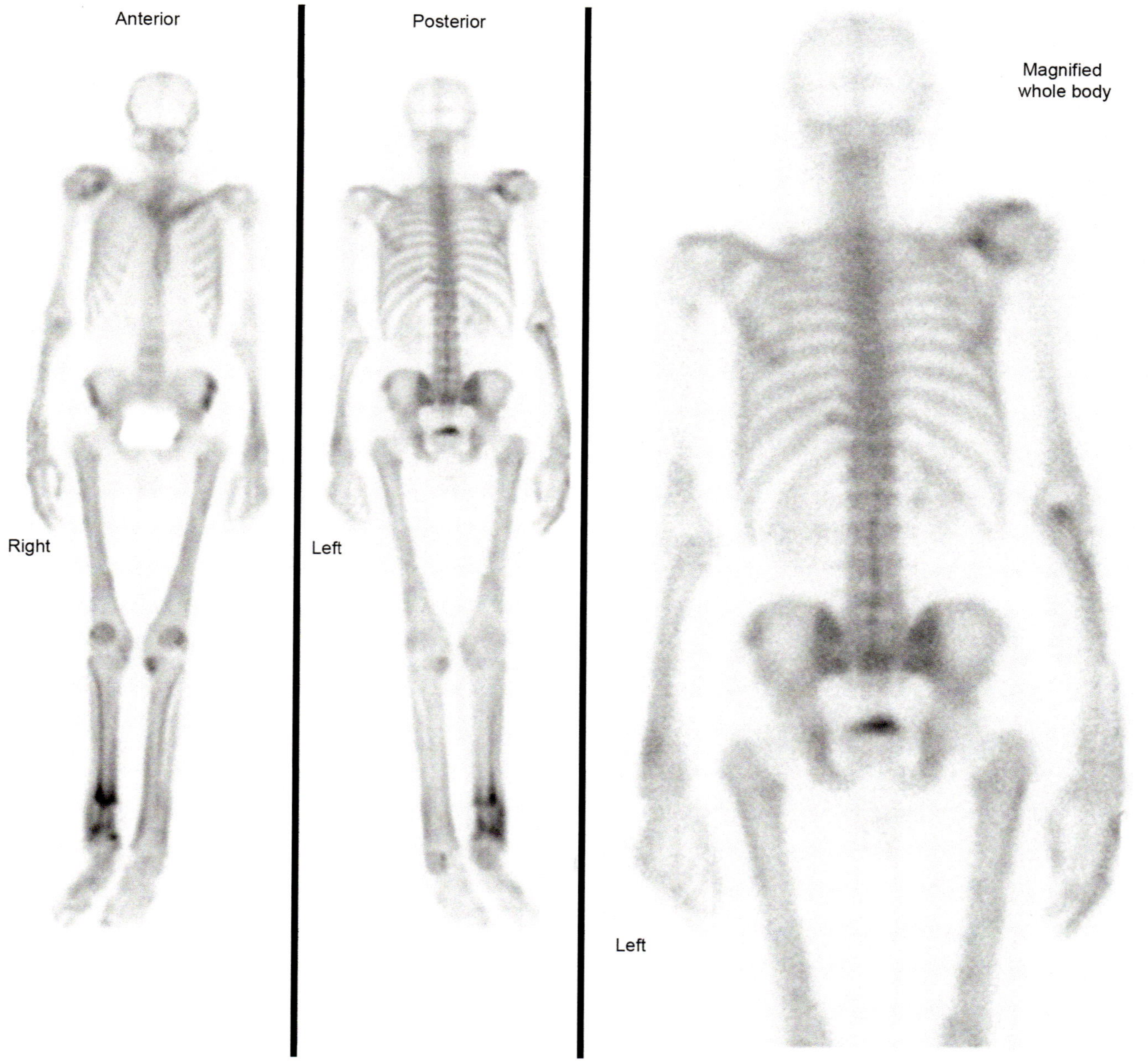

Fig. 1: Whole body 99mTc-Methyl diphosphonate bone scan images demonstrate diffuse periosteal uptake in tram track pattern, characteristic of hypertrophic osteoarthropathy. Focal uptake seen in the right distal tibia is at the site of known fracture.

superior iliac spine turned out to be due to degenerative disease, correlating with a spur seen on the concurrent CT scan.

Main Teaching Points

- Hypertrophic osteoarthropathy is a characteristic periosteal change which can be seen in lung cancer. Lung cancer can easily invade the vasculature and cause arterial metastases. These tumor emboli can reach the distal extremities and result in appendicular involvement. Periosteal changes are most often seen as linear, parallel "track" uptake in the medial and lateral margins of the long bones, but may be patchy or show skip areas.
- The activity may decrease after treatment of the underlying disease. Primary treatment and symptomatic relief for pain related to hypertrophic osteoarthropathy are the most widely reported therapy regimen.

REFERENCE

1. Nguyen S, Hojjati M. Review of current therapies for secondary hypertrophic pulmonary osteoarthropathy. Clin Rheumatol. 2011;30(1):7-13.

CASE 17: ASSESSMENT OF OSTEOMYELITIS

Brief History

A 70-year-old diabetic male with right ankle Charcot's joint on plain film is referred for bone scan along with bone marrow and White blood cell (WBC) scan for assessment of suspected osteomyelitis.

Findings

Bone scan shows increased uptake in proximal right tarsal bones, including right calcaneus, talus and cuboid bones in all three phases. WBC and bone marrow scan demonstrate concurrent right calcaneal uptake consistent with marrow reactivation. No evidence of infection is seen.

Main Teaching Points

- Lesions that can mimic osteomyelitis on three phase skeletal scintigraphy include Charcot's joint, osteoarthritis, gout, fracture, stress fracture, osteonecrosis (healing), osteotomy, complex regional pain syndrome (reflex sympathetic dystrophy).
- Indium-111 (In-111) WBC scintigraphy supplemented by visual comparison with concurrent Tc-99m sulfur colloid bone marrow imaging is used to identify infection within the marrow-containing skeleton. Typically, a pattern of increased In-111 WBC uptake and lack of Tc-99m sulfur colloid uptake in the corresponding distribution and/or intensity (discordant uptake pattern) is suggestive of infection. Concordant uptake, such as in this case, is suggestive of mere marrow redistribution without superimposed infection.

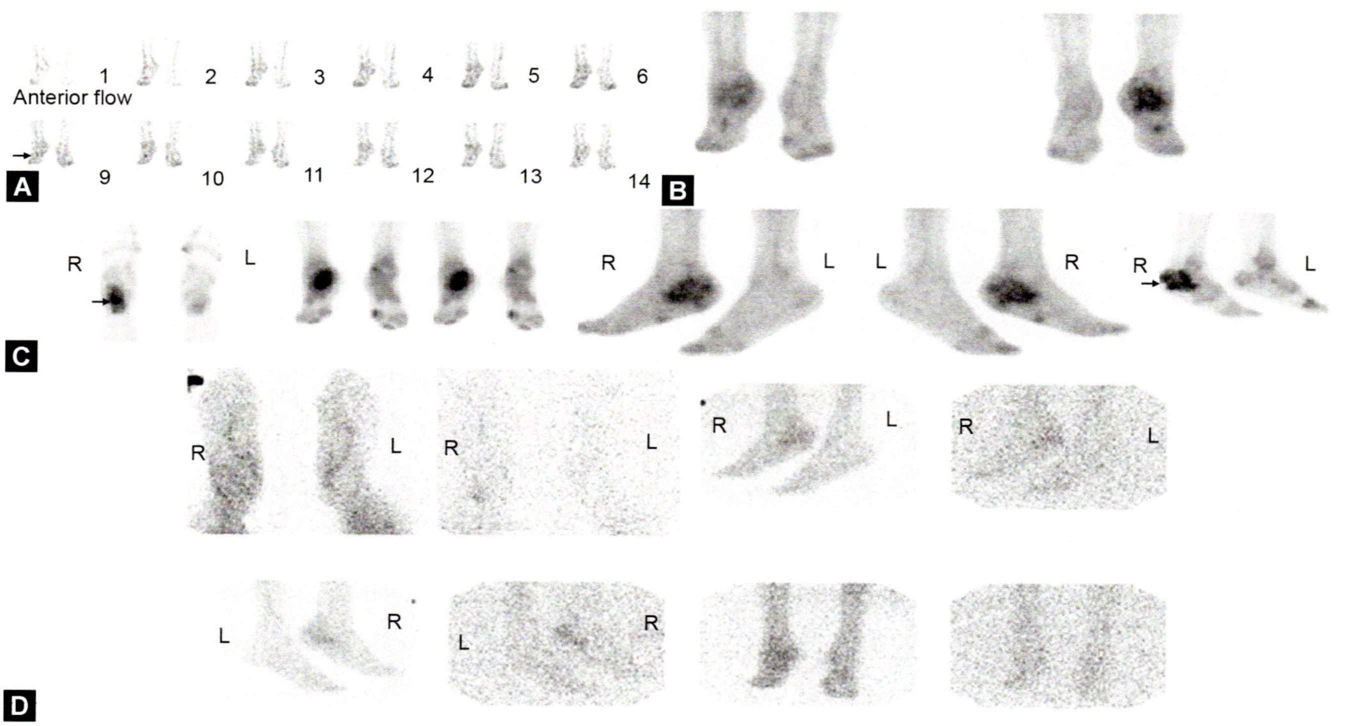

Figs. 1A to D: Triple phase 99mTc-Methyl diphosphonate bone scan images (A-Angiographic phase, B-Blood pool images and C-delayed phase) demonstrate increased radiotracer uptake in the right ankle in all three phases of bone scan, indicative of either neuropathic joint or osteomyelitis. 99m Tc bone marrow and 111In WBC scan images (D) demonstrate radiotracer uptake of similar configuration and intensity in the right ankle, compatible with bone marrow reactivation. These findings exclude osteomyelitis.

REFERENCE

1. Palestro CJ, Love C. Radionuclide imaging of musculoskeletal infection: conventional agents. Semin Musculoskelet Radiol. 2007;11(4):335-52.

CASE 18: ASSESSMENT OF SUSPECTED ACUTE PYELONEPHRITIS

Brief History

A 6-year-old male with no prior history of urinary tract infection (UTI) undergoes evaluation for acute pyelonephritis on dimercaptosuccinic acid (DMSA) scan. An ultrasound of the kidneys on the same day was negative.

Findings

Posterior and posterior oblique pinhole images from a Tc-99m DMSA scan show multiple foci of decreased or absent radiotracer activity. In the given clinical context, the findings are consistent with acute pyelonephritis. Cortical defects represent postinflammatory renal scarring.

Main Teaching Point

- Tc-99m DMSA scans detect acute pyelonephritis in 50–64% of children with first-time episode of UTI, and renal cortical scarring in 11–18% of children on follow-up. Vesicoureteral reflux is associated with a higher incidence of pyelonephritis (relative risk 1.5) and renal scarring (relative risk 2.6).

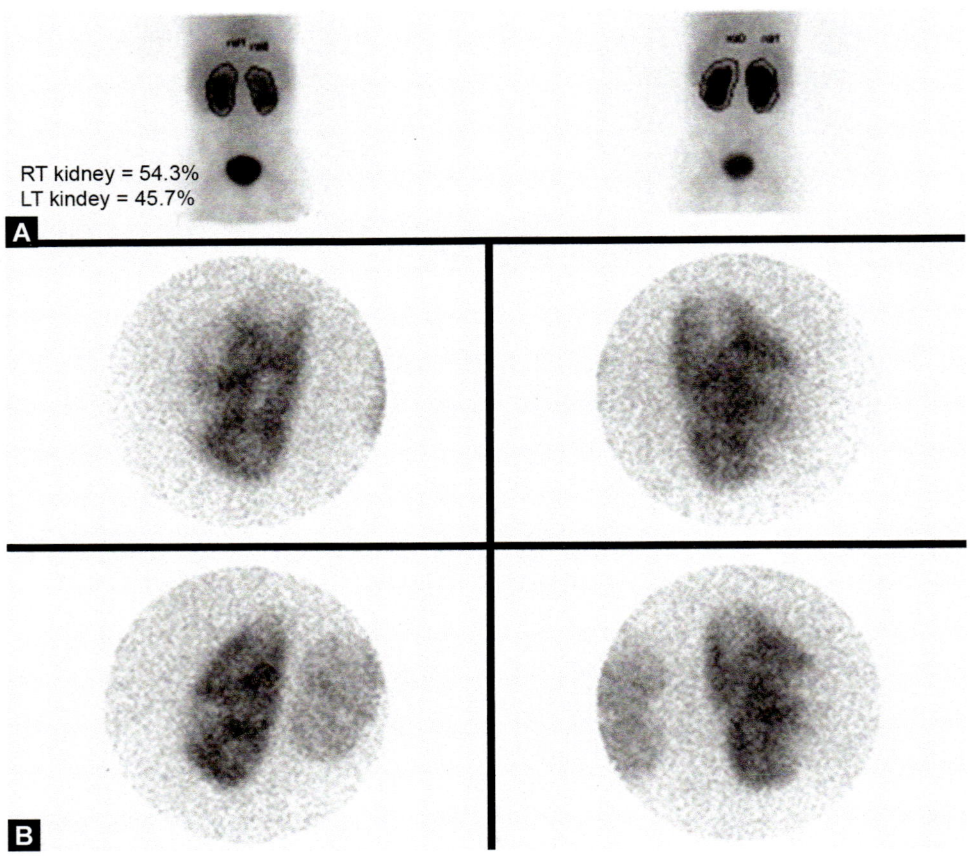

Figs. 1A and B: Planar (A) and pinhole (B) images of Tc-99m DMSA scan. Multiple photopenic defects are seen in both renal parenchyma. The overall renal architecture is preserved. The findings are compatible with acute pyelonephritis.

REFERENCE

1. Shaikh N, Ewing AL, Bhatnagar S, et al. Risk of renal scarring in children with a first urinary tract infection: a systematic review. Pediatrics. 2010;126(6):1084-91.

CASE 19: ASSESSMENT OF RISING TG LEVELS STATUS POSTRADIOIODINE ABLATION

Brief History

A 45-year-old female with history of thyroid carcinoma status post Iodine-131 (I-131) ablation is referred for radioiodine scan for evaluation of rising Tg levels.

Findings

The whole body I-131 scan is negative for recurrence. However, ^{18}F Fluorodeoxyglucose-positron emission tomography (FDG-PET) demonstrates hypermetabolism in right-sided cervical and superior mediastinal lymph nodes consistent with recurrence of dedifferentiated thyroid carcinoma. Therefore, the I-131 scan alone led to a false-negative result but correct diagnosis was made possible by the addition of FDG-PET/CT examination.

Main Teaching Point

- Fluorodeoxyglucose-positron emission tomography is performed in patients with thyroid cancer status post total thyroidectomy with rising Tg levels but unremarkable iodine scan. The sensitivity and specificity of FDG-PET are 60–94% and 20–90%, respectively, in patients with high Tg levels but negative I-131 scans. However, FDG-PET can fail to detect well differentiated thyroid cancers that concentrate iodine in a phenomenon known as "flip flop".

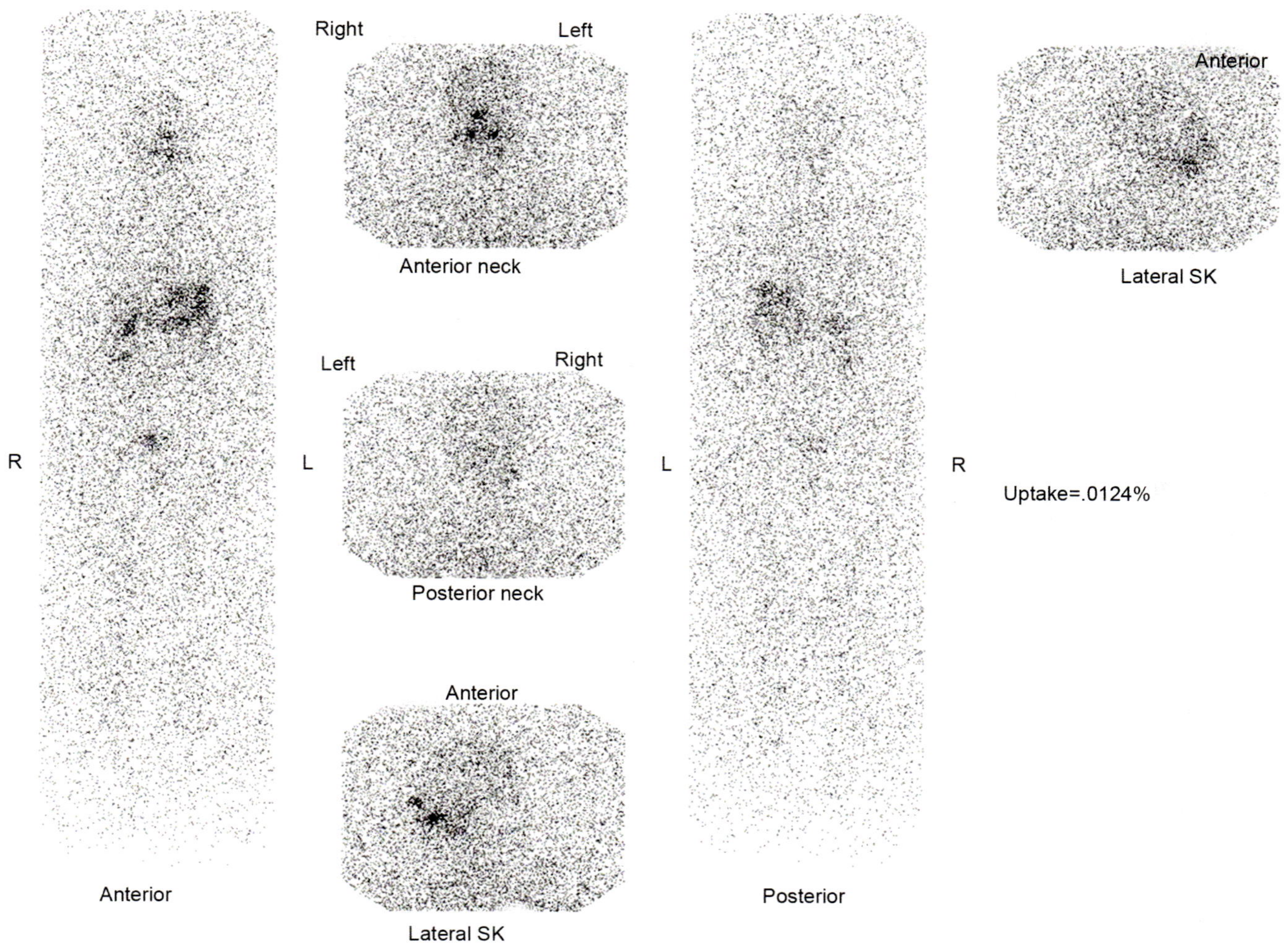

Fig. 1: Whole body and spot images of head and neck from ^{131}I Na scan demonstrating expected radiotracer uptake in the oropharynx and salivary glands. Expected radiotracer excretion is seen in the stomach, large colon and in the urinary bladder. No abnormal radiotracer uptake is seen to indicate recurrence.

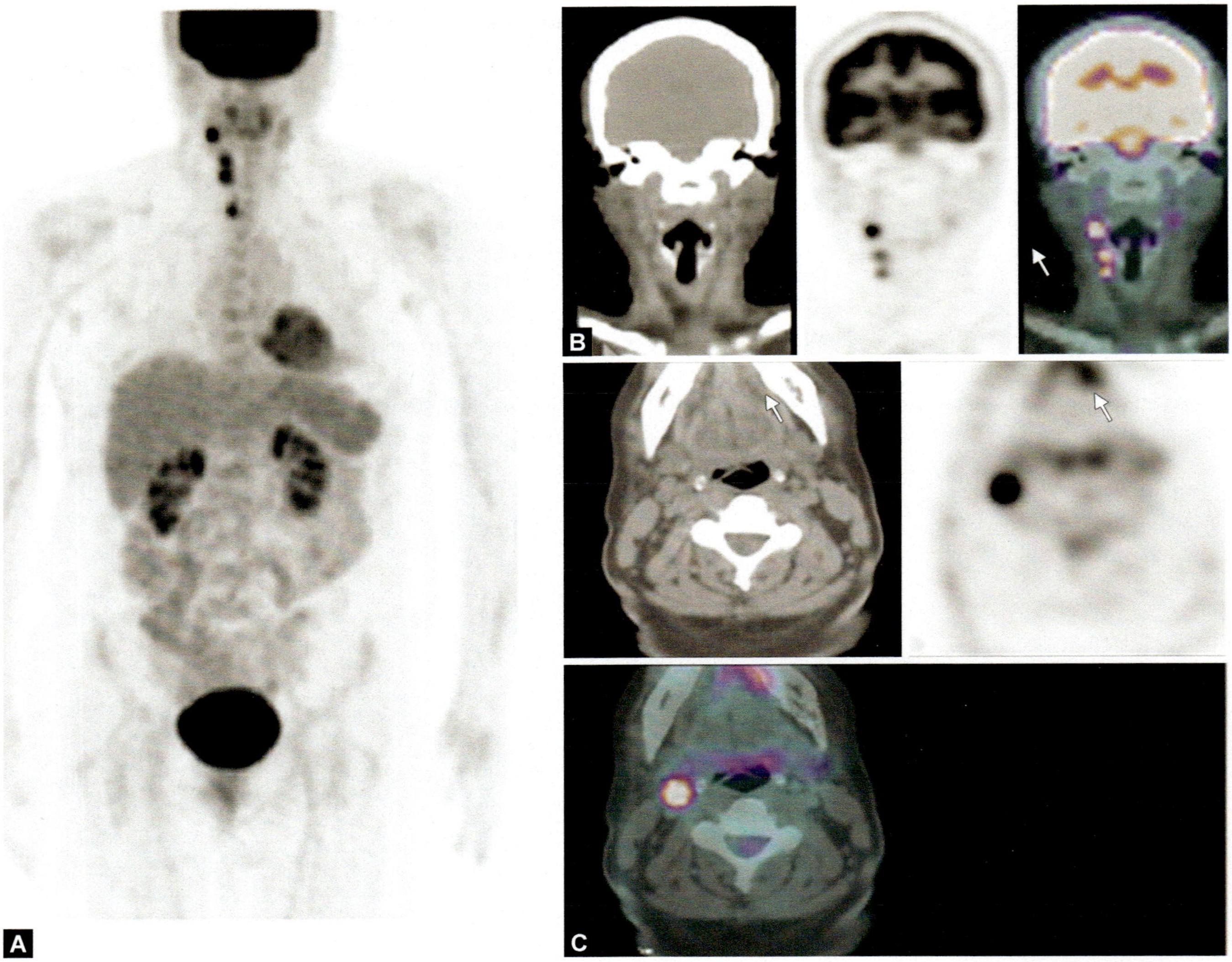

Figs. 2A to C: Whole body (A), CT, PET and fused images in coronal projection (B) and transaxial (C) projection with ^{18}F FDG PET/CT scan demonstrate foci of increased radiotracer uptake in the right level II and level III lymph node stations of the neck (arrows), reflective of lymph node metastasis. A small focus of increased radiotracer uptake was seen in the thyroid bed, in the right paratracheal region (arrow head), indicative of local recurrence.

REFERENCE

1. Khan N, Oriuchi N, Higuchi T, et al. PET in the follow-up of differentiated thyroid cancer. Br J Radiol. 2003;76(910): 690-5.

CASE 20: EVALUATION OF GASTROINTESTINAL HEMORRHAGE

Brief History

A 58-year-old man presents with bleeding per rectum.

Findings

Tc99-m tagged red blood cell (RBC) scan demonstrates a serpentine region of uptake that turned out to be an arteriovenous malformation (AVM) producing a jejunal hemorrhage. The central distribution and serpentine accumulation of hemorrhage indicates hemorrhage within the small bowel.

Main Teaching Point

- A positive scintigraphic study for GI hemorrhage is characterized by accumulation of tracer activity outside the normal blood pool. Although both Tc-99m labeled RBC and Tc-99m sulfur colloid have been used for detection of bleed, Tc-99m RBC, in contrast to sulfur colloid imaging, offers the added advantage of extended duration of imaging beyond first 30–40 minutes. However, continuous dynamic imaging is essential as focal extravasation on a single delayed spot imaging confirms the presence of bleeding but does not help to localize the site of bleeding. Localization of bleeding site is crucial in determining next management steps, whether surgery or interventional procedure.

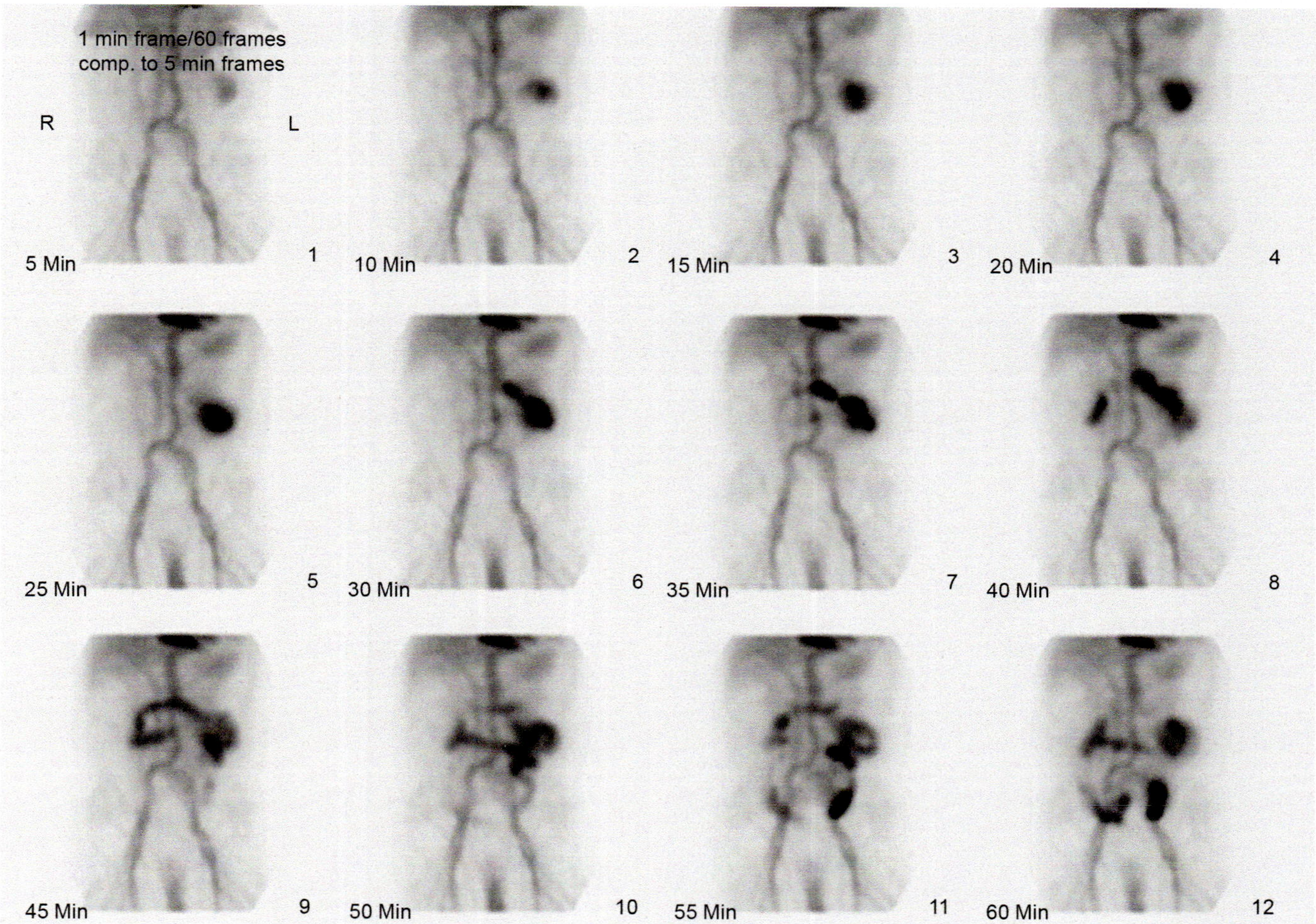

Fig. 1: Dynamic images of gastrointestinal bleeding scan performed with Tc-99m labeled red blood cells demonstrate prompt radiotracer uptake in the left upper abdomen. In subsequent images, the radiotracer activity traverse across the midline in serpentine fashion. The central location of active bleeding site and subsequent migration of activity across the midline are characteristics of small intestinal bleeding.

REFERENCE

1. Howarth DM. The role of nuclear medicine in the detection of acute gastrointestinal bleeding. Semin Nucl Med. 2006;36(2):133-46.

CASE 21: ASSESSMENT OF METABOLIC BONE DISEASE

Brief History

A 35-year-old woman with end-stage renal disease on dialysis recently diagnosed with breast cancer is referred for evaluation of suspected metastatic disease.

Findings

Tc-99m methylene diphosphonate (MDP) whole body bone scan shows uniform markedly increased skeletal tracer uptake relative to the soft tissues with concurrent decreased or absent renal uptake. Tracer uptake in the skull is even more intense relative to the remainder of the skeleton.

Main Teaching Points

- A superscan is defined as a bone scan with marked skeletal uptake relative to the soft tissues. In the setting of a primary neoplasm, a superscan is highly suspicious for diffuse osseous metastases correlating with widespread osteoblastic activity. A bone scan is less sensitive in detecting lytic lesions that do not incorporate MDP, such as those from renal, thyroid or lung cancer.
- However, superscan is not specific for metastatic disease as it may also be seen in the setting of metabolic bone disease including hyperparathyroidism, renal osteodystrophy, Paget's disease, and in myeloproliferative disorders such as lymphoma, leukemia, myelofibrosis and Waldenstrom's macroglobulinemia.

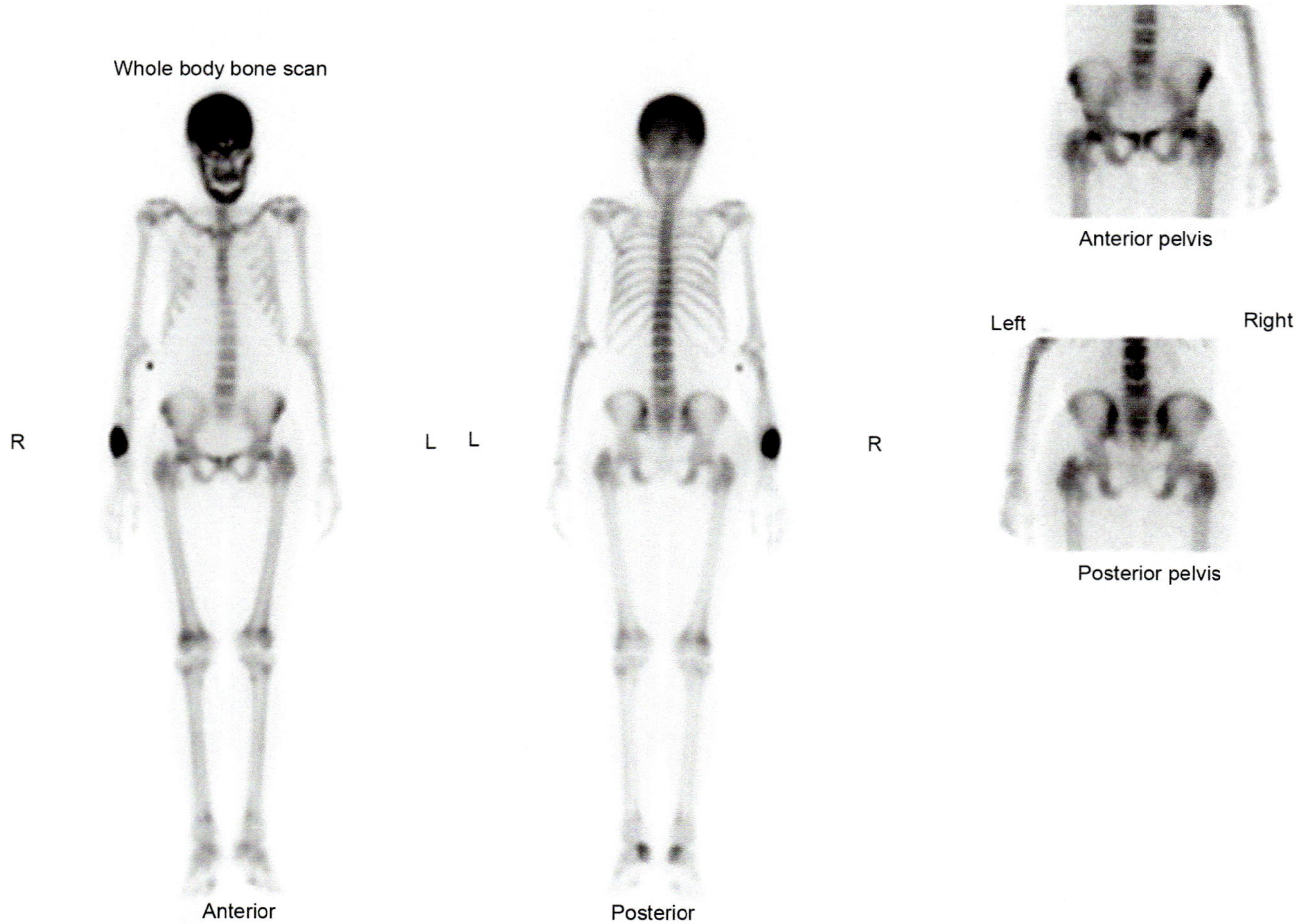

Fig. 1: Whole body 99mTc-Methyl diphosphonate (MDP) images demonstrate diffusely increased radiotracer uptake in the axial and appendicular skeleton in uniform pattern. There is minimal soft tissue uptake and no evidence of radiotracer excretion in the kidneys and urinary bladder. The findings are compatible with "Superscan". Uniform increase in radiotracer uptake and involvement of the axial and appendicular skeleton are characteristics of "Superscan" from metabolic bone disease.

- Fluorodeoxyglucose-positron emission tomography is used in conjunction with bone scintigraphy in detection of skeletal metastases. Single-photon emission computed tomography (SPECT) provides further improved contrast resolution by localizing the site of uptake in the facet joints (which makes degenerative disease more likely) as opposed to pedicles (which makes metastatic disease more likely).

REFERENCE

1. Buckley O, O'Keeffe S, Geoghegan T, et al. Tc-99m bone scintigraphy superscans: a review. Nucl Med Commun. 2007;28(7):521-7.

CASE 22: ASSESSMENT OF CHRONIC HYDRONEPHROSIS

Brief History

A 46-year-old woman with history of renal stone.

Findings

Contrast-enhanced axial computed tomography (CT) image demonstrates a massively dilated right renal collecting system with associatedparenchymal atrophy consistent with long-standing ureteropelvic junction (UPJ) obstruction. Tc-99m mercaptoacetyltriglycin (MAG3) scan shows absent right renal flow and absent right nephrogram activity.

Main Teaching Point

- Chronic obstruction at the UPJ can lead to hydronephrosis and chronic renal failure. Both Tc-99m diethylenetriaminepentaacetate (DTPA) and Tc-99m dimercaptosuccinic acid (DMSA) are used to assess relative renal functions. Although Tc-99m DMSA static scintigraphy is the most reliable method for calculating renal function, DMSA is useful for renogram curve acquisition and glomerular filtration rate (GFR) calculation. Complete absence of flow and function, as seen in this case, would preclude any invasive approaches to mitigate obstruction.

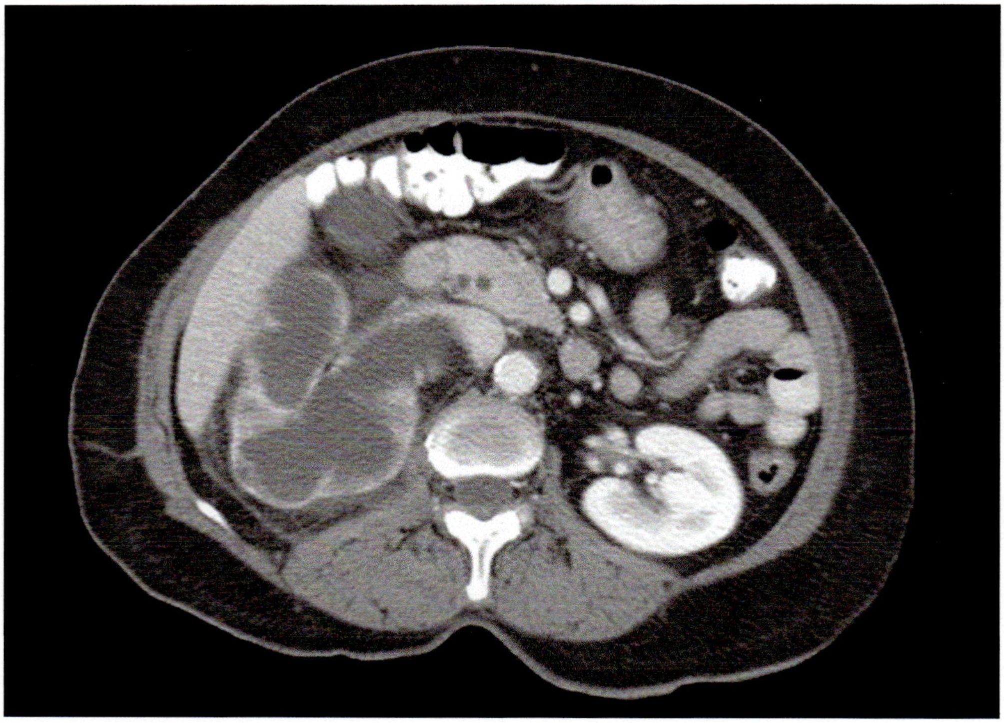

Fig. 1: Contrast-enhanced axial CT image demonstrates a massively dilated right renal collecting system with associated parenchymal atrophy consistent with long-standing ureteropelvic junction (UPJ) obstruction.

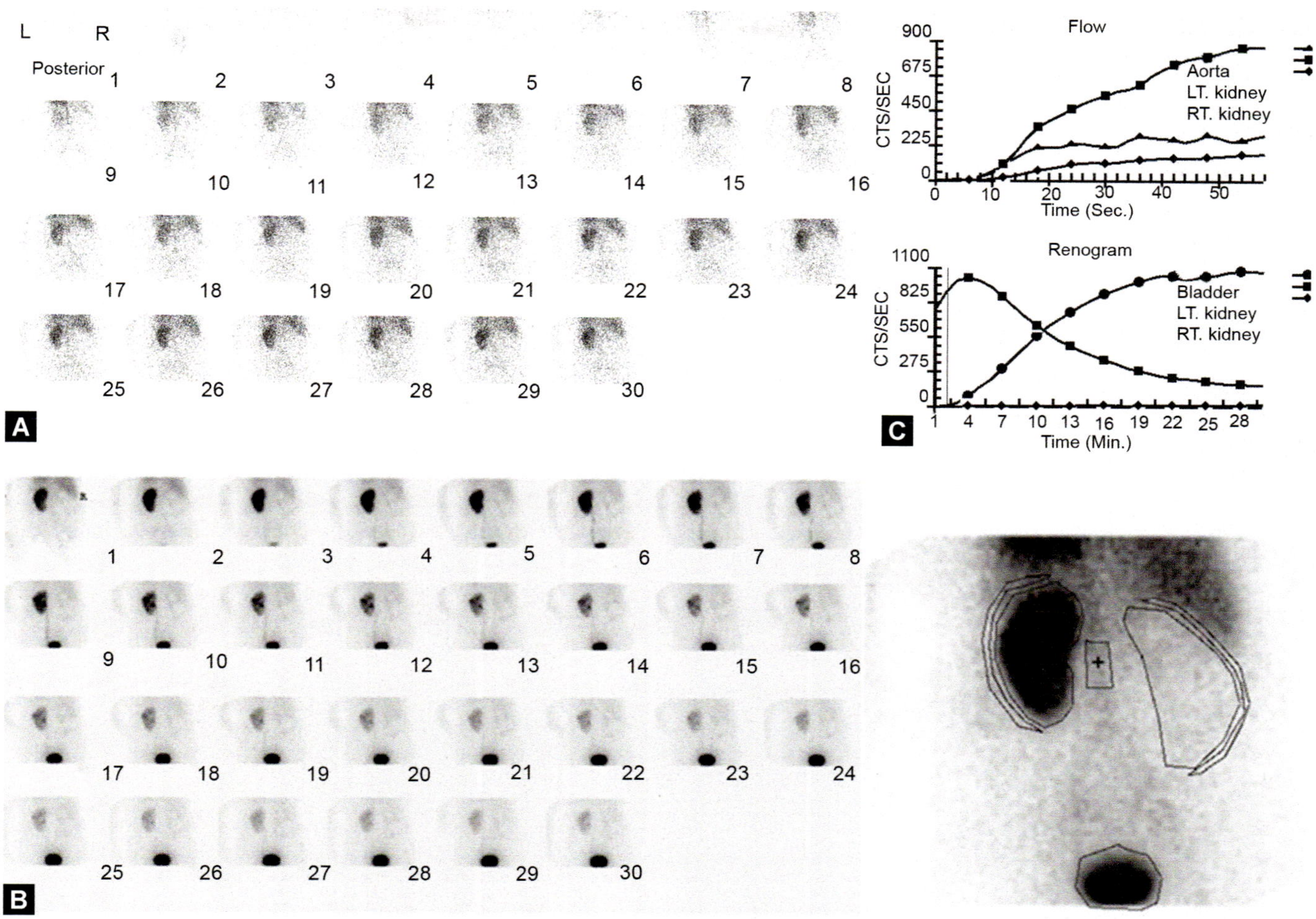

Figs. 2A to C: F-0 Diuretic renography with Tc-99m MAG-3 in posterior projection. Radionuclide angiographic images (A) demonstrate prompt flow to the left kidney and absence of blood flow to the right kidney. Function phase images (B) demonstrate normal cortical transit and prompt excretion of radiotracer from the left kidney. There is no radiotracer uptake in the right kidney. The findings are compatible with loss of function in the right kidney from long-standing ureteropelvic junction obstruction. Renogram (C) also demonstrates similar findings.

REFERENCE

1. Yalçın H, Ozen A, Günay EC, et al. Can Tc-99m DTPA be Used in Adult Patients in Evaluation of Relative Renal Function Measurement as the Reference Tc-99m DMSA Method? Mol Imaging Radionucl Ther. 2011;20(1):14-8.

CASE 23: ASSESSMENT FOR SUSPECTED DELAYED GASTRIC EMPTYING

Brief History

A 55-year-old man with diabetes presents with early satiety.

Findings

Gastric emptying study is performed after oral administration of Tc-99m Sulfur Colloid labeled test meal containing two scrambled eggs and two slices of toasted bread. The images are acquired every hour for total of 4 hours in the anterior and posterior projections. Region-of-interest is drawn around the stomach in the anterior and posterior projections. The geometric mean is obtained from the counts from region of interest and a time activity curve is plotted with obtained geometric mean. In general, retention of >10% of administered activity at four hours indicates delayed gastric emptying.

Reference Range		
Time Point	Lower Normal Limit for Gastric Retention	Upper Normal Limit for Gastric Retention
0 min	A lower value suggests rapid gastric emptying	A greater value suggests delayed gastric emptying
0.5 h	70%	
1 h	30%	90%
2 h		60%
3 h		30%
4 h		10%

Values are the 95th percentile confidence interval.

Main Teaching Point

- Gastroparesis is defined as delayed gastric emptying in the absence of mechanical obstruction leading to symptoms of nausea, vomiting, abdominal pain, and early satiety. Gastroparesis is often associated with diabetes, gastric surgery, or neuromuscular disorders that involve the gastric myenteric plexus. Idiopathic gastroparesis accounts for as many as 40% of total gastroparesis cases, which poses a treatment challenge for symptom relief.

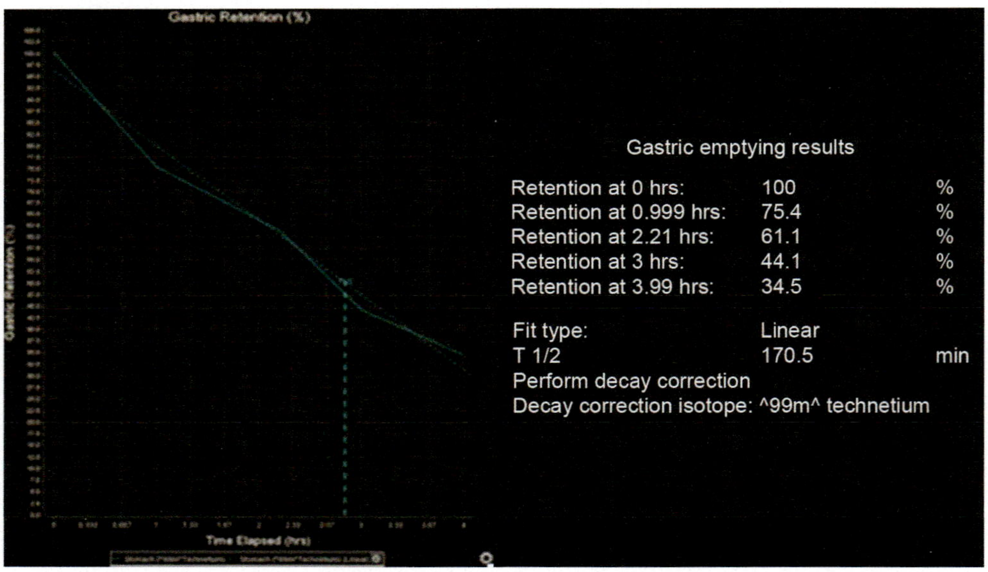

Fig. 1: Time activity curve of Geometric mean obtained from gastric emptying study performed after oral administration of Tc-99m Sulfur Colloid labeled test meal demonstrate significant retention of radiotracer in the stomach.

REFERENCE

1. Am J Gastroenterol. 2008 Mar;103(3):753-63. Epub 2007 Nov 19. Consensus recommendations for gastric emptying scintigraphy: a joint report of the American Neurogastroenterology and Motility Society and the Society of Nuclear Medicine. Abell TL1, Camilleri M, Donohoe K, Hasler WL, Lin HC, Maurer AH, McCallum RW, Nowak T, Nusynowitz ML, Parkman HP, Shreve P, Szarka LA, Snape WJ Jr,Ziessman HA; American Neurogastroenterology and Motility Society and the Society of Nuclear Medicine.

CASE 24: ASSESSMENT OF LOW BACK PAIN IN A YOUNG PATIENT

Brief History

A 15-year-old boy presents with low back pain.

Findings

Tc-99m methylene diphosphonate (MDP) whole body and Single-photon emission computed tomography (SPECT) imaging of the lumbar spine demonstrate increased tracer uptake in the bilateral L5 pars interarticularis, left greater than right, consistent spondylolysis with right-sided likely reactive uptake.

Main Teaching Points

- Spondylolysis is a common cause of low back pain in young athletes characterized by a unilateral or bilateral defect in the pars interarticularis of the vertebral body. The vast majority of defects occur at L5. Risk factors for spondylolisthesis include occult spina bifida and family history. Bilateral spondylolysis produces spondylolisthesis or vertebral body slippage whereas unilateral spondylolysis may cause reactive changes in the contralateral pars interarticularis.
- Scintigraphic bone scan can differentiate between acute spondylolysis and chronic nonunion: increased uptake at the pars articularis suggests osteoblastic activity and healing potential whereas an absence of increased uptake suggests chronic nonunion and decreased healing potential.

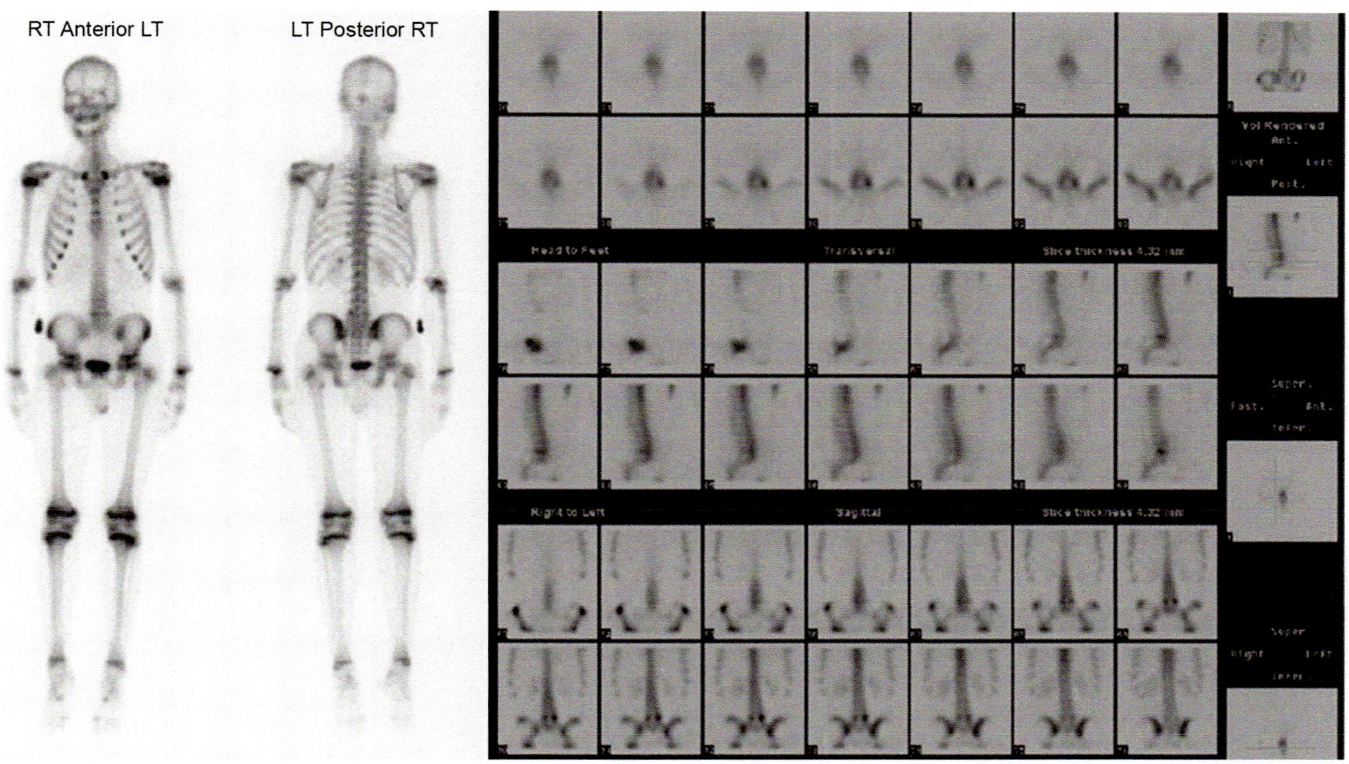

Fig. 1: Whole body 99mTc-Methyl diphosphonate (MDP) images (A) demonstrate increased radiotracer uptake in the right and left L5 posterior element, greater on the left side. SPECT images of the lumbar spine (B) localizes this uptake in both L5 pars interarticularis, greater on the left side. The findings are compatible with left L5 spondylolysis and reactive uptake in the right L5 pars interarticularis.

REFERENCE

1. Foreman P, Griessenauer CJ, Watanabe K, et al. L5 spondylolysis/spondylolisthesis: a comprehensive review with an anatomic focus. Childs Nerv Syst. 2013;29(2):209-16.

CASE 25: EVALUATION OF ABDOMINAL PAIN FOLLOWING RENAL TRANSPLANTATION

Brief History

A 43-year-old man status postrenal transplant undergoes a diethylenetriaminepentaacetate (DTPA) renal scan for evaluation of abdominal pain.

Findings

Prior ultrasound demonstrated free fluid in the pelvis. Tc-99m DTPA renal scan demonstrates abnormal activity in the pelvis outside the collecting system consistent with a urine leak.

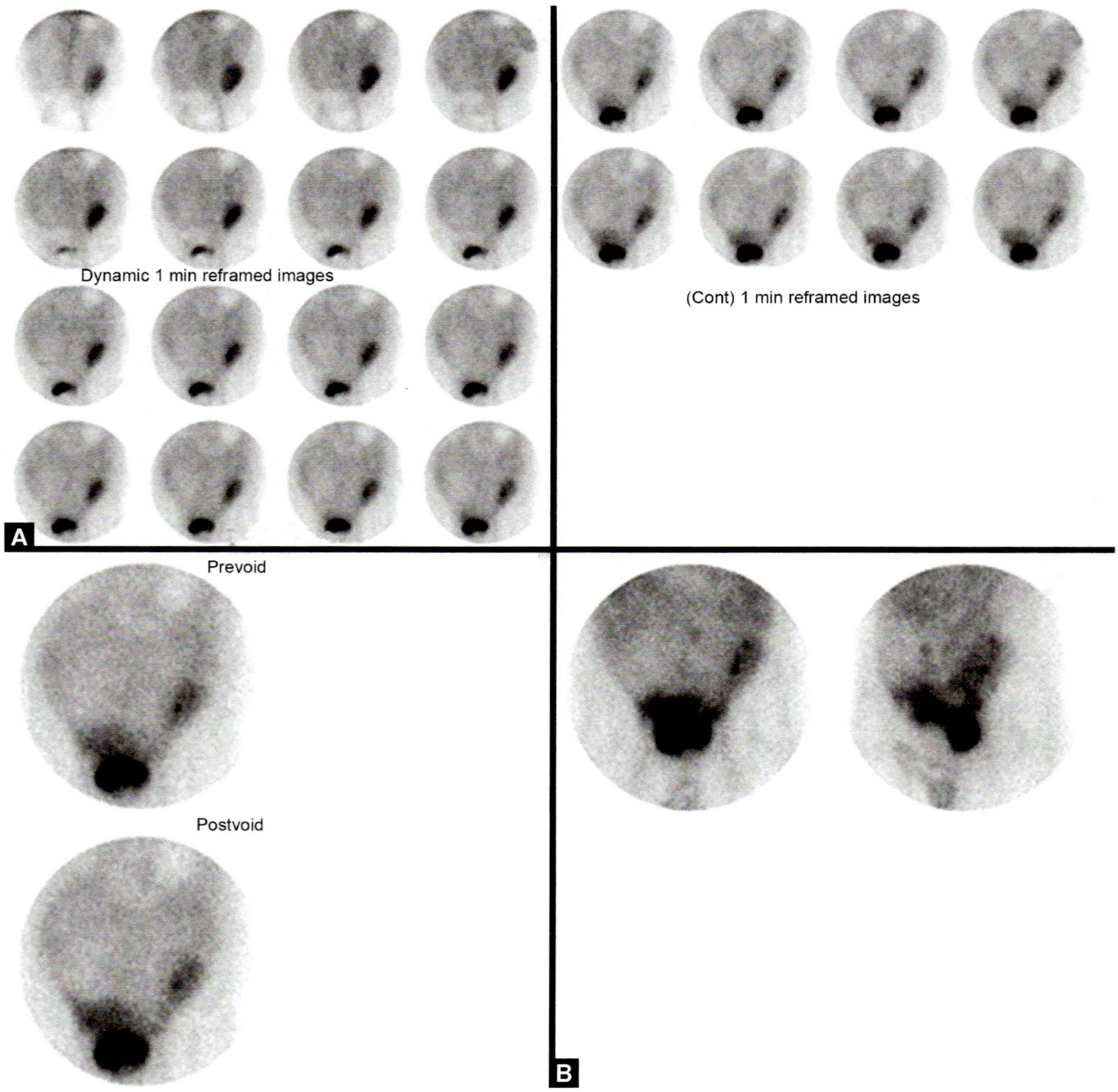

Figs. 1A and B: Tc-99m DTPA renal scan demonstrates prompt uptake, normal cortical transit and expected excretion of radiotracer from the renal transplant in the left iliac fossa and abnormal extravasation of radiotracer activity in the right lower pelvis, superior to the dome of the urinary bladder. Delayed spot images in the anterior and right lateral decubitus position (B) demonstrate layering of activity in the right lower pelvis. The findings are compatible with post-transplant urine leak from anastomotic failure.

Main Teaching Points

- Urine leak occurs with an incidence of 3% following renal transplantation and is diagnosed on scintigraphy by visualization of tracer accumulation outside the expected region of the kidneys, ureters and bladder. A urinoma may appear as an initial photopenic region adjacent to the kidney with subsequent tracer fill-in that does not extend beyond the border of that region. Alternatively, a urinoma may produce progressive tracer accumulation confined to a region adjacent to the kidney without regional photopenia.
- The differential for post-transplant perirenal photopenia on a scintigraphic renal scan includes hematoma, seroma, abscess, or lymphocele. Clinical correlation and cytologic analysis may be required for definitive diagnosis.

REFERENCE

1. Sfakianaki E, Sfakianakis GN, Georgiou M, et al. Renal scintigraphy in the acute care setting. Semin Nucl Med. 2013;43(2):114-28.

CASE 26: ASSESSMENT OF RIGHT UPPER QUADRANT PAIN

Brief History

A 44-year-old woman with right upper quadrant pain. A prior same-day ultrasonography was negative for acute cholecystitis and cholelithiasis.

Findings

Hepatobiliary scintigraphy demonstrates no gallbladder emptying on sequential images with gallbladder ejection fraction (EF) of less than 10%. Administration of cholecystokinin (CCK) resulted in an EF of 9% consistent with biliary dyskinesia. Time-activity curve shows little change in counts over 30 minutes of image acquisition, consistent with decreased gallbladder EF.

Main Teaching Points

- Cholecystokinin-hepatobiliary iminodiacetic acid is a standard of radionucleotide imaging for diagnosis of biliary dyskinesia, also referred to as chronic acalculous cholecystitis. Tc-99m labeled hepatobiliary iminodiacetic acid (HIDA) is taken up by the liver and excreted into the biliary system. CCK is then administered to stimulate gallbladder contraction. An abnormally low gallbladder EF following CCK infusion is consistent with biliary dyskinesia.
- The Society of Nuclear Medicine Practice Guidelines for Hepatobiliary Scintigraphy reports the following recommendations: nothing by mouth for 4–6 hours prior to the study; withholding opiates or other drugs that affect gallbladder contraction; injection of 3–5 mCi Tc-99m mebrofenin or disofenin; imaging acquisition over 60 minutes; slow infusion of 0.02 μg/kg CCK over 60 minutes; calculation of gallbladder EF where a threshold of less than 38% is considered abnormal.

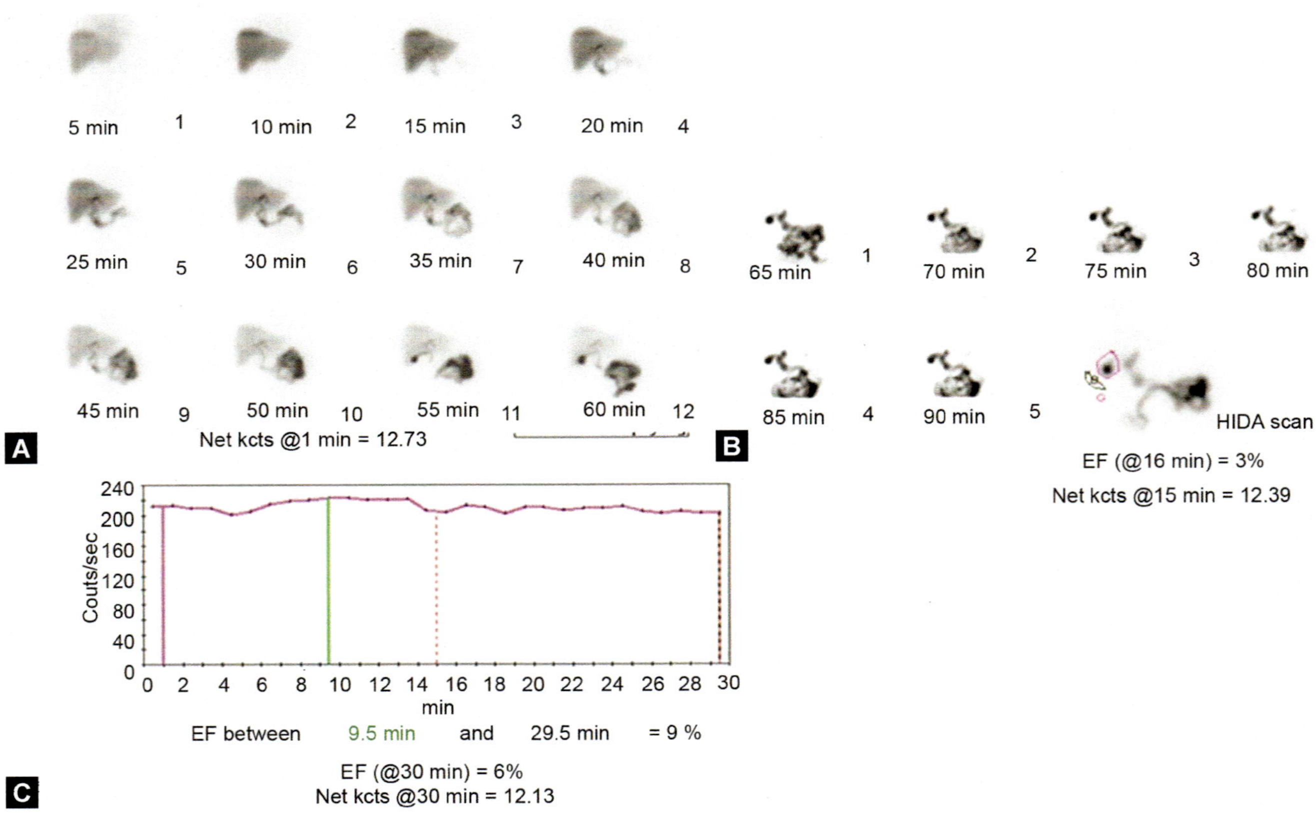

Figs. 1A to C: First hour dynamic images (A) of hepatobiliary scintigraphy demonstrates prompt excretion of radiotracer in the gall bladder and in small intestine. Post cholecystokinin images (B) demonstrate no gallbladder emptying on sequential images with gallbladder ejection fraction (EF) of less than 10%. Administration of cholecystokinin (CCK) resulted in an EF of 9% consistent with biliary dyskinesia. Time-activity curve (C) shows little change in counts over 30 minutes of image acquisition, consistent with decreased gallbladder EF.

REFERENCE

1. Richmond BK, DiBaise J, Ziessman H. Utilization of cholecystokinin cholescintigraphy in clinical practice. J Am Coll Surg. 2013;217(2):317-23.

CASE 27: ASSESSMENT OF RENAL ECTOPIA AND ASSOCIATED COMPLICATIONS

Brief History

A 45-year-old man presents with flank pain.

Findings

Noncontrast computed tomography (CT) scan shows renal crossed fused ectopia (horseshoe kidney) with a nonobstructive calculus in the lower pole of the right kidney. mercaptoacetyltriglycin (MAG3) renal scan demonstrates prompt cortical clearance of radiotracer activity without abnormal retention in the collecting system and is therefore negative for obstruction.

Main Teaching Point

- Crossed fused ectopia is the most common congenital genitourinary fusion anomaly with an incidence of 1 in 400–600 individuals and is characterized by renal malrotation, ectopia and vascular changes. Although usually asymptomatic, clinical symptoms of crossed fused ectopia include abdominal pain, nausea and vomiting secondary to associated renal and ureteral pathologies. The course of the ureter across the isthmus, the association with congenital ureteral stricture, and the variable arterial supply predispose individuals with crossed fused ectopia to hydronephrosis, pyelonephritis and nephrolithiasis.

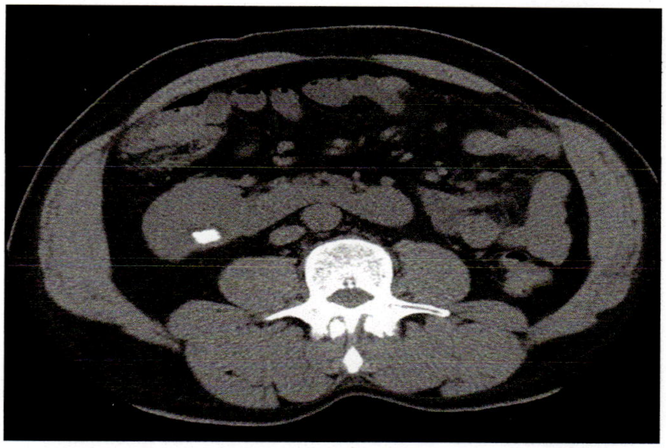

Fig. 1: Noncontrast CT scan shows renal crossed fused ectopia with a nonobstructive calculus in the lower pole of the right kidney.

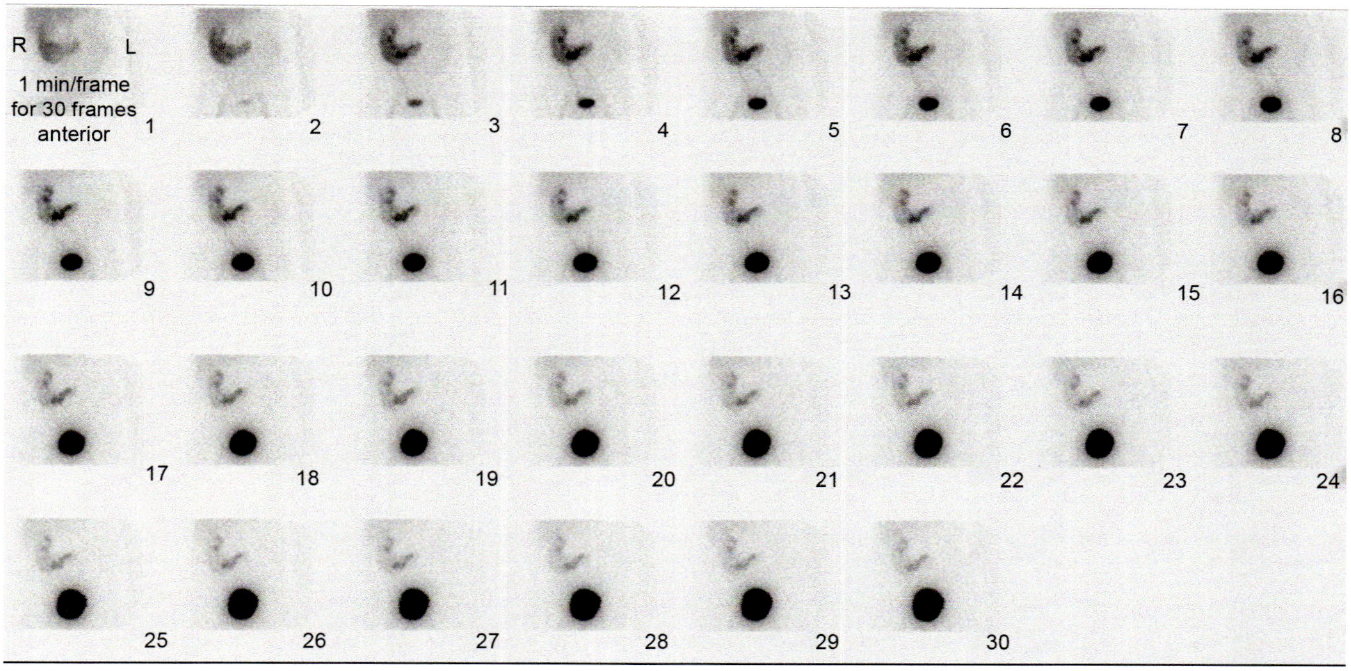

Fig. 2: Tc-99m MAG3 renal scan obtained in anterior projection demonstrates prompt cortical clearance of radiotracer activity without abnormal retention in the collecting system and is therefore negative for obstruction. The right kidney has unusual shape and lower pole crosses the midline. The left kidney is not seen in its normal location.

REFERENCE

1. Natsis K, Piagkou M, Skotsimara A, et al. Horseshoe kidney: a review of anatomy and pathology. Surg Radiol Anat. 2014;36(6):517-26.

CASE 28: ASSESSMENT OF SHORTNESS OF BREATH

Brief History

A 33-year-old woman with human immunodeficiency virus/acquired immunodeficiency syndrome (HIV/AIDS) underwent whole body Gallium scan to evaluate for shortness of breath.

Findings

Radiograph of the chest demonstrates diffuse patchy airspace opacities including a near-confluent region in the right upper lung. Whole body Gallium-citrate scan reveals diffuse increased uptake which is more intense than liver in the right upper lung zone and left upper/mid lung zone. Intensity of Gallium uptake in the right mid lung zone is as intense as that in the liver.

Main Teaching Points

- Gallium is an iron analog which binds to transferrin and lactoferrin receptors in regions of increased inflammation and metabolic activity. A variety of clinical conditions produce diffuse bilateral increased pulmonary uptake on Gallium-citrate scan. The most common etiologies include sarcoidosis, pulmonary fibrosis, interstitial pneumonia, *Pneumocystis carinii* pneumonia, tuberculosis, lymphoma and primary lung cancer.
- Diffuse pulmonary uptake of Gallium is a nonspecific finding observed in a number of pulmonary pathologies. The value of Gallium scintigraphy lies in its sensitivity where abnormal increased uptake should prompt further diagnostic evaluation. One grading system compares intensity of uptake in the lungs to that in the liver (Grade IV: lung more intense than liver; Grade III: as intense; Grade II: less intense; Grade I: faint uptake, and Grade 0: no uptake).

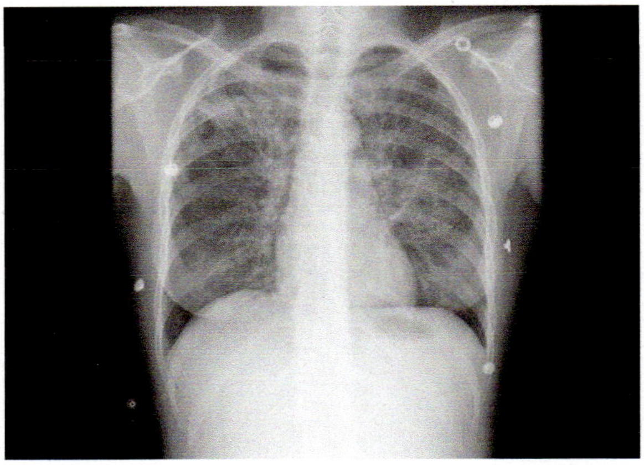

Fig. 1: Radiograph of the chest demonstrates diffuse patchy airspace opacities including a near-confluent region in the right upper lung.

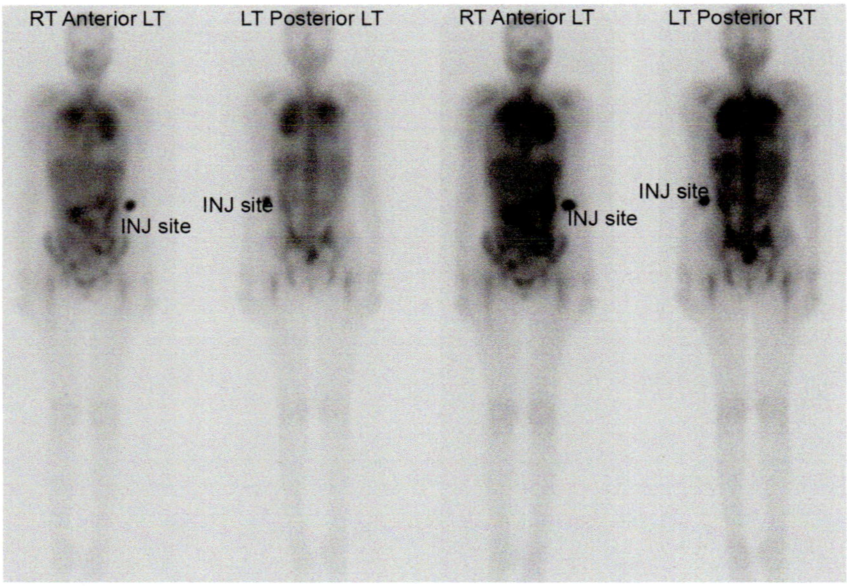

Fig. 2: Whole body 67Ga Citrate scan reveals diffuse increased pulmonary uptake which is more intense than liver in the right upper lung zone and left upper/mid lung zone. Intensity of Gallium uptake in the right mid lung zone is as intense as that in the liver.

REFERENCE

1. Schuster DM, Alazraki N. Gallium and other agents in diseases of the lung. Semin Nucl Med. 2002;32(3):193-211.

CASE 29: ASSESSMENT OF DIFFUSE SKELETAL METASTASES

Brief History

A 64-year-old woman with breast cancer undergoes evaluation for skeletal metastases.

Findings

Tc-99m methylene diphosphonate (MDP) whole body bone scan with focal spot views of the pelvis and skull demonstrates diffuse increased skeletal radiotracer uptake consistent with a "superscan".

Main Teaching Points

- Bone scintigraphy detects osteoblastic activity which may not yet be evident on other imaging modalities. A superscan is characterized by diffuse increased skeletal radiotracer uptake relative to soft tissue with significantly reduced or absent renal activity.
- Pathologies that produce a superscan include metabolic disorders such as Paget's disease hyperparathyroidism, hypertrophic osteodystrophy, metastatic disorders commonly secondary to breast or prostate cancer. Whereas metastatic disease typically demonstrates a patchy heterogeneous appearance involving the central axial and appendicular skeleton, metabolic disease typically exhibit a homogeneous diffuse increased tracer uptake throughout the skeleton. Occasionally, however, diffuse metastatic skeletal disease with large tumor burden may manifest a pattern of diffuse homogenous increased tracer uptake.

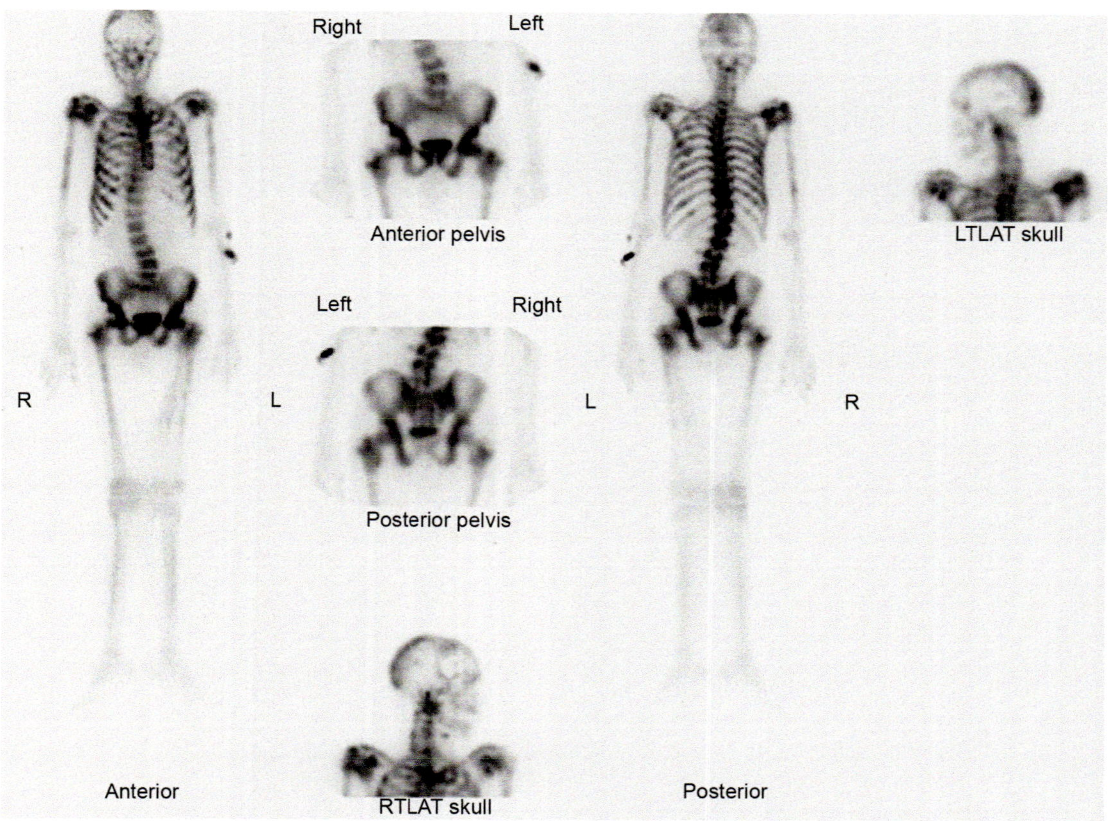

Fig. 1: Whole body 99mTc-Methyl diphosphonate (MDP) images demonstrate diffusely increased radiotracer uptake in heterogeneous pattern in the central skeleton, including the skull, the spine, the ribs, the pelvis and proximal long bones. There is minimal soft tissue and renal uptake. The radiotracer excretion is seen in the urinary bladder. The findings are compatible with "Superscan". Heterogeneous pattern of radiotracer uptake and involvement of the central skeleton are characteristics of "Superscan" from metastatic disease.

REFERENCE

1. Love C, Din AS, Tomas MB, et al. Radionuclide bone imaging: an illustrative review. Radiographics. 2003;23(2):341-58.

CASE 30: ASSESSMENT OF UNCONTROLLED HYPERTENSION

Brief History

A 56-year-old woman with uncontrolled hypertension undergoes whole body I-123 metaiodobenzylguanidine (MIBG) scan.

Findings

Noncontrast computed tomography (CT) demonstrates a homogenous left adrenal gland mass. I-123 whole body MIBG scan shows increased uptake in the left adrenal gland consistent with a pheochromocytoma.

Main Teaching Point

- Metaiodobenzylguanidine, an analog of noradrenaline, localizes to tumors arising from adrenal tissue. I-123 MIBG is the imaging modality of choice for the detection of pheochromocytomas with reported 99% sensitivity. The I-123 MIBG protocol requires prior blockade of iodine uptake in the thyroid gland with potassium chloride or SSKI as well as discontinuation of drugs such as calcium channel blockers and tricyclic antidepressants that affect MIBG uptake.

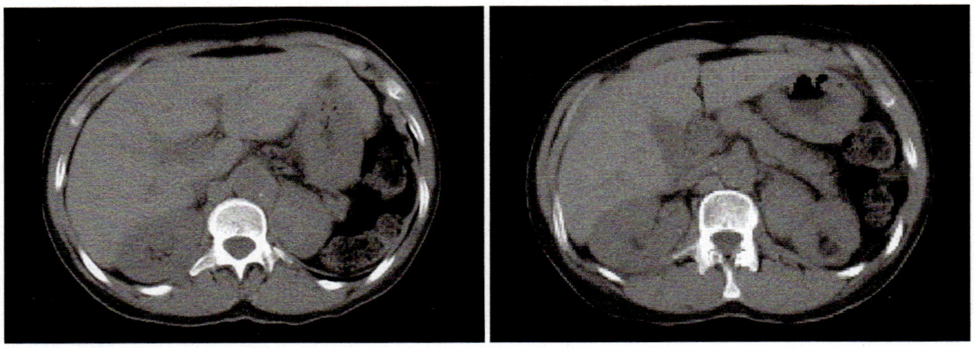

Fig. 1: Noncontrast CT demonstrates a homogenous left adrenal gland mass.

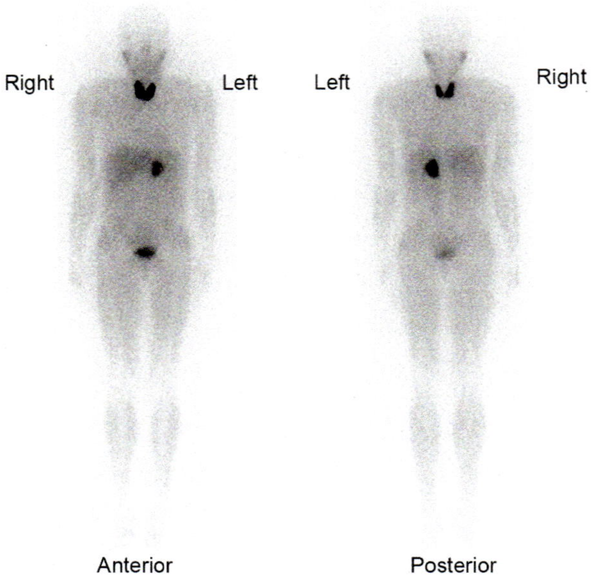

Fig. 2: I-^{123} whole body MIBG scan demonstrates expected radiotracer uptake in the liver and thyroid gland. Faint radiotracer uptake is seen in the myocardium. Abnormally increased uptake seen in the left adrenal gland compatible with a pheochromocytoma.

REFERENCE

1. Brink I, Hoegerle S, Klisch J, et al. Imaging of pheochromocytoma and paraganglioma. Fam Cancer. 2005;4(1):61-8.

CASE 31: EVALUATION OF BRAIN DEATH

Brief History

A 25-year-old man status post motor vehicle accident (MVA) undergoes brain perfusion scan to evaluate for brain death.

Findings

Tc-99m HMPAO scan demonstrates absence of radiotracer activity in the intracranial vasculature.

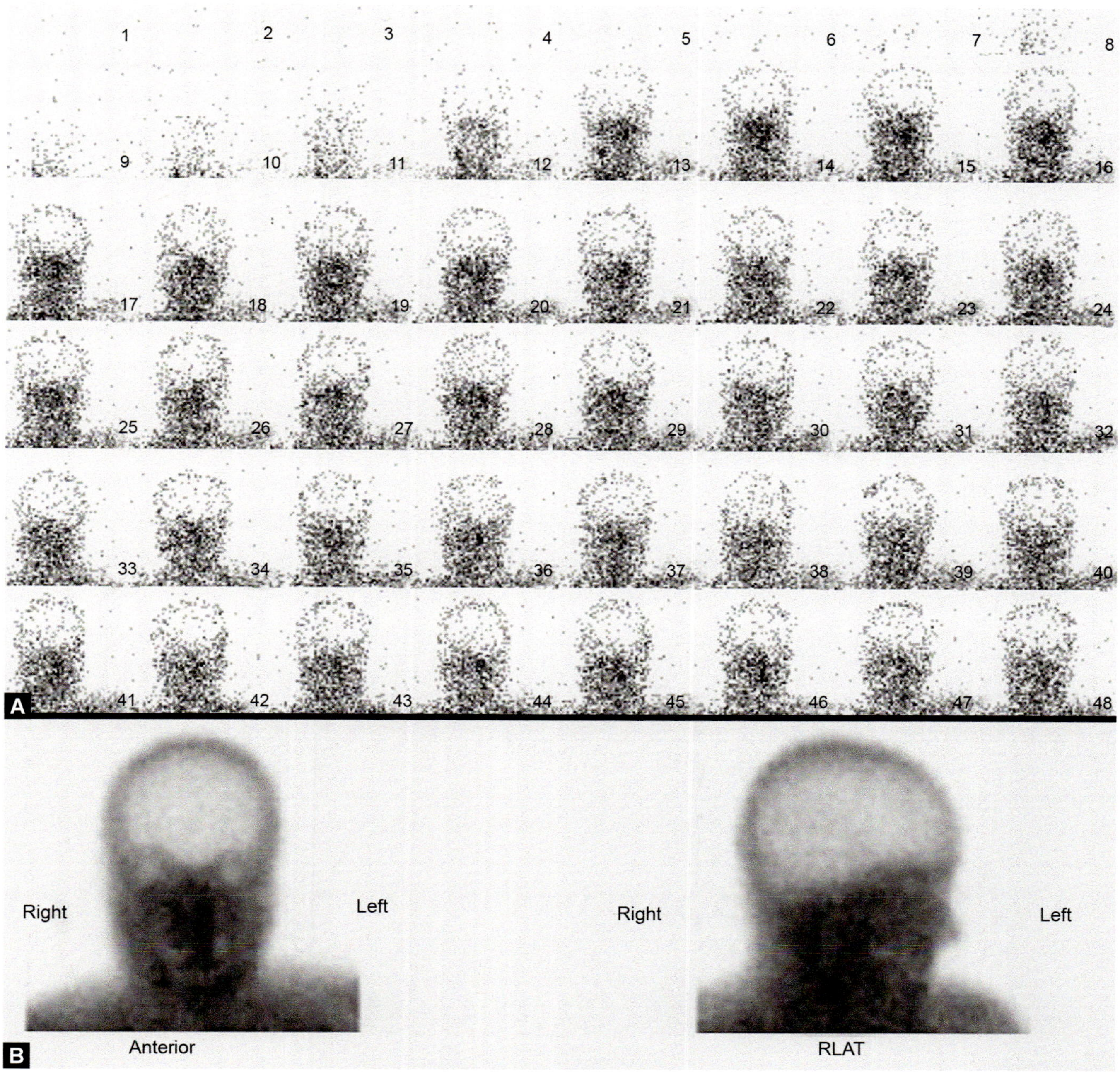

Figs. 1A and B: Tc-99m HMPAO scan. A dynamic angiographic images of the skull in anterior projection demonstrate intact perfusion in the external carotid artery distribution and absence of perfusion in the internal carotid artery territory. The static images in anterior projection (A) and in the right lateral projection (B) demonstrate absence of intracranial perfusion.

Main Teaching Points

- The clinical manifestations of brain death are absent cranial nerve function, lack of central respiratory drive, and absent response to noxious stimuli. Tc-99m HMPAO is an ancillary examination which can shorten the time interval between replicate physical examinations, or replace components of the physical examination in cases such as facial trauma, vital sign instability, or medication-induced coma.
- Tc-99m HMPAO is a lipophilic compound, which readily traverses the blood brain barrier. Traumatic brain injury results in cerebral edema with resultant increase in intracranial pressure. The diminished antegrade blood flow to the brain exacerbates ischemic injury, which produces further increase in intracranial pressure. Failure to visualize radiotracer activity in the intracranial arteries or veins is compatible with brain death.

REFERENCE

1. Zuckier LS, Sogbein OO. Brain perfusion studies in the evaluation of acute neurologic abnormalities. Semin Nucl Med. 2013;43(2):129-38.

CASE 32: ASSESSMENT OF DELAYED VISUALIZATION OF GALLBLADDER

Brief History

A 35-year-old man admitted in the intensive care unit on total parenteral nutrition presents with abdominal pain.

Findings

Tc-99m Mebrofenin hepatobiliary scintigraphy demonstrates prompt uptake in the liver, rapid clearance of cardiac blood pool, prompt excretion in the bowel but nonvisualization of gallbladder at 1 hour. After morphine augmentation, radiotracer activity within the gallbladder is visualized.

Main Teaching Points

- Biliary scintigraphy is the imaging modality of choice in the evaluation of gallbladder function. It is also used in conjunction with ultrasound and computed tomography (CT) examinations in the assessment of suspected acute cholecystitis. Normal gallbladder is visualized by 60 minutes on a hepatobiliary iminodiacetic acid (HIDA) scan and produces an EF of greater than 35%.
- Delayed visualization of gallbladder activity after 60 minutes, or visualization of gallbladder after morphine administration to cause contraction of the sphincter of Oddi, can be seen in cases of chronic cholecystitis, peptic ulcer disease, hepatitis, pancreatitis, or gallbladder neoplasms, and occasionally in the setting of low oral intake/chronic fasting, prolonged hospitalization/intensive unit care.

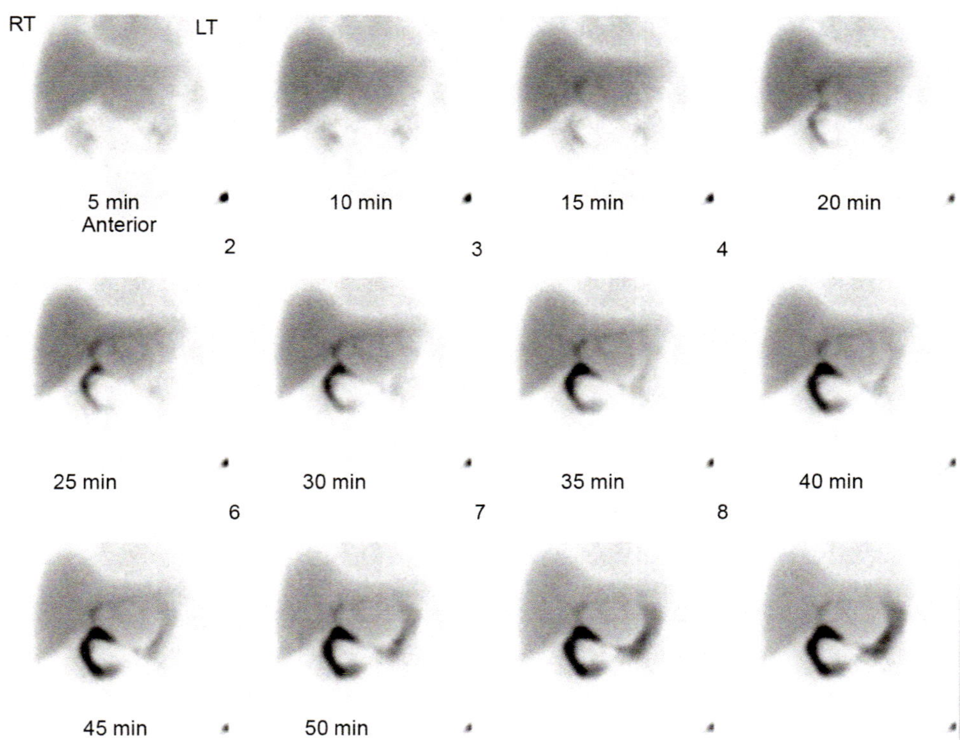

Fig. 1: Dynamic images of Tc-99m Mebrofenin hepatobiliary scintigraphy demonstrates prompt uptake in the liver, slightly delayed clearance of cardiac blood pool, prompt excretion in the bowel but nonvisualization of gallbladder at 1 hour.

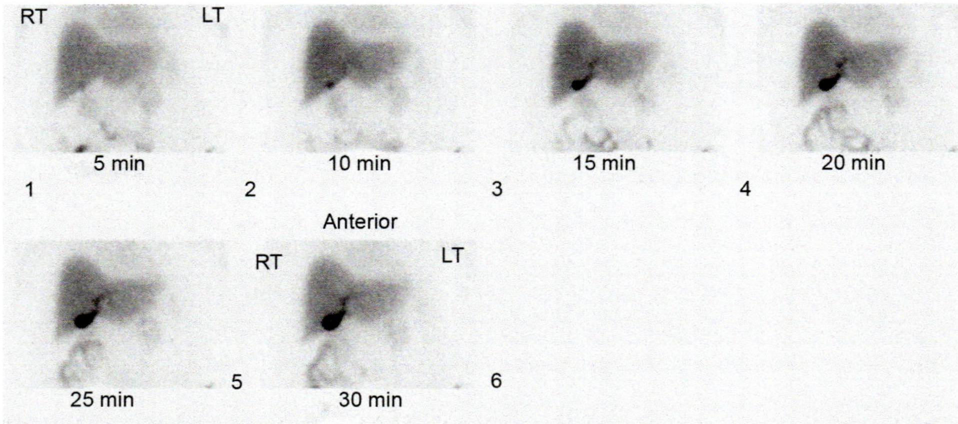

Fig. 2: Additional 30 minute dynamic images obtained after morphine augmentation. Radiotracer activity is promptly visualized within the gallbladder. The findings exclude acute cholecystitis.

REFERENCE

1. O'Connor OJ, Maher MM. Imaging of cholecystitis. AJR Am J Roentgenol. 2011;196(4):W367-74.

CASE 33: ASSESSMENT OF CHRONIC URINARY OBSTRUCTION

Brief History

A 15-year-old boy with vesicoureteral reflux undergoes evaluation for renal function.

Findings

Dimercaptosuccinic acid renal scan reveals a small atrophic left kidney with heterogeneous decreased tracer uptake and multiple photopenic defects, consistent with chronic renal scarring.

Main Teaching Point

- Chronic obstructive uropathy leads to hydronephrosis and eventual renal atrophy and cortical scarring. Recovery of renal function in patients with unilateral obstructive uropathy and a normal contralateral kidney has been shown to depend on preoperative renographic clearance and perfusion of the affected kidney. A renographic GFR of less than 10 mL/min/1.73m^3 indicates irreversible damage, while improvement in renal function can be expected after relief of obstruction in cases above this threshold.

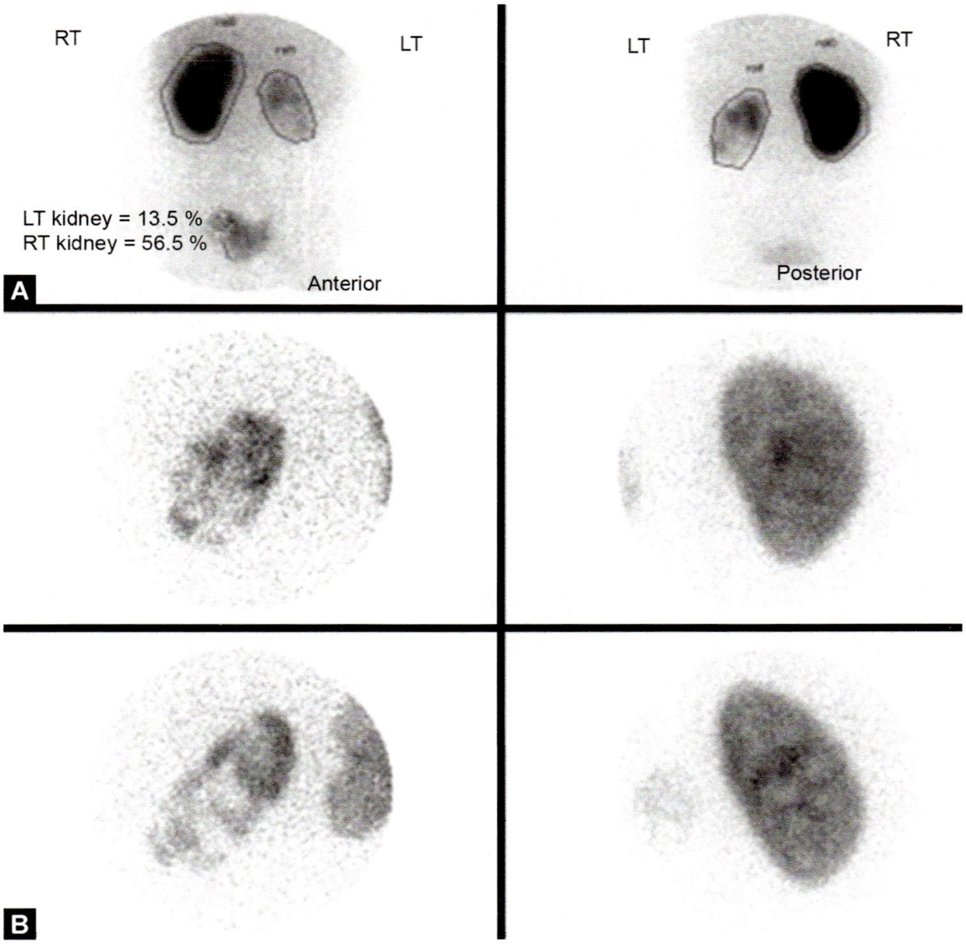

Figs. 1A and B: Planar (A) and pinhole (B) images of Tc-99m DMSA scan. Multiple photopenic defects are seen in left renal parenchyma with loss of renal architecture. The left kidney appears smaller and atrophic. The findings are compatible with chronic pyelonephritis/scarring. The radiotracer uptake in the right kidney is normal.

REFERENCE

1. Khalaf IM, Shokeir AA, El-Gyoushi FI, et al. Recoverability of renal function after treatment of adult patients with unilateral obstructive uropathy and normal contralateral kidney: a prospective study. Urology. 2004;64(4):664-8.

CASE 34: ASSESSMENT OF DIFFUSE RENAL UPTAKE ON BONE SCAN

Brief History

A 35-year-old man with human immunodeficiency virus (HIV) undergoes a whole body bone scan.

Findings

Whole body bone scan reveals bilateral diffuse increased renal uptake, more intense than usually seen and confined to the renal cortical distribution.

Main Teaching Points

- Nonosseous accumulation of Tc-99m methylene diphosphonate (MDP) is observed in a number of inflammatory, ischemic, neoplastic, traumatic and hormonal disorders. Bilateral diffuse increased renal uptake can result from ischemic injury that leads to calcium deposition in injured tissue. Temporary occlusions of the renal arteries have been shown to increase serum calcium concentration and causes Tc-99m MDP uptake in the renal parenchyma.
- Other etiologies that produce diffuse increased renal uptake on bone scan include hypercalcemia, dehydration, sickle cell anemia, nephrocalcinosis and administration of antineoplastic agents.

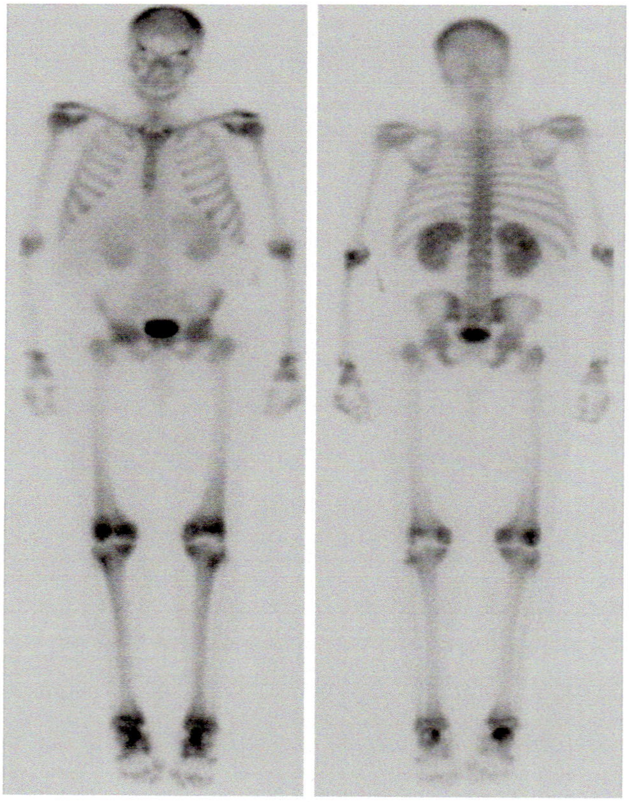

Fig. 1: Whole body 99mTc-Methyl diphosphonate (MDP) images reveals bilateral diffuse increased renal uptake, more intense than usually seen and confined to the renal cortical distribution.

REFERENCE

1. Peller PJ, Ho VB, Kransdorf MJ. Extraosseous Tc-99m MDP uptake: a pathophysiologic approach. Radiographics. 1993; 13(4):715-34.

CASE 35: ASSESSMENT OF HYPERCALCEMIA AND HYPERPARATHYROIDISM

Brief History

A 49-year-old woman with hypercalcemia and hyperparathyroidism is referred for evaluation of a parathyroid adenoma.

Findings

Tc-99m sestamibi scan shows a focus of intense radiotracer uptake in the anterior mediastinum that persists on delayed imaging consistent. Subsequent imaging with computed tomography (CT) scan revealed a mediastinal mass and surgical resection was consistent with an ectopic parathyroid adenoma.

Main Teaching Points

- The parathyroid glands originate from the dorsal endoderm of the third and fourth pharyngeal pouches and lose their parapharyngeal connections by the seventh week of gestation. The superior pair of parathyroid glands descends with the superior pole of the thyroid gland from the base of the tongue, and migrates to the junction of the upper and middle third of the thyroid gland posteriorly in 75% of the population. In the remaining population, they are located posterior to the upper pole of the thyroid gland, intrathyroidal, or retroesophageal.
- The inferior pair of parathyroid glands migrates caudally with the thymus and demonstrates a more variable distribution. In approximately 40% of the population, they are located near the lower poles of the thyroid gland. However, the inferior parathyroid glands can be found anywhere from above the carotid bifurcation to the mediastinum. Planar imaging alone is often sufficient in the assessment of ectopic parathyroid adenoma. Single-photon emission computed tomography (SPECT) and SPECT/CT aid significantly in the assessment of parathyroid adenoma, particularly when localized in their usual expected anatomic distribution.

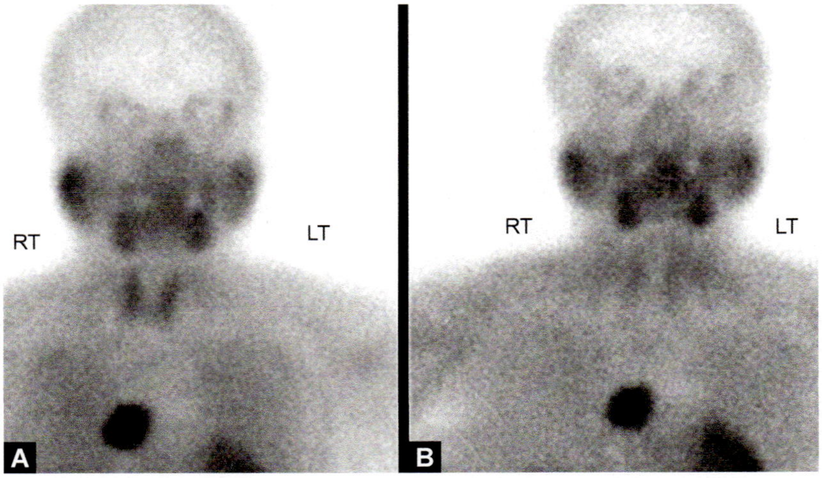

Figs. 1A and B: Early (A) and washout/delayed (B) images of Tc-99m sestamibi scan demonstrate a focus of intense radiotracer uptake in the anterior mediastinum that persists on delayed imaging consistent with ectopic parathyroid adenoma.

REFERENCE

1. Palestro CJ, Tomas MB, Tronco GG. Radionuclide imaging of the parathyroid glands. Semin Nucl Med. 2005;35(4): 266-76.

CASE 36: ASSESSMENT OF BACK PAIN

Brief History

A 65-year-old diabetic status post right above knee amputation presents with back pain.

Findings

Whole body Gallium scan reveals radiotracer accumulation in the lower thoracic spine compatible with discitis.

Main Teaching Points

- Gallium citrate localize to sites of infection via binding to transferrin in regions of vascular permeability, binding to lactoferrin which exhibits antimicrobial activity, and via direct uptake into bacteria through siderophores. Gallium citrate Single-photon emission computed tomography (SPECT) improves the sensitivity and specificity of bone scans in evaluating for discitis and represents an alternative to MR. The sensitivity and specificity of Gallium citrate SPECT are 91% and 92% respectively, compared to 91% and 77% with MR.
- Interpretation of positive Gallium-citrate result in the postoperative setting is challenging given the likelihood of a false-positive finding due to inflammation at the site of surgery. In general, greater intensity and/or distribution of gallium relative to the bone scan favors discitis rather than nonspecific inflammatory process.

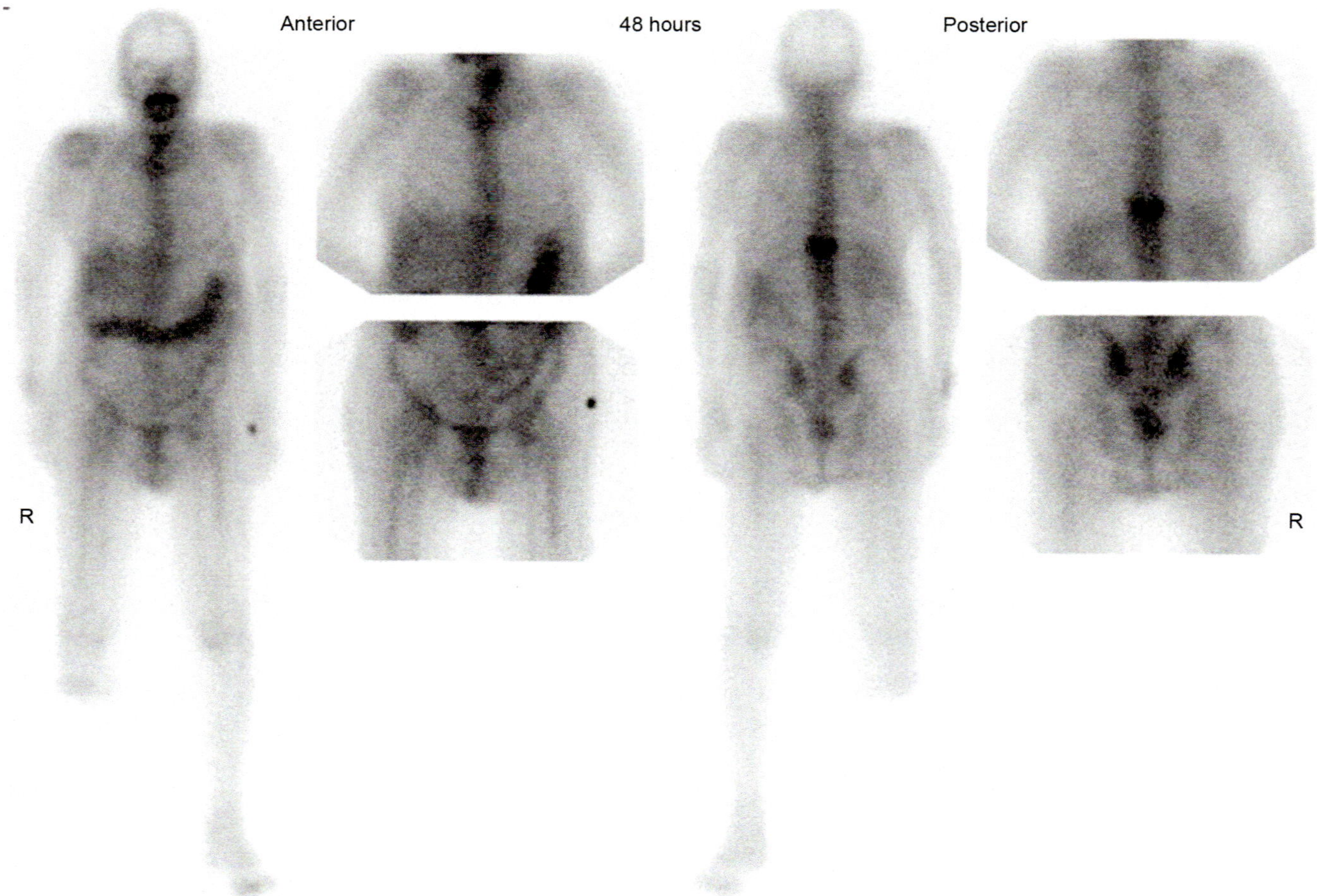

Fig. 1: Whole body 67Ga Citrate scan reveals that patient is status post right above knee amputation. Abnormal radiotracer accumulation in the intervertebral disc space of the lower thoracic spine is compatible with discitis.

REFERENCE

1. Treglia G, Focacci C, Caldarella C, et al. The role of nuclear medicine in the diagnosis of spondylodiscitis. Eur Rev Med Pharmacol Sci. 2012;16 Suppl 2:20-5.

CASE 37: ASSESSMENT OF HYPERPARATHYROIDISM

Brief History

A 57-year-old man presents with biochemical recurrence of hyperparathyroidism.

Findings

Early Tc-99m sestamibi imaging demonstrates homogenous thyroid uptake. Delayed image reveals a focus of persistent radiotracer activity in the region of the left lower pole of the thyroid. In the given clinical context, this is consistent with a parathyroid adenoma.

Main Teaching Points

- Scintigraphic imaging of parathyroid adenomas relies on the observation that Tc-99m sestamibi in general demonstrates earlier washout from thyroid tissue than from abnormal parathyroid tissue.
- Exceptions include parathyroid lesions that do not retain sestamibi or thyroid tissue (particularly thyroid adenoma) that does not demonstrate early washout and demonstrate pattern of persistent uptake. Other causes of a false-positive sestamibi scan include solitary thyroid nodule, thyroid carcinoma and lymphadenopathy. Additional imaging with pertechnetate and iodine which accumulate in thyroid lesions will reduce the rate of false positive sestamibi results. False negative results include parathyroid adenomas that express P-glycoprotein and consequently do not retain sestamibi in the delayed images.

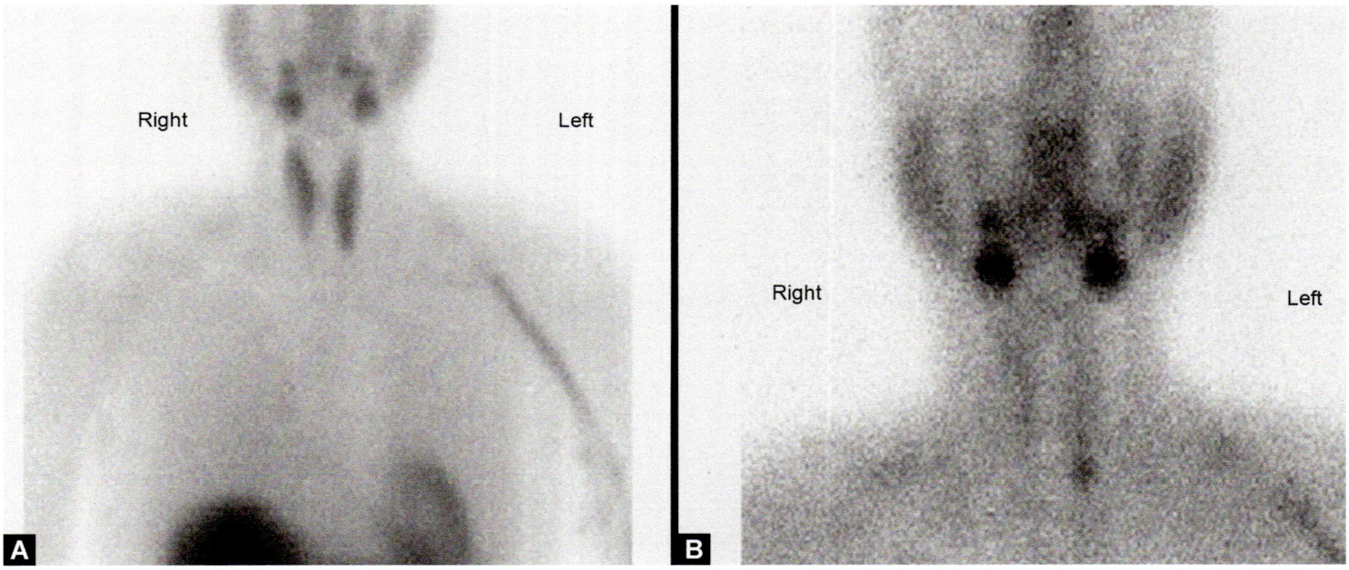

Figs. 1A and B: Early Tc-99m sestamibi image(A) demonstrates homogenous thyroid uptake. Delayed image (B) reveals complete washout of radiotracer from the thyroid gland and a focus of persistent radiotracer activity in the region of the left lower pole of the thyroid. In appropriate clinical context, this is consistent with a parathyroid adenoma.

REFERENCE

1. Palestro CJ, Tomas MB, Tronco GG. Radionuclide imaging of the parathyroid glands. Semin Nucl Med. 2005;35(4): 266-76.

CASE 38: ASSESSMENT OF INTRACRANIAL MASS LESION IN THE SETTING OF HUMAN IMMUNODEFICIENCY VIRUS (HIV)

Brief History

A 33-year-old man with HIV presents with altered mental status.

Findings

Axial MRI shows a heterogeneously-enhancing right periventricular mass. Thallium-201 scan shows intense tracer uptake corresponding to the mass.

Main Teaching Points

- The most common causes of central nervous system (CNS) mass lesions in HIV patients are infection with *Toxoplasma gondii*, primary lymphoma, followed less commonly by progressive multifocal leukoencephalopathy (PML), tuberculosis, and *Cryptococcus* or other opportunistic infections. The combination of thallium and Gallium imaging of intracranial tumors can improve diagnostic specificity in differentiating tumors from nonmalignant lesions in patients with HIV.
- Lesions that are thallium-positive and Gallium-positive include lymphoma, glioma and PML. Comparing intensity of thallium uptake in the target lesion to the corresponding contralateral site improves specificity for prediction of malignancy. Lesions that are thallium-negative but Gallium-positive include intracranial infections secondary to tuberculosis, *Cryptococcus*, and bacterial infections. Finally, infarction is thallium-negative and Gallium-negative. Thallium scans should be performed prior to Gallium scans in order to avoid compton scatter from the higher energy Ga-67 photons.

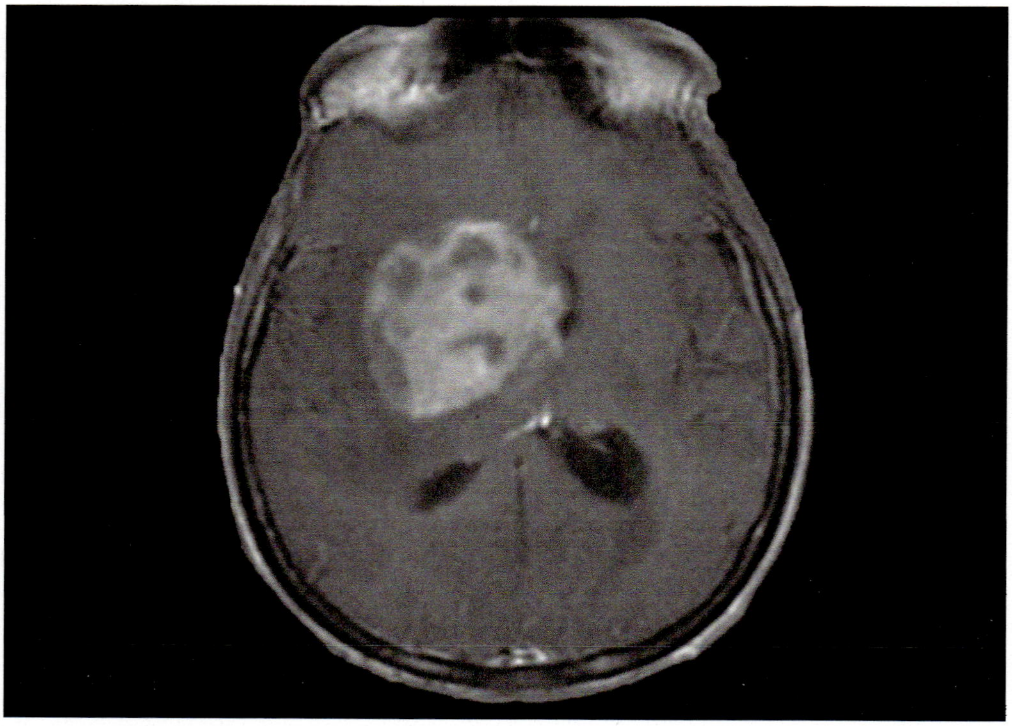

Fig. 1: Axial MRI shows a heterogeneously-enhancing right periventricular mass.

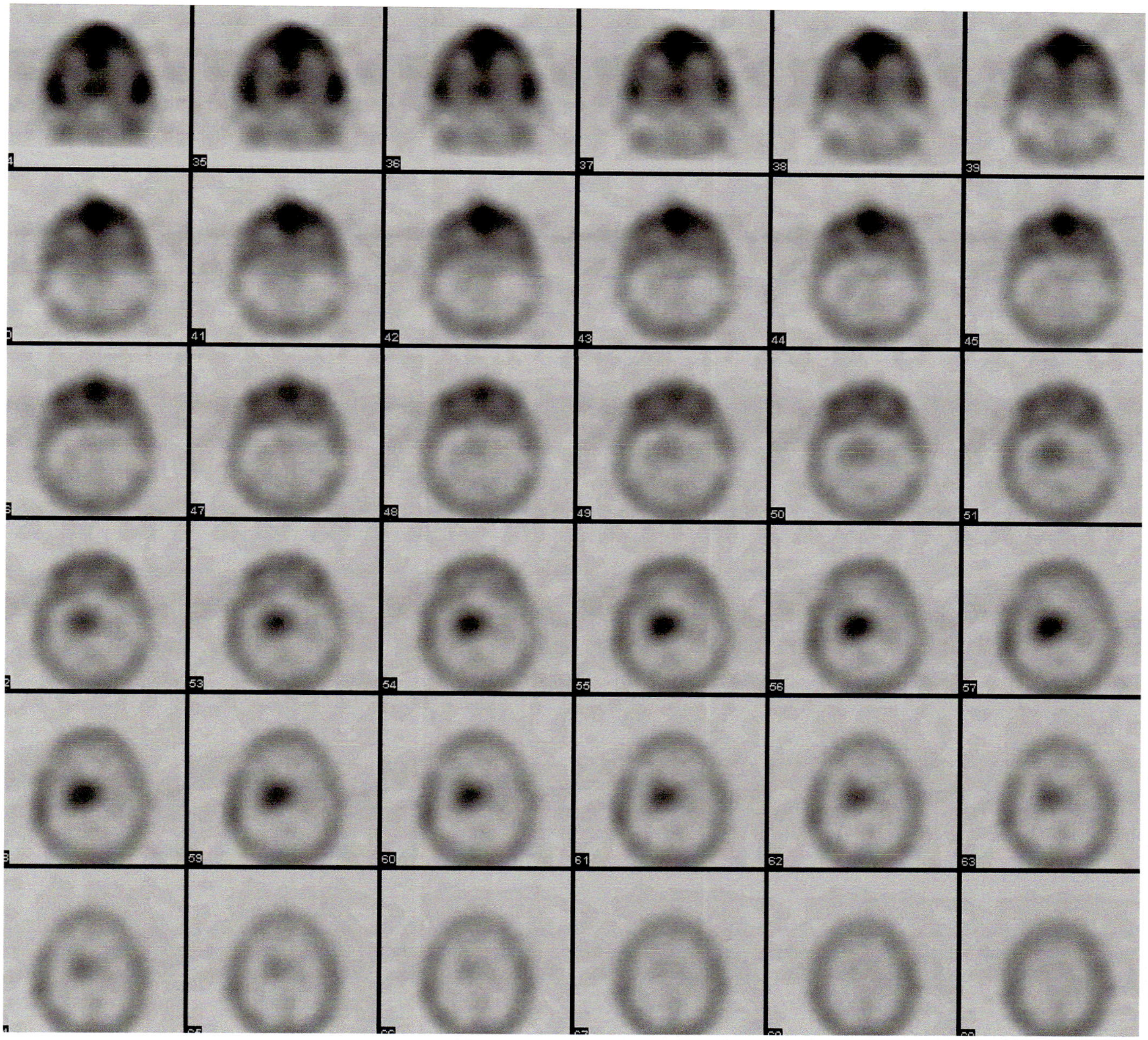

Fig. 2: Thallium-201 SPECT images of the brain demonstrate scan intense tracer uptake corresponding to the right periventricular mass. The target to background(contralateral brain) ratio is 3.3. The findings are compatible with central nervous system (CNS) lymphoma in an immunocompromised patient.

REFERENCES

1. Robert Young, Munir Ghesani, Nolan Kagetsu et al. lesion size determines accuracy of thallium-201 brain single-photon emission tomography in differentiating between intracranial malignancy and infection in AIDS patients. Am J Neuroradiol. 2005;26:1973-9.
2. Lee VW, Antonacci V, Tilak S, et al. Intracranial mass lesions: sequential thallium and Gallium scintigraphy in patients with AIDS. Radiology. 1999;211(2):507-12.

CASE 39: ASSESSMENT OF HIP PAIN

Brief History

A 24-year-old female is referred for hip radiograph and bone scintigraphy for evaluation of right hip pain.

Findings

Single frontal hip radiograph demonstrates a well-circumscribed lucency in the right ilium with a narrow zone of transition. Triple phase bone scan shows increased flow and blood pool uptake in the right ilium. Delayed phase imaging demonstrates a rim of increased uptake with central photopenia consistent with an aneurysmal bone cyst.

Main Teaching Point

- Scintigraphic bone scan is sensitive to bony remodeling due to either malignant or benign processes. Benign bone lesions that demonstrate increased radiotracer uptake include aneurysmal bone cyst, eosinophilic granuloma, fibrous dysplasia, and enchondroma. While infection can have a similar pattern of uptake on bone scan the plain radiograph is characteristic of a benign process. Correlation with plain radiographs and other imaging modalities is important to differentiate benign from malignancy etiologies.

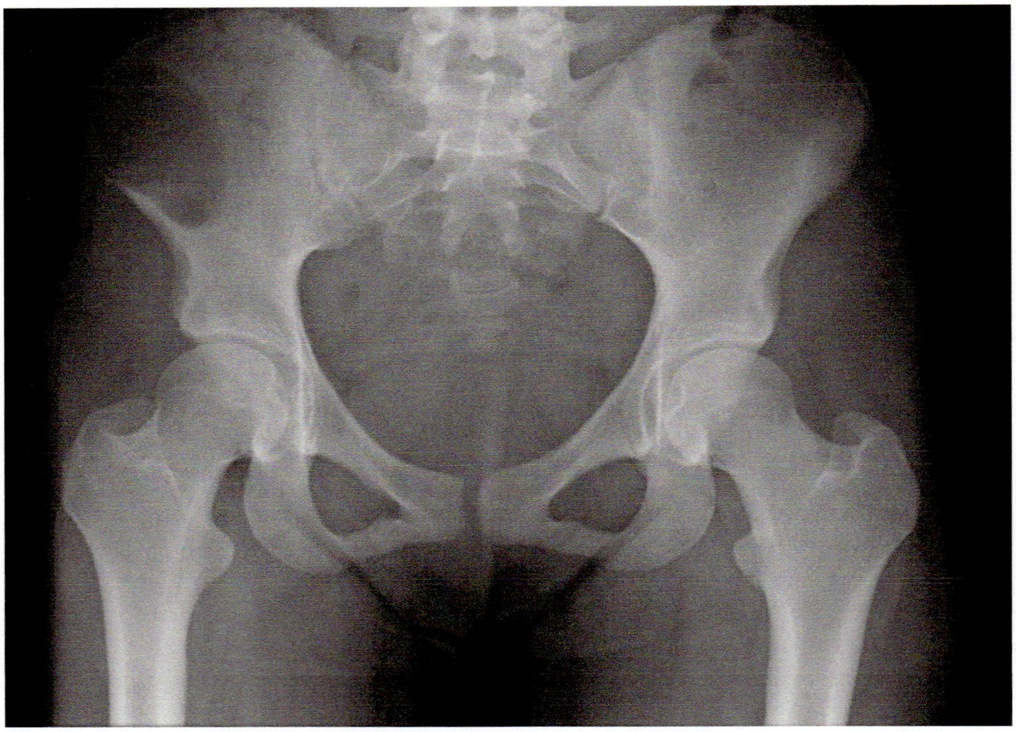

Fig. 1: Single frontal hip radiograph demonstrates a well-circumscribed lucency in the right ilium with a narrow zone of transition.

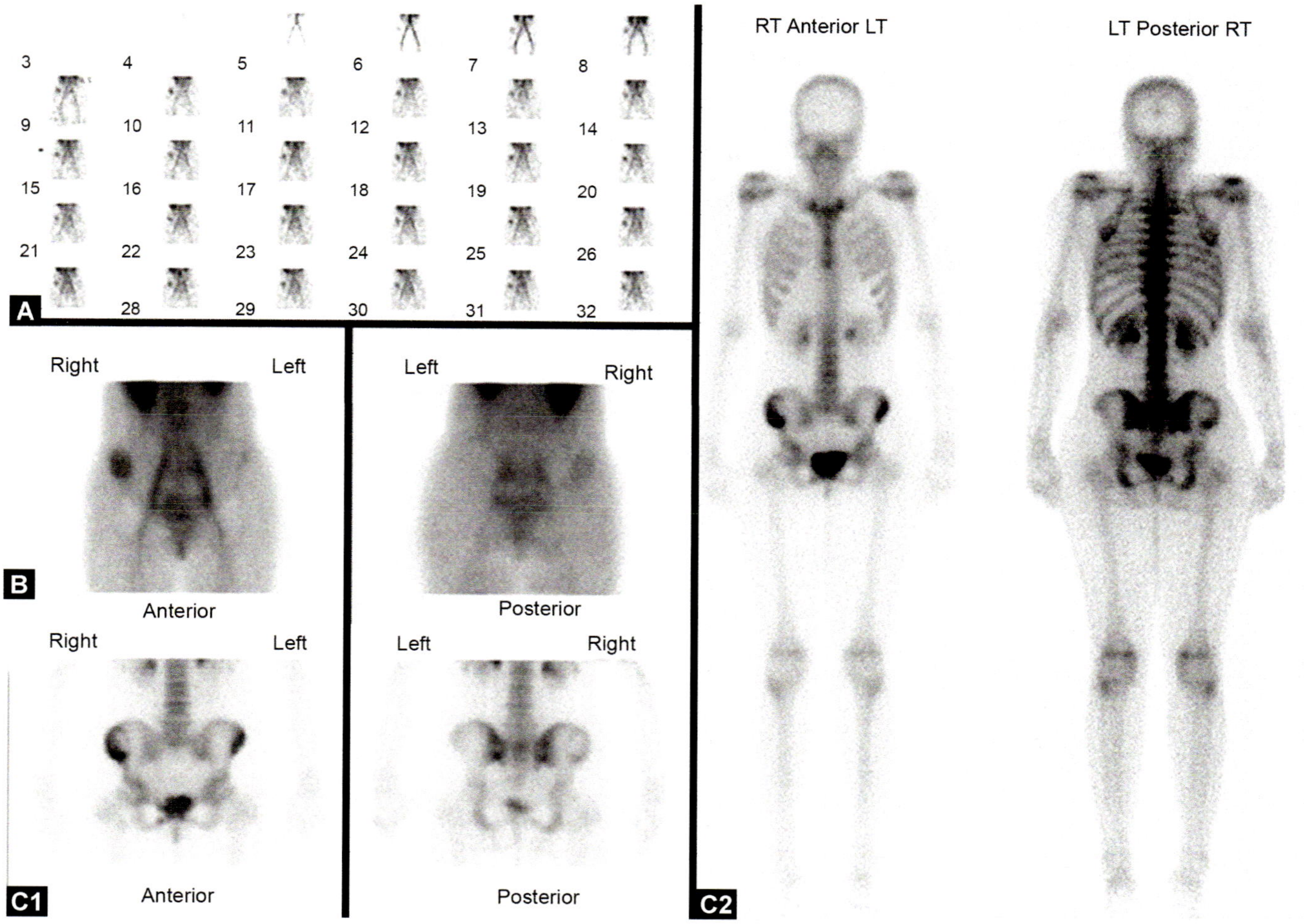

Figs. 2A to C: Triple phase bone scan shows increased flow in angiographic images (A) and hyperemia in blood pool images (B) in the right ilium. Delayed phase images (C1 and C2) demonstrate a rim of increased uptake with central photopenia, the findings can be seen in an aneurysmal bone cyst.

REFERENCE

1. Zhang Y, Zhao C, Liu H, et al. Multiple metastasis-like bone lesions in scintigraphic imaging. J Biomed Biotechnol. 2012;2012:957364.

CASE 40: ASSESSMENT FOR METASTATIC NEUROENDOCRINE NEOPLASM

Brief History

A 62-year-old man with small bowel obstruction is diagnosed with carcinoid of the small bowel on laparotomy.

Findings

Indium-111 octreotide scan shows uptake in the right paramedian mid abdomen which on axial computed tomography (CT) was correlated, localizing to a mesenteric lymph node.

Main Teaching Points

- Octreotide binds to the SSTRs of a wide variety of neuroendocrine tumors including carcinoid, paraganglioma, gastrinoma, insulinoma and medullary carcinoma. Five different subtypes of human somatostatin receptors have been identified (SSTR1–SSTR5). The commercially available radiopharmaceutical In-111 octreotide binds with high affinity to the SSTR2 and SSTR5 subtypes, to a lesser extent to SSTR3, and not at all to SSTR1 or SSTR4.
- Normal uptake of octreoscan occurs in the thyroid gland, liver, gallbladder, spleen, kidneys and bladder. The kidneys retain considerable radiotracer and appear quite intense even on delayed imaging, which

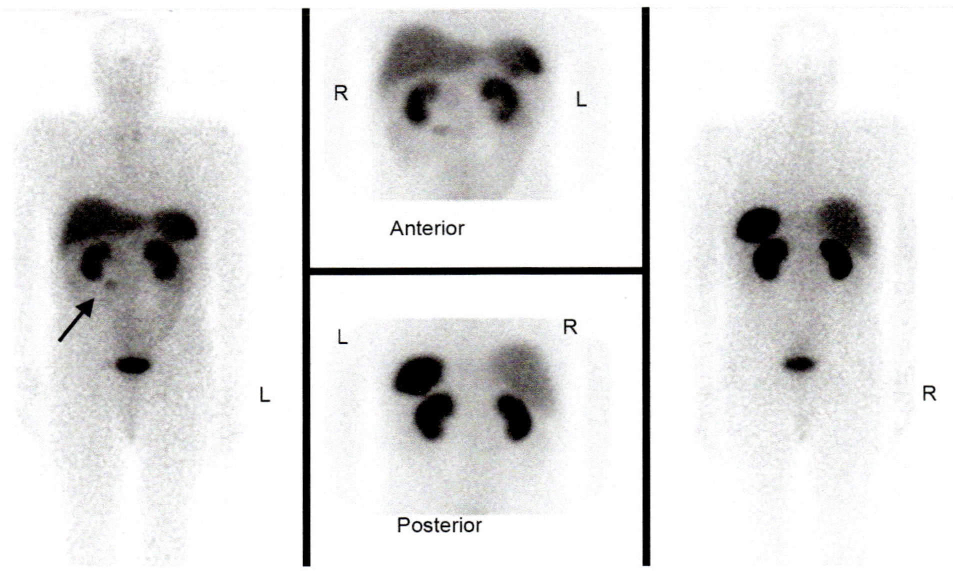

Fig. 1: Indium-111 octreotide scan reveals a focus of abnormal radiotracer uptake in the right paramedian mid abdomen, inferomedial to the lower pole of right kidney (arrow).

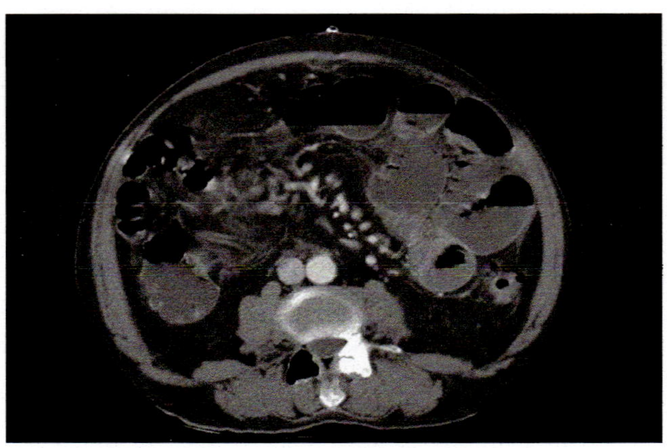

Fig. 2: Contrast enhanced axial CT demonstrated a right mesenteric lymph node. The findings were confirmed by removal of the lymph node with intraoperative localization using gamma probe.

poses a diagnostic challenge in detecting perirenal lesions. Bowel uptake should be absent or should be in a low grade, non-focal pattern on the 4-hour images. Approximately 80–90% of neuroendocrine tumors are visible by 4 hours, although ideal imaging interpretation is at 24 hours due to decreased background activity. Single-photon emission computed tomography (SPECT) imaging further aids in the assessment/localization of abnormal foci of uptake. The presence of skeletal activity on octreoscans is abnormal.

REFERENCE

1. Pepe G, Moncayo R, Bombardieri E, et al. Somatostatin receptor SPECT. Eur J Nucl Med Mol Imaging. 2012;39 Suppl 1:S41-51.

CASE 41: ASSESSMENT OF VENTRICULOPERITONEAL (VP) SHUNT PATENCY

Brief History

A 40-year-old man with intracranial neoplasm undergoes a VP shunt study for patency.

Findings

111 In diethylenetriaminepentaacetate (DTPA) ventricular shunt study in a patient with a VP shunt shows normal reflux of radiolabeled cerebrospinal fluid (CSF) from the shunt to the intracranial ventricular circulation, the shunt tube, and the normal spilling of radiolabeled CSF into the peritoneal cavity, confirming shunt patency.

Main Teaching Points

- The main indication for VP shunt placement is treatment of hydrocephalus. VP shunt malfunction include obstruction, shunt fracture, migration and infection. Clinical symptoms, such as nausea, vomiting, lethargy, headache and coma, should raise the suspicion for VP shunt malfunction and prompt computed tomography

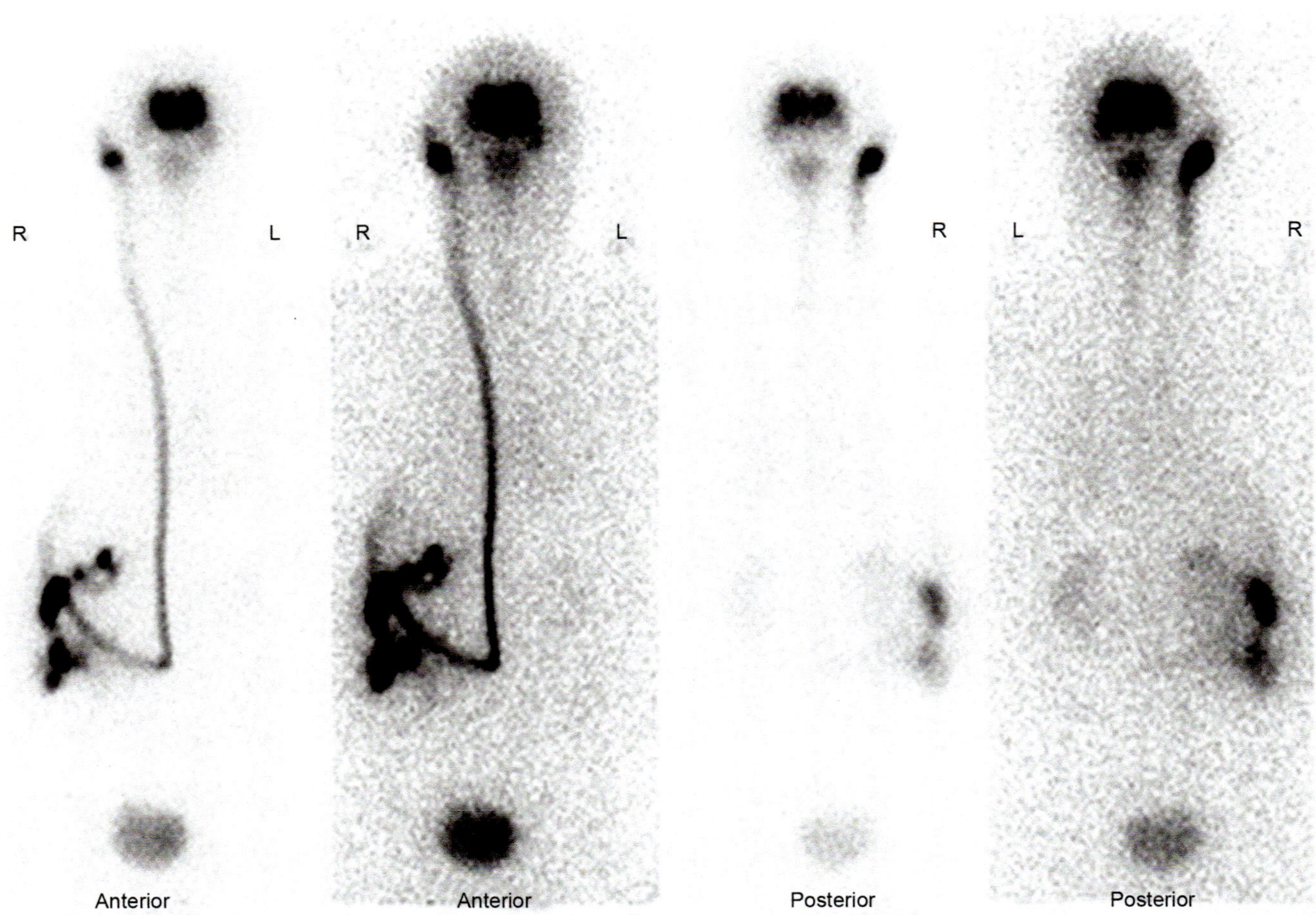

Fig. 1: ^{111}In DTPA ventricular shunt study. The radiotracer was injected in the shunt reservoir. The images display a normal reflux of radiolabeled cerebrospinal fluid (CSF) from the shunt to the intracranial ventricular circulation (proximal limb) and the shunt tube (distal limb) and the normal spilling of radiolabeled CSF into the peritoneal cavity, confirming shunt patency.

(CT) evaluation of ventricular size. Scintigraphic shunt study can be performed in cases of stable ventricular size or in cases where prior comparison is not available.

- In a patent, VP shunt, there is normal reflux of radiolabeled CSF into the proximal ventricular system as well as spillage distally into the peritoneal cavity. Nonvisualization of activity in the lateral ventricles suggests shunt obstruction proximal to the reservoir while nonvisualization of the distal tip suggests obstruction distal to the reservoir.
- Meningitis, subarachnoid hemorrhage, or trauma produces obstruction of CSF at the arachnoid granulations leading to communication hydrocephalus. Obstruction at the ventricles, foramen of Monroe, cerebral aqueduct, fourth ventricle, and outflow tracts due to tumor, inflammation/infection, or intraventricular hemorrhage produces noncommunicating hydrocephalus.

REFERENCE

1. Sivaganesan A, Krishnamurthy R, Sahni D, et al. Neuroimaging of ventriculoperitoneal shunt complications in children. Pediatr Radiol. 2012;42(9):1029-46.

CASE 42: EVALUATION OF SOLITARY COLD THYROID NODULE

Brief History

A 69-year-old female presents with a large palpable thyroid nodule.

Findings

Iodine-123 scan shows a large heterogeneous cold thyroid nodule occupying the right thyroid lobe.

Main Teaching Points

- Thyroid nodules are palpated in 4–8% in the adult population and detected in 13–67% under ultrasonography. Although thyroid cancers account for only 1% of all malignancies in the general population, they occur in about 5–15% of all thyroid nodules. With regards to likelihood of malignancy within a given thyroid nodule, there is a bimodal age-related peak of higher incidence, the first peak in teens and 20's, and the second peak after 50–55 years of age. Malignancy is found in less than 2% of hot solitary thyroid nodules and in 10–15% of cold solitary thyroid nodules. The differential diagnosis for a cold thyroid nodule includes hypofunctioning adenoma, colloid cyst and thyroid carcinoma.
- Extracapsular growth or metastatic growth is similar in nodules greater than or less than 10 mm. Therefore, suspicious nodules should undergo biopsy regardless of size. However, there is an ongoing controversy regarding the optimal management of thyroid nodules less than 1 cm in size.

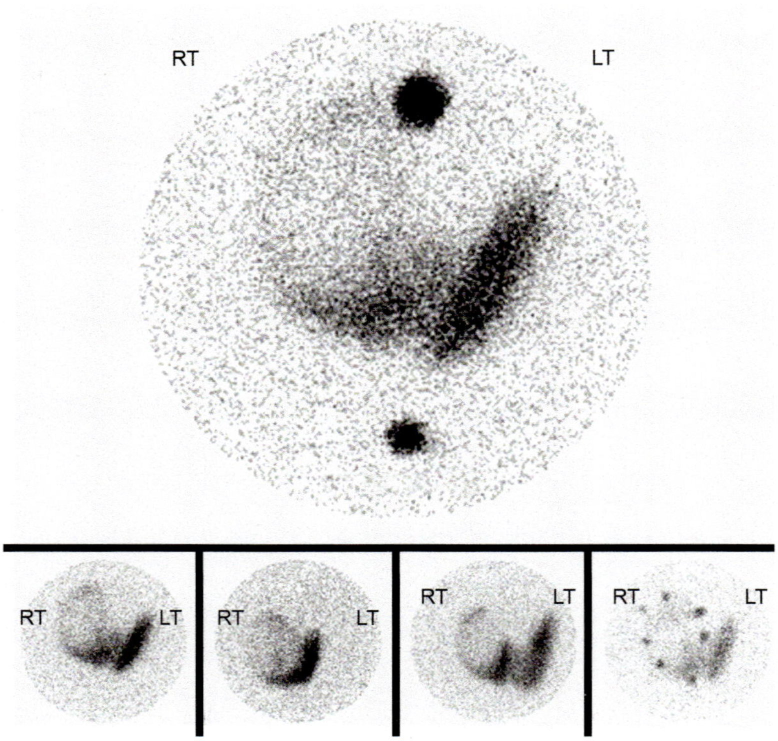

Fig. 1: ^{123}I Na thyroid scan illustrates a large heterogeneous cold thyroid nodule occupying the right thyroid lobe.

REFERENCE

1. Yeung MJ, Serpell JW. Management of the solitary thyroid nodule. Oncologist. 2008;13(2):105-12.

CASE 43: ASSESSMENT OF SSTR POSITIVE TUMORS

Brief History

A 45-year-old female presents with headaches.

Findings

Indium-111 pentetreotide scan demonstrates a focus of increased uptake in the left skull base which correlates with an enhancing mass adjacent to the left cavernous sinus on the coronal postcontrast T1 weight MR image.

Main Teaching Points

- Indium-111 pentetreotide scan detects a wide variety of neuroendocrine and non neuroendocrine tumors with potential metastases. In-111 pentetreotide is a conjugate of octreotide, a somatostatin analog that binds to SSTRs expressed in neuroendocrine tumors such as pheochromocytoma, neuroblastoma, gastrinoma, insulinoma, glucagonoma, carcinoid, medullary thyroid carcinoma, paraganglioma, pituitary adenoma, and others. Non-neuroendocrine tumors detected on In-111 pentetreotide scan include well-differentiated astrocytoma, meningioma, lymphoma, renal cell carcinoma, breast carcinoma, and others.
- Indium-111 pentetreotide scan allows determination of SSTR status in order to evaluate prognosis with octreotide therapy. It also offers the advantage of detecting distant metastases not evident on CT or MR. Although radiotracer uptake is seen as early as 4 hours after injection, the optimal time for localization of tumors is at 24 hours or later after injection.

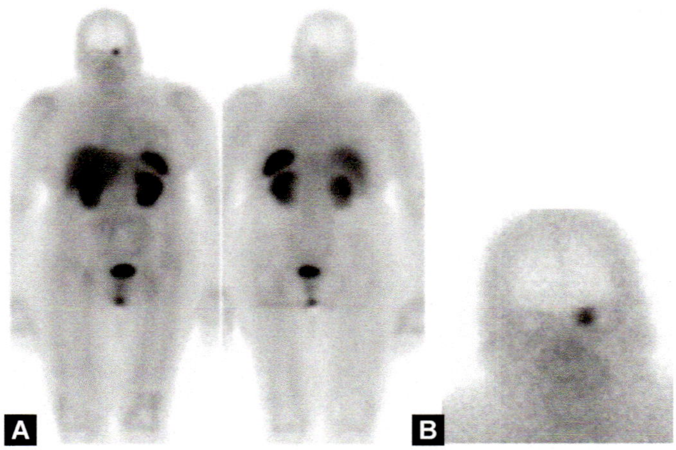

Figs. 1A and B: Whole body (A) and anterior spot images (B) of 11Indium pentetreotide scan demonstrate a focus of increased uptake in the left skull base.

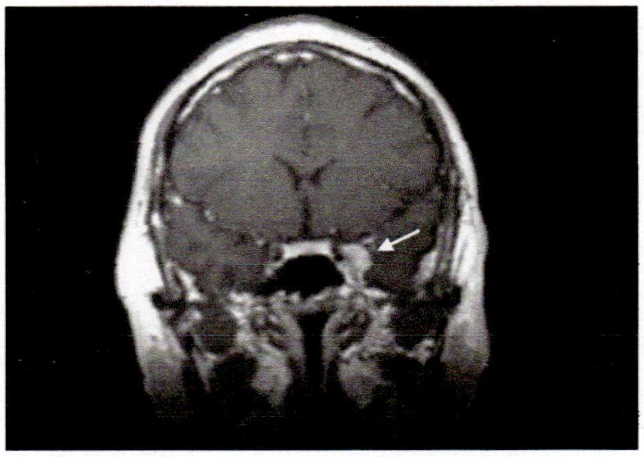

Fig. 2: Coronal post-contrast T1 weighted MR image demonstrate enhancing mass adjacent to the left cavernous sinus.

REFERENCE

1. Balon HR, Goldsmith SJ, Siegel BA, et al. Procedure guideline for somatostatin receptor scintigraphy with (111) In-pentetreotide. J Nucl Med. 2001;42(7):1134-8.

CASE 44: ASSESSMENT OF BILIARY OBSTRUCTION IN NEONATES

Brief History

A 4-week-old female who appeared normal at birth developed progressive jaundice at week 3. A hepatobiliary iminodiacetic acid (HIDA) scan to evaluate biliary tree patency was performed.

Findings

There is persistent retention of tracer in the liver which may be seen with neonatal jaundice versus biliary atresia. However, static image of the abdomen image after 24 hours demonstrates absence of radiotracer in the bowel, consistent with biliary atresia.

Main Teaching Points

- Biliary atresia is characterized by inflammatory sclerosis and obliteration of extrahepatic and intrahepatic bile ducts. Treatment involves surgery (palliative hepatic portoenterostomy or Kasai procedure) and subsequent liver transplantation.
- Biliary atresia must be differentiated from neonatal hepatitis and cholestasis. Clinical features of biliary atresia include jaundice after full-term birth that persists after 2 weeks, hepatomegaly, and hyperbilirubinemia. In contrast, infants with idiopathic neonatal hepatitis or cholestasis are often preterm and/or small for gestational age. Pretreatment with phenobarbitone (5 mg/kg/day for 7 days) induces cytochrome P450, which facilitates biliary excretion in the bowel, thereby improving specificity of bowel nonvisualization for the diagnosis of biliary atresia.

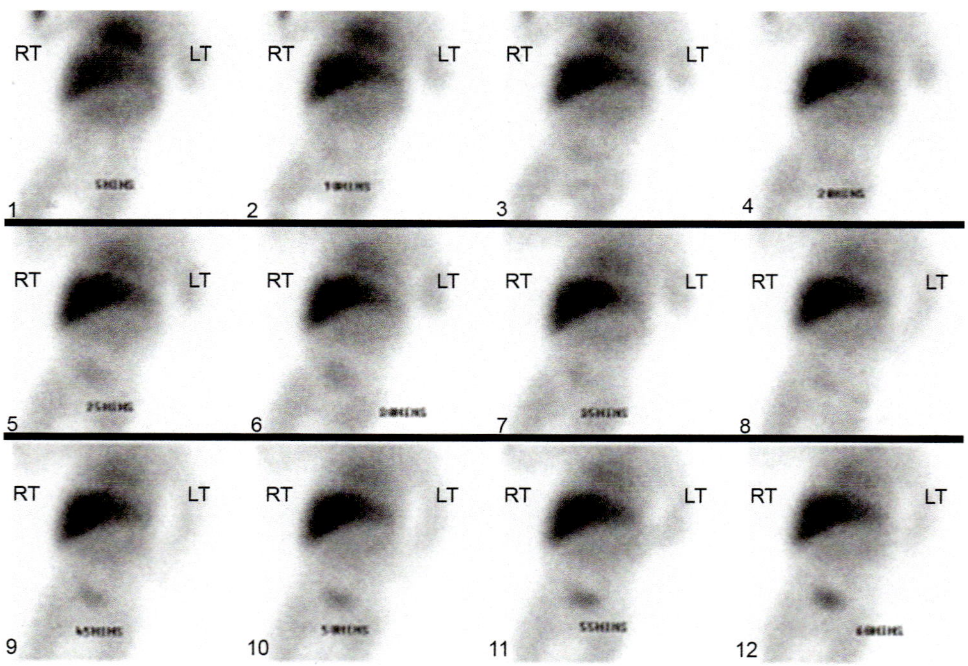

Fig. 1: Sequential dynamic images of Tc-99m Mebrofenin hepatobiliary scintigraphy exhibit persistent retention of tracer in the liver and no radiotracer excretion in the intestinal track which may be seen with neonatal jaundice versus biliary atresia. However, static image of the abdomen image after 24 hours demonstrates absence of radiotracer in the bowel. The findings are concerning for biliary atresia.

REFERENCE

1. Jensen MK, Biank VF, Moe DC, et al. Percutaneous transhepatic cholecysto-cholangiography and liver biopsy in infants with persistent jaundice: can a combination of PTCC and liver biopsy reduce unnecessary laparotomy? Pediatr Radiol. 2012;42(1):32-9.

CASE 45: ASSESSMENT OF LYTIC BONY LESIONS

Brief History

A 60-year-old woman with computed tomography (CT) findings of lytic lesions in the spine and pelvis is referred for a whole body bone scan.

Findings

The bone scan is negative for metastatic disease. Uptake in the right parasternal region is within the central line is where patient was injected.

Main Teaching Point

- Over 90% of bone metastasis distribute to the red marrow. In adult, red marrow is found in the axial skeleton and the proximal portions of the humeri femurs. Tc-99m MDP binds to regions of osteoblastic activity instead of to the tumor itself. Sensitivity of bone scan is low for bone tumors that are predominantly lytic, such as multiple myeloma and renal cell carcinoma, as well as those which are contained in the marrow such as lymphoma.

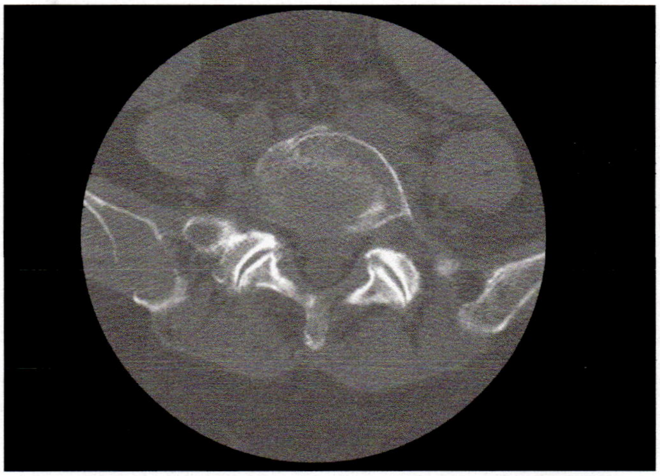

Fig. 1: Axial CT images through the iliac crest demonstrate a lytic lesion in the right posterior iliac crest.

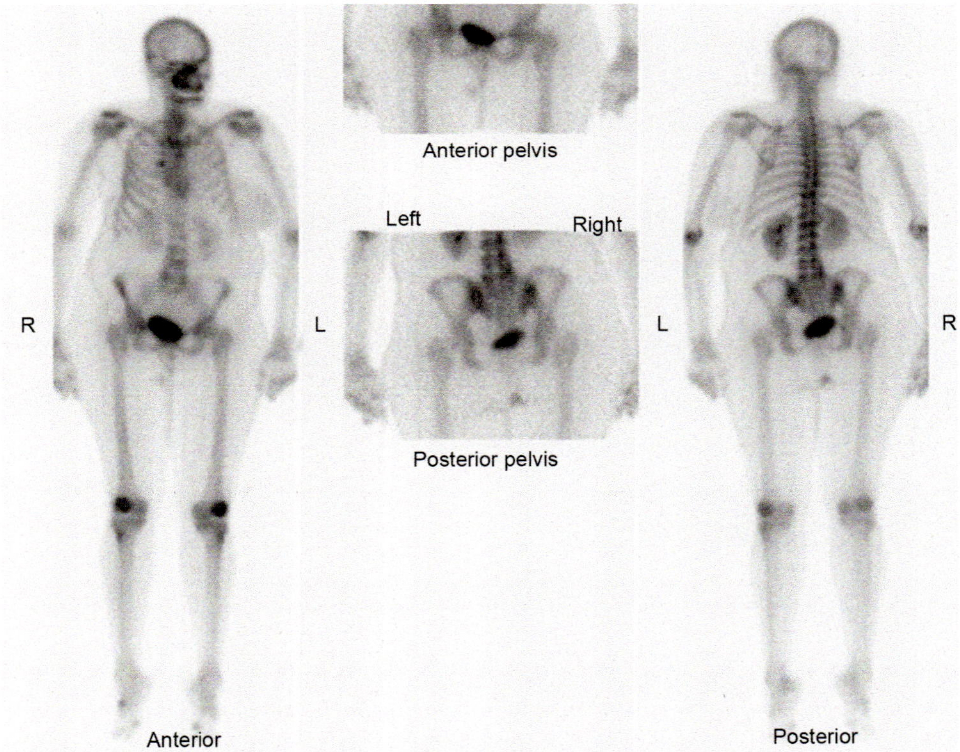

Fig. 2: Whole body 99mTc-Methyl diphosphonate (MDP) images demonstrate focal radiotracer uptake at the tip of the central line in the right parasternal region. No abnormal uptake in the right iliac crest or elsewhere.

REFERENCE

1. Abdelrazek S, Szumowski P, Rogowski F, et al. Bone scan in metabolic bone diseases. Nucl Med Rev Cent East Eur. 2012;15(2):124-31.

CASE 46: ASSESSMENT OF THYROIDITIS

Brief History

A 45-year-old female with history of neck pain/swelling and palpitations is referred for I-123 thyroid scan.

Findings

There is a minimal iodine uptake in the thyroid gland in a patient with 24-hour radioiodine uptake measuring 1.5%. There is no history of recent high iodine load (such as CT scan with intravenous contrast). Therefore, the finding in the given clinical context favors the diagnosis of thyroiditis.

Main Teaching Point

- Subacute thyroiditis can is a painful condition with local symptoms such as pain and swelling of the neck and systemic manifestations such as palpitations, tachycardia, etc. Increased erythrocyte sedimentation rate (ESR) is often observed in the testing of lab panels, so is high T3/T4 and suppressed to non-detectable thyroid-stimulating hormone (TSH). Thyroiditis can also occur in the setting of postpartum state although local symptoms are typically absent in this setting.

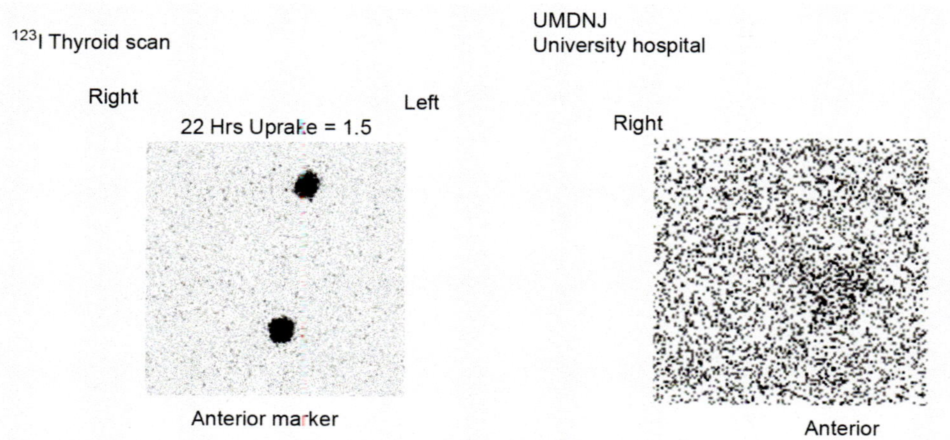

Fig. 1: Iodine 123 thyroid scan exhibits minimal iodine uptake in the thyroid gland in with 24-hour radioiodine uptake measuring at 1.5%. There is no history of recent high iodine load (such as CT scan with intravenous contrast). Therefore, the finding in the given clinical context favors the diagnosis of thyroiditis.

REFERENCE

1. Pearce EN, Farwell AP, Braverman LE. Thyroiditis. N Engl J Med. 2003;348(26):2646-55.

CASE 47: ASSESSMENT OF INFECTION/INFLAMMATION WITH WBC SCAN

Brief History

A 30-year-old male with postoperative abdominal pain and leukocytosis is referred for a whole body white blood cell (WBC) scan to evaluate for infection.

Findings

A focus of increased radiotracer uptake in the mid-pelvis is consistent with infection/inflammation. Correlative CT scan showed a focal abscess, which was drained and the patient received antibiotics. Follow-up CT scan demonstrated diverticular abscess in the sigmoid colon and colonic diverticulosis. Patient was treated with antibiotics.

Main Teaching Points

- Leukocytes labeled with In-111 8-hydroxyquinoline (oxine) is routine used for whole body WBC scan. Ideally the patient's leukocyte count should be more than 5000/m^3 although diagnostic scintigraphy can often be performed with patient counts as low as 3000/mm^3. Typical labeling efficiency ranges from 75–90%.
- Activity outside the expected normal distribution of leukocytes suggests infection. Focal abnormal Indium WBC uptake in the abdomen is considerably more specific than gallium uptake for the diagnosis of focal infection.

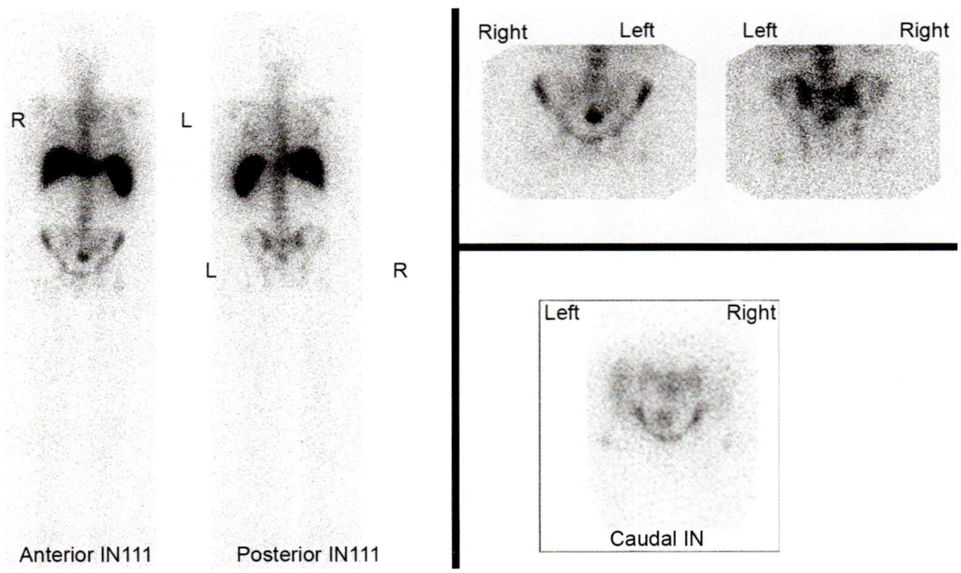

Fig. 1: Whole body In-111 Oxime labeled WBC scan displays a focus of increased radiotracer uptake in the mid-pelvis, superior to the expected location of urinary bladder, compatible with active infection.

REFERENCE

1. Ballinger JR, Gnanasegaran G. Radiolabelled leukocytes for imaging inflammation: how radiochemistry affects clinical use. Q J Nucl Med Mol Imaging. 2005;49(4):308-18.

CASE 48A: EVALUATION OF OSTEOMYELITIS

Brief History

A 55-year-old man stepped on a nail 2 weeks ago, now presents with right foot swelling, pain and fever.

Findings

Triple phase bone scan shows focal hyperemia in the right foot. Plain film showed diffuse soft tissue swelling but no signs of osteomyelitis. On delayed phase images, there is focally increased radiotracer uptake in the distal right third metatarsal, compatible with osteomyelitis.

Main Teaching Point

- Scintigraphic bone scans are commonly used for evaluation of osteomyelitis and demonstrate abnormal pattern before plain-film changes are visualized. The triple phase bone scan consists of an arterial flow phase during injection of bone seeking radiopharmaceutical such as Tc-99m methylene diphosphonate (MDP), a blood pool image obtained within 5 minutes of injection, and a delayed image obtained at 2–3 hours when soft tissue uptake clears and relatively more bone localization of the tracer occurs. Osteomyelitis demonstrates increased activity in all three phases. In contrast, cellulitis generally produced increased uptake in flow and blood pool phases, but demonstrates normal or decreased uptake on the delayed images. In the appropriate setting, specificity of the bone scan can be improved by addition of In-111 white blood cell (WBC) scan and sulfur colloid bone marrow scan.

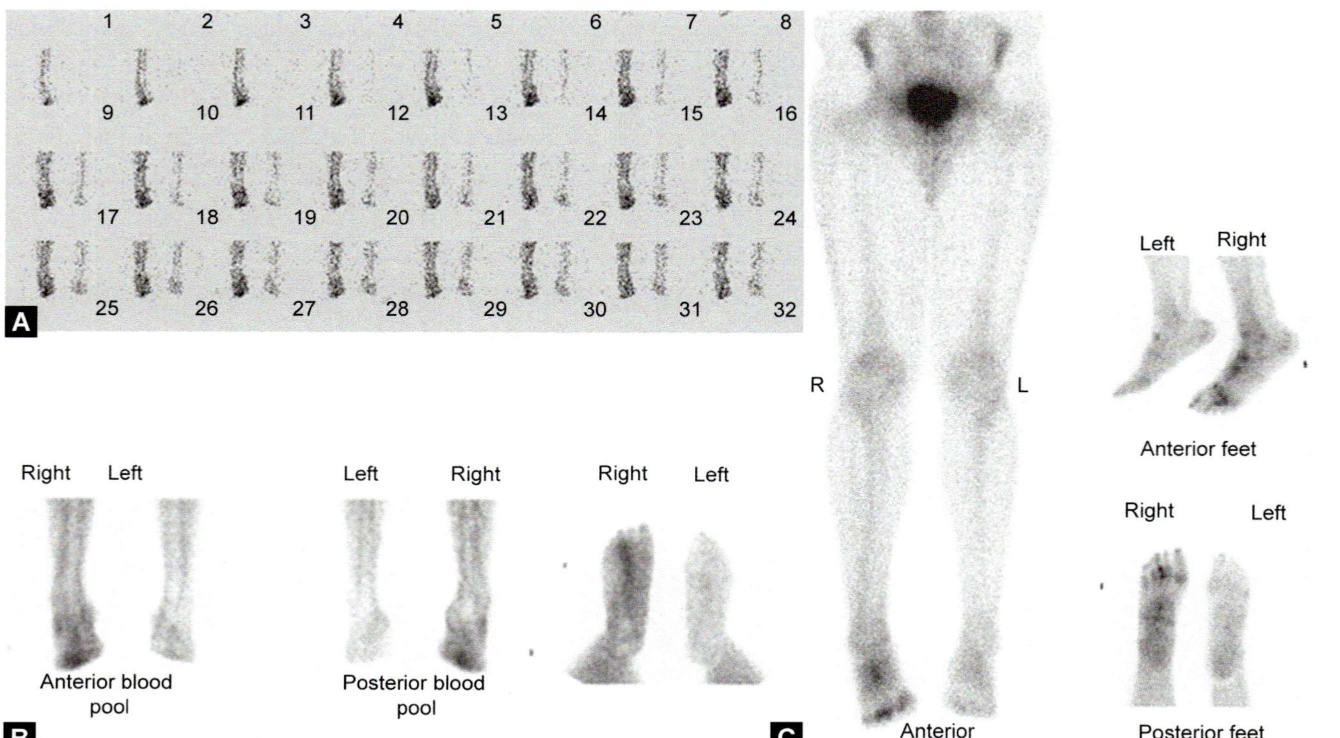

Figs. 1A to C: 99mTc-Methyl diphosphonate (MDP) triple phase bone scan images demonstrate increased blood flow in angiographic phase (A) and hyperemia in blood pool phase (B) in the entire right foot. Delayed images (C) demonstrate increased radiotracer uptake in the right third proximal phalanx compatible with osteomyelitis. Mildly increased radiotracer uptake seen in all the bones of right foot is likely from increased blood flow to the entire right foot.

REFERENCE

1. Schauwecker DS. The scintigraphic diagnosis of osteomyelitis. AJR Am J Roentgenol. 1992;158(1):9-18.

CASE 48B: EVALUATION OF OSTEOMYELITIS

Brief History

A 60-year-old diabetic patient with history of surgical debridement who presents with pain and swelling.

Findings

Top row: Bone scan. *Middle row*: White blood cell (WBC) scan after changing the dressing. *Bottom row*: Sulfur colloid scan. Increased uptake in bone scan and WBC scan in the right great toe but not in sulfur colloid scan is compatible with osteomyelitis.

Main Teaching Point

- Indium-111 labeled WBC scan is performed to evaluate osteomyelitis in cases where an abnormal triple phase bone scan is equivocal for osteomyelitis versus post-surgical change. In-111 WBC localizes to areas of infection and inflammation in the acute setting. To improve the specificity of In-111 WBC scan, a Tc-99m sulfur colloid scan is performed to delineate the extent of marrow replacement. Osteomyelitis is diagnosed by identifying any discrepancy in marrow activity between the In-111 WBC scan and sulfur colloid scan.

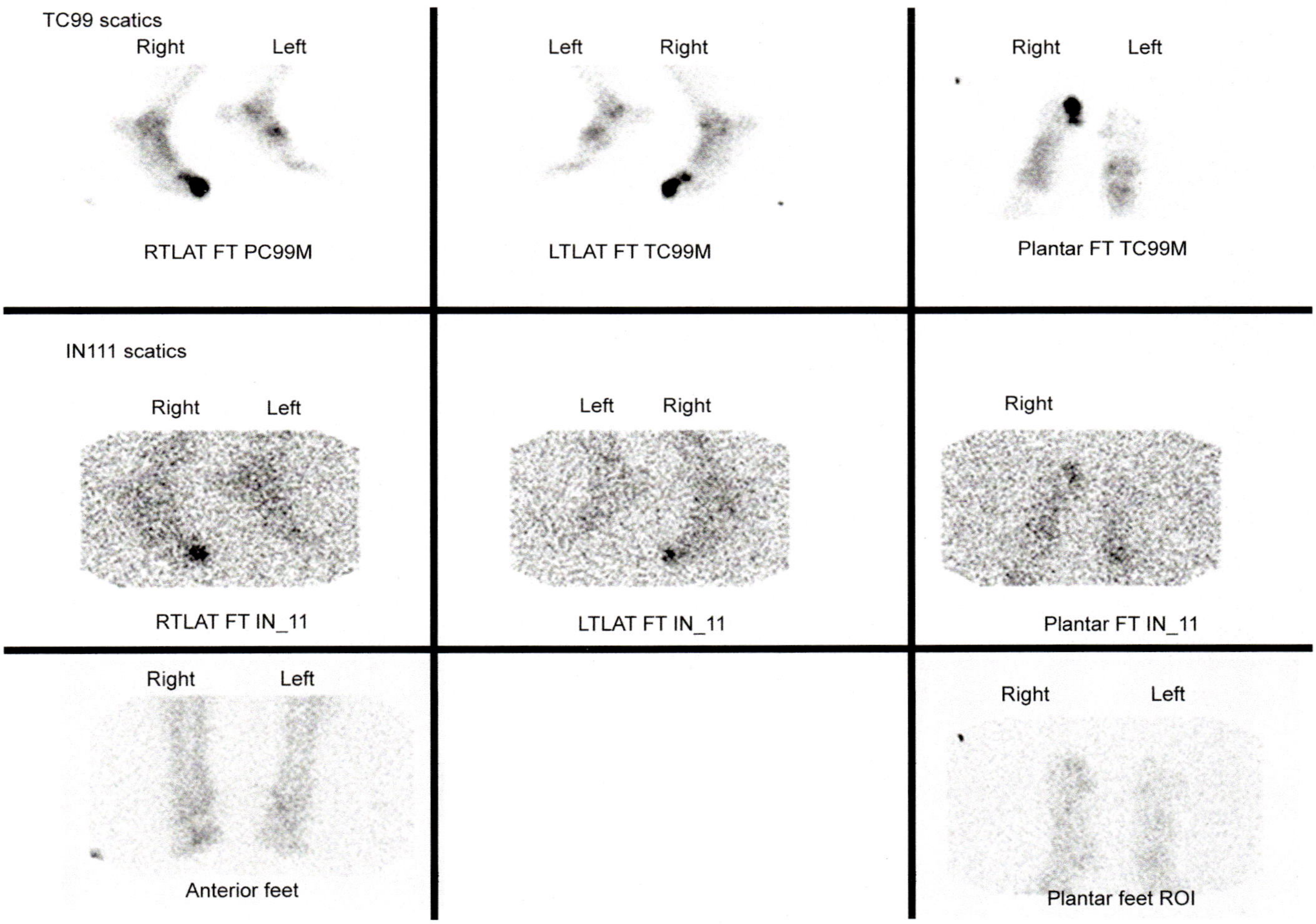

Fig. 1: Top row: Tc 99m-Methyl diphosphonate (MDP) Bone scan. Middle row: 111In-WBC scan after changing the dressing. Bottom row: Tc-99m Sulfur colloid scan. Increased uptake in bone scan and WBC scan in the right great toe but not in sulfur colloid scan is compatible with osteomyelitis.

REFERENCE

1. Schauwecker DS. The scintigraphic diagnosis of osteomyelitis. AJR Am J Roentgenol. 1992;158(1):9-18.

CASE 49: ASSESSMENT OF THYROID CANCER METASTASES

Brief History

A 53-year-old female status post I-131 ablation for thyroid carcinoma for follow-up evaluation.

Findings

Whole body post therapy I-131 scan demonstrates residual thyroid uptake at midline. Focus of uptake in the left neck may correspond to lymph node activity. There is right lung metastasis. Activity in the liver is reflective of metabolized radioiodinated Tg (which in this case is due to its localization in thyroid cancer metastases.

Main Teaching Points

- Radioiodine is sensitive in detecting differentiated thyroid carcinoma; however it normally accumulates in a number of organs which should not be mistaken to represent metastatic disease. The thyroid conjugates free iodine into thyroid hormone, decreasing the circulating free iodine pool. Unconjugated iodine is either excreted by the kidneys or to a lesser extent excreted by the bowel.
- Normal hepatic uptake is expected post I-131 therapy as thyroid hormone deconjugation occurs in the liver at approximately 7–10 days.

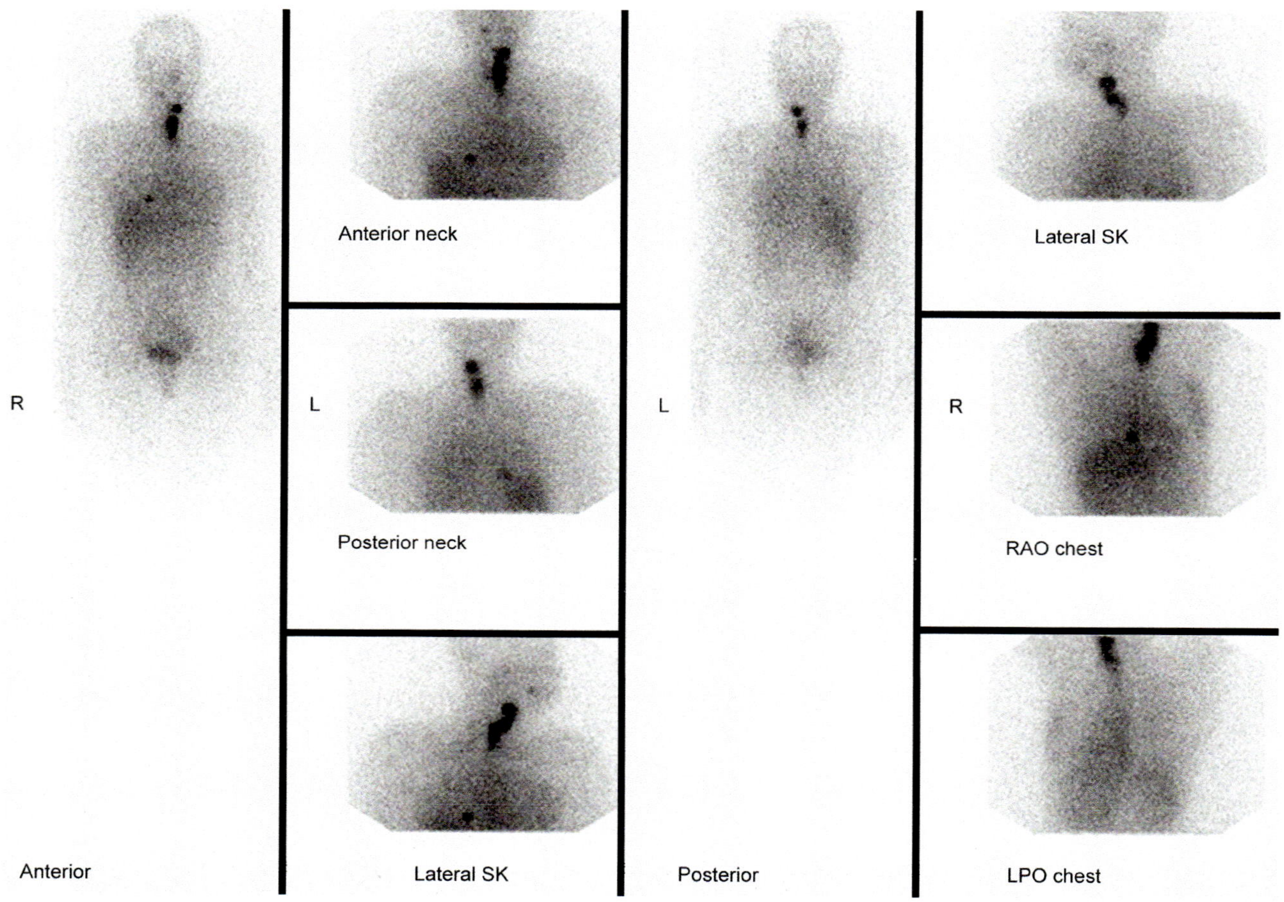

Fig. 1: Whole body post therapy I-^{131} scan demonstrates residual thyroid uptake at midline. Focus of uptake in the left neck may correspond to lymph node activity. There is right lung metastasis. Activity in the liver is reflective of metabolized radioiodinated Tg (which in this case is due to its localization in thyroid cancer metastases.

REFERENCE

1. Oh JR, Ahn BC. False-positive uptake on radioiodine whole-body scintigraphy: physiologic and pathologic variants unrelated to thyroid cancer. Am J Nucl Med Mol Imaging. 2012;2(3):362-85.

CASE 50: EVALUATION OF HYPERTHYROIDISM

Brief History

A 35-year-old female presents with symptoms of hyperthyroidism.

Findings

There is a solitary toxic nodule in the right thyroid lobe that suppresses activity in the remainder of the gland.

Main Teaching Point

- Radioiodine ablation is the mainstay of treatment for hyperfunctioning thyroid adenomas. The administered dose is dependent on nodule size, and usually ranges from 10–30 mCi. Postablation hypothyroidism may occur due to uptake by normal thyroid tissue or excessive administered dose. Radioiodine ablation for Grave's disease typically involves administering either a fixed dose of 5–15 mCi– (18.5 to 55.5 MBq) of I-131 or a dose calculated based upon gland size and percent uptake at 24 hours. Postablation hypothyroidism more often occurs after treatment of Graves' disease compared to hyperfunctioning adenoma.

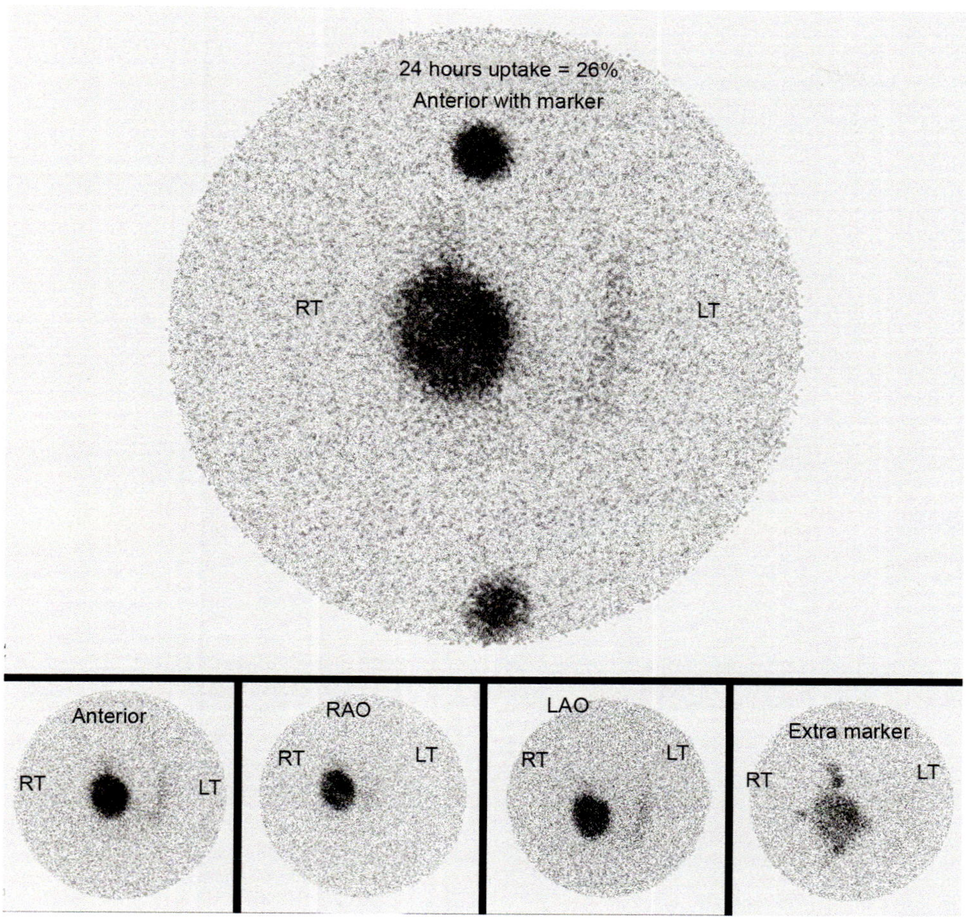

Fig. 1: 123 Iodine thyroid scan: solitary toxic nodule in the right thyroid lobe that suppresses activity in the remainder of the gland.

REFERENCE

1. Pacini F, Burroni L, Ciuoli C, et al. Management of thyroid nodules: a clinicopathological, evidence-based approach. Eur J Nucl Med Mol Imaging. 2004;31(10):1443-9.

CASE 51: EVALUATION OF RENAL ANOMALIES

Brief History

A normal 3-year-old child was found to have a congenital renal anomaly.

Findings

A MAG3 renal scan demonstrates a horseshoe kidney with normal perfusion and renal clearance.

Main Teaching Points

- Horseshoe kidney is the most common congenital renal anomaly which occurs in 1 out of 400–600

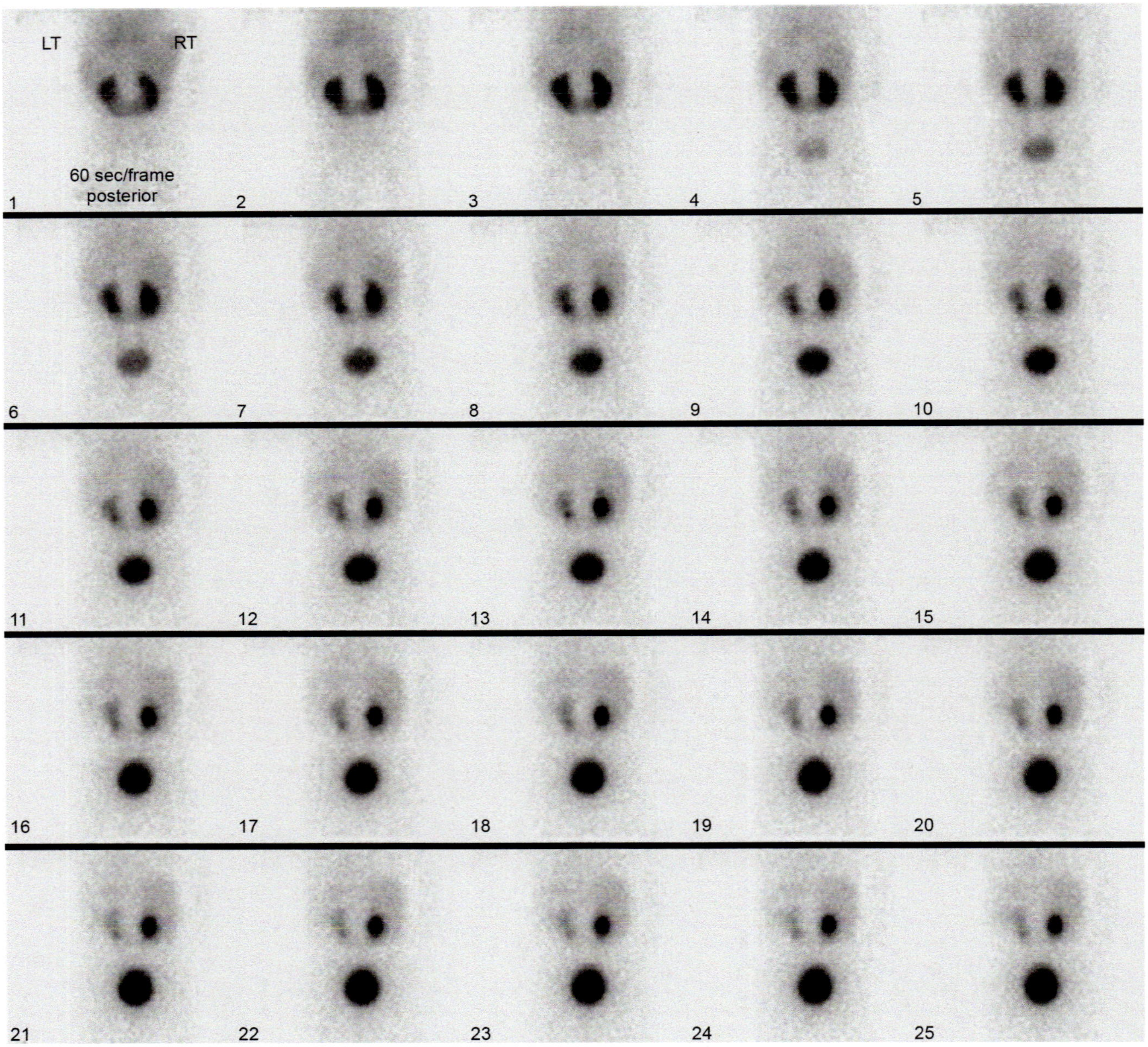

Fig. 1: Tc-99m MAG3 renal scan obtained in anterior projection demonstrates a horseshoe kidney with normal perfusion and renal clearance. Retention of radiotracer in the left renal pelvis without evidence of obstruction.

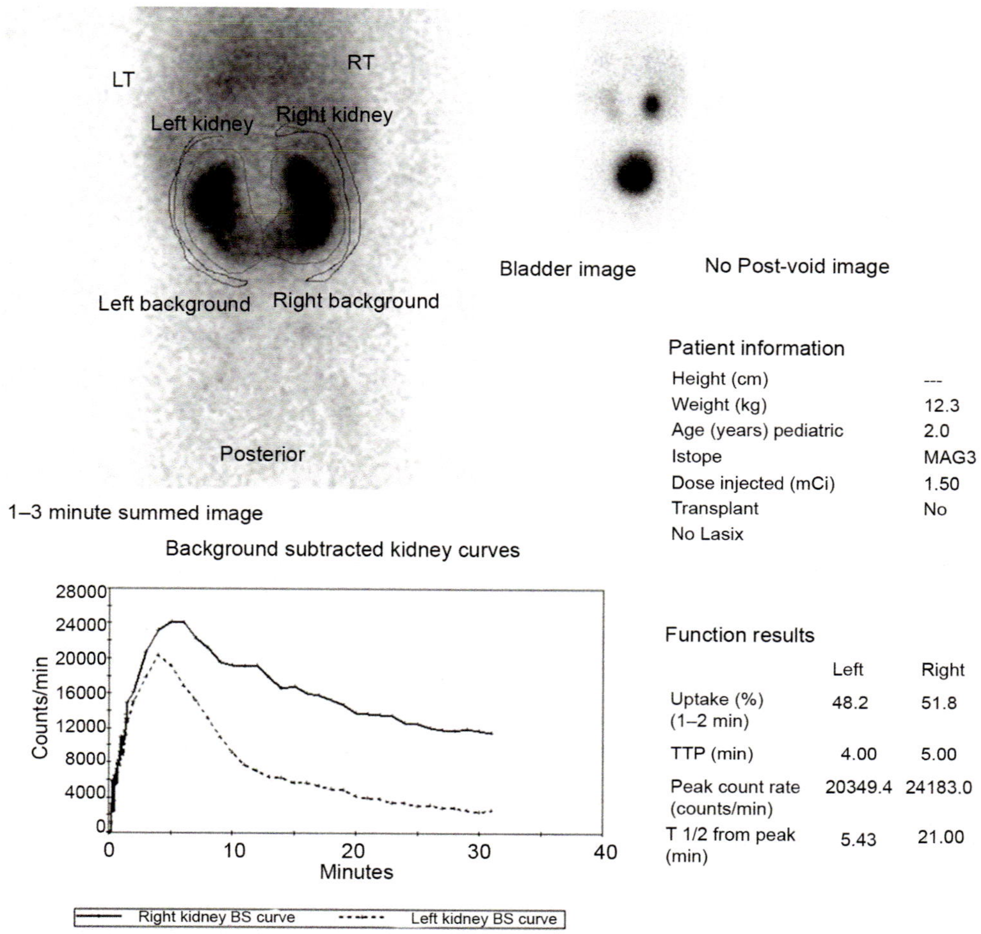

Fig. 2: Tc-99m MAG3 renal scan obtained in anterior projection demonstrates a horseshoe kidney with normal perfusion and renal clearance. Retention of radiotracer in the left renal pelvis without evidence of obstruction.

individuals. It is characterized by renal ectopia most commonly consisting of two fused renal tissue connected at the lower poles by an isthmus. For assessment of horseshoe kidneys an anterior image is added to the standard posterior projection protocol to evaluate the isthmus.

- Horseshoe kidneys are usually asymptomatic; however symptoms of abdominal pain radiating to the lower lumbar region as well as nausea and vomiting have been reported. Congenital anomalies associated with horseshoe kidneys include Down syndrome, Edward syndrome, and Turner syndrome.

REFERENCE

1. Natsis K, Piagkou M, Skotsimara A, et al. Horseshoe kidney: a review of anatomy and pathology. Surg Radiol Anat. 2014; 36(6):517-26.

CASE 52: EVALUATION OF RENAL UPTAKE ON GALLIUM SCAN

Brief History

A 50-year old man with abnormal renal function tests.

Findings

Whole body Gallium scan acquired at 48 hours demonstrates abnormal bilateral increased renal uptake.

Main Teaching Points

- Gallium-citrate binds to the transferrin, an inflammatory marker released in regions of increased blood flow and vascular permeability. Approximately 10–20% of Gallium is excreted by the kidneys, producing faint renal activity on early imaging. However, accumulation of radiotracer activity in the kidneys beyond 24 hours is abnormal, and raises the possibility of infection and/or inflammation of the kidneys.
- The differential diagnosis for intense renal uptake includes pyelonephritis, vasculitis, amyloidosis, renal parenchymal lymphoma and renal malakoplakia.

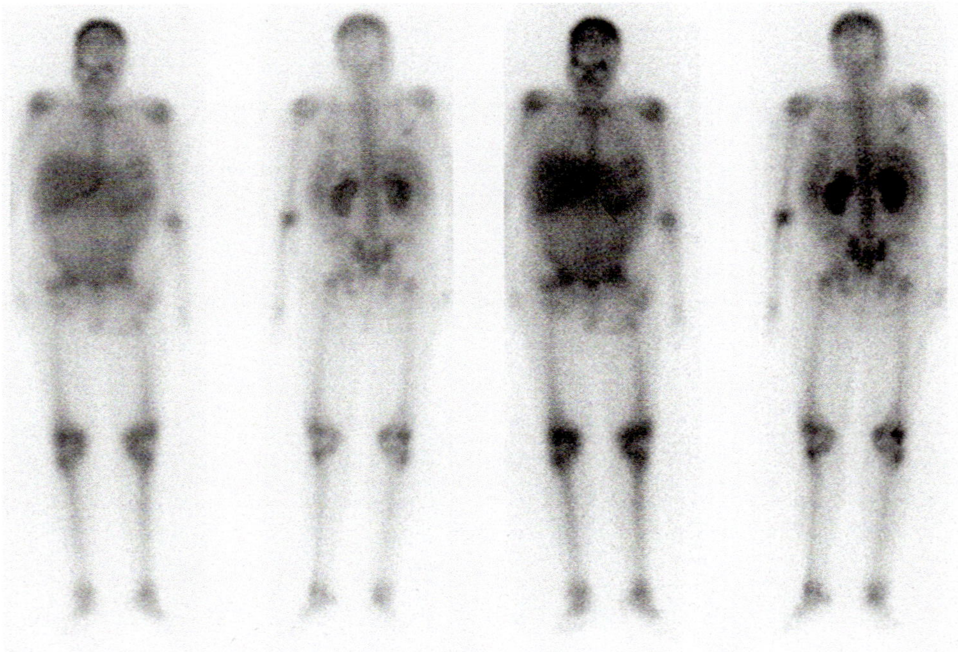

Fig. 1: Whole body 67Ga Citrate scan acquired at 48 hours demonstrates abnormal radiotracer uptake in both renal parenchyma. Otherwise, there is expected radiotracer uptake liver, spleen and in the bone marrow.

REFERENCE

1. Houston TK 2nd, Peacock JE Jr, Appel RG, et al. Gallium-67-citrate scanning of renal parenchymal malacoplakia. J Nucl Med. 1998;39(8):1454-7.

CASE 53: ASSESSMENT OF CARDIAC EJECTION FRACTION

Brief History

A 60-year-old man on Adriamycin presents with shortness of breath.

Findings

Top: Initial Multigated equilibrium angiocardiography (MUGA) scan shows an EF of 56%. *Bottom*: 4 months after receiving Adriamycin, the EF decreased to 45%.

Main Teaching Point

- Cardiotoxicity is a major side-effect of many antineoplastic agents. Anthracycline-based chemotherapy agents or breast cancer, for instance, has been associated with a 5-year incidence of chronic heart failure in up to 3% of patients, and that the combination of anthracyclines and taxanes leads to increased cardiotoxicity. Herceptin, used in the treatment of breast carcinoma, is also shown to result in cardiotoxicity, therefore requiring monitoring of left ventricular ejection fraction (LVEF) during therapy.

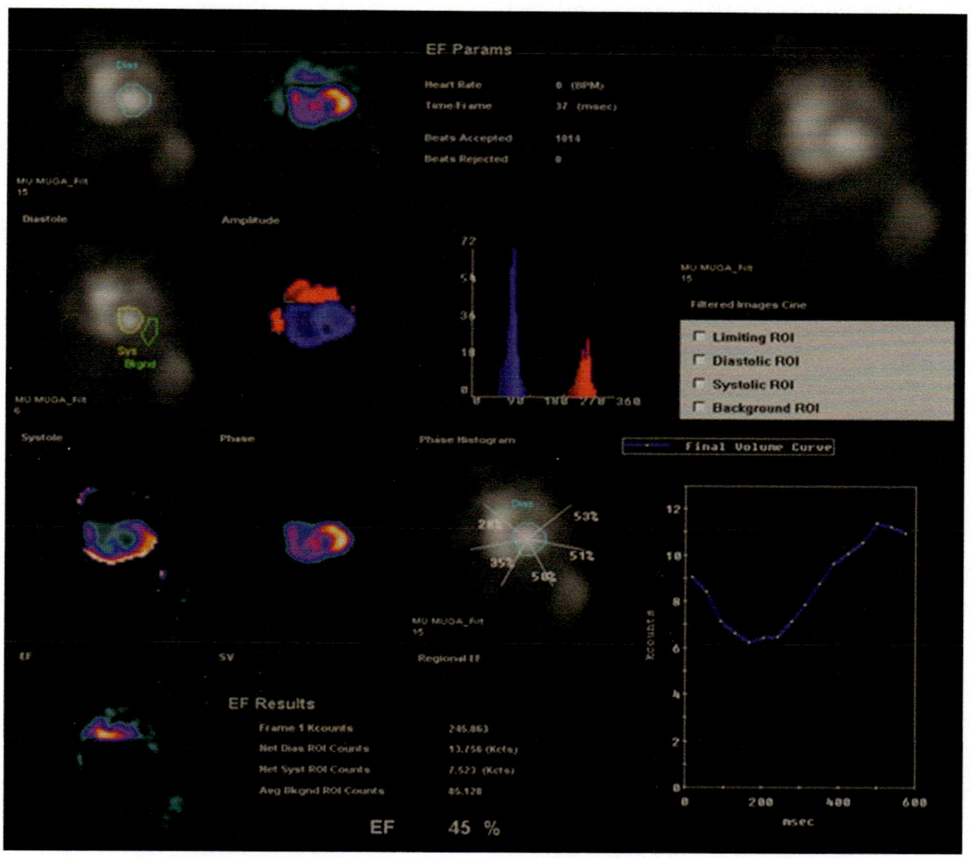

Fig. 1: Multigated cardiac blood pool study obtained following intravenous administration of Tc-99m labeled red blood cell (RBC). Follow-up study after six cycles of Adriamycin demonstrating left ventricular ejection fraction of 45%.

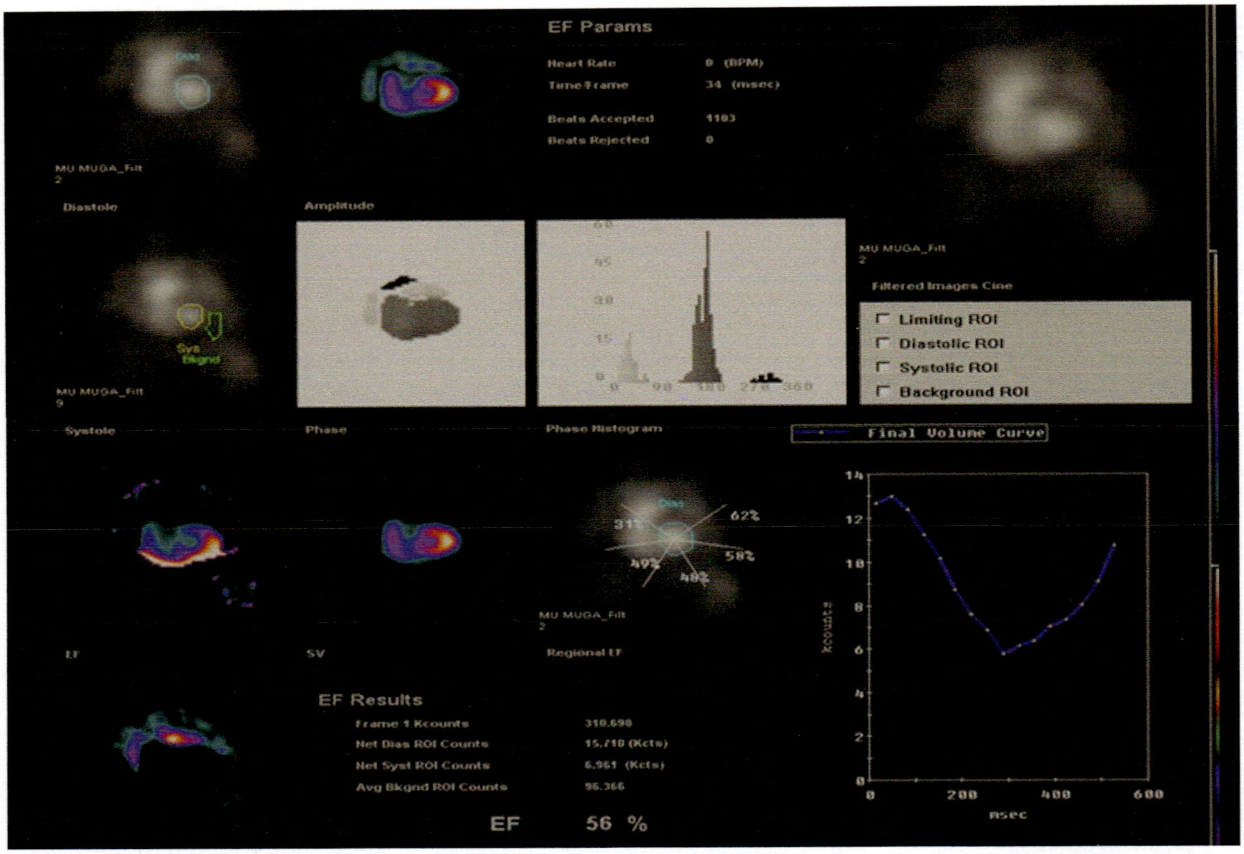

Fig. 2: Multigated cardiac blood pool study obtained following intravenous administration of Tc-99m labeled RBC. Base line study prior to starting chemotherapy demonstrating left ventricular ejection fraction of 56%.

- Serial MUGA scan is the gold standard noninvasive imaging study to evaluate LVEF in order to identify clinically-occult ventricular dysfunction which may meet criteria for altering or discontinuing chemotherapy regimens.

REFERENCE

1. de Geus-Oei LF, Mavinkurve-Groothuis AM, Bellersen L, et al. Scintigraphic techniques for early detection of cancer treatment-induced cardiotoxicity. J Nucl Med Technol. 2013;41(3):170-81.

CASE 54: EVALUATION OF LIVER METASTASES

Brief History

A 75-year-old woman with a gastrinoma presents with abdominal pain and abnormal liver function tests.

Findings

Whole body octreotide scan demonstrates abnormal uptake in the hepatic dome consistent with metastasis. Sulfur colloid scan reveals photopenic defects in the same region representing nonfunctioning liver tissue.

Main Teaching Points

- Octreotide binds to the SSTRs of neuroendocrine tumors such as gastrinoma, carcinoid, insulinoma and medullary carcinoma. Approximately 80–90% of neuroendocrine tumors are visible by 4 hours, although ideal imaging interpretation is at 24 hours due to decreased background activity.
- Normal uptake of octreoscan occurs in the thyroid gland, liver, gallbladder, spleen, kidneys and bladder. However, focal heterogeneous increased uptake such as that in the liver in this patient is consistent with metastasis. Sulfur colloid scan confirms nonfunctioning liver tissue.

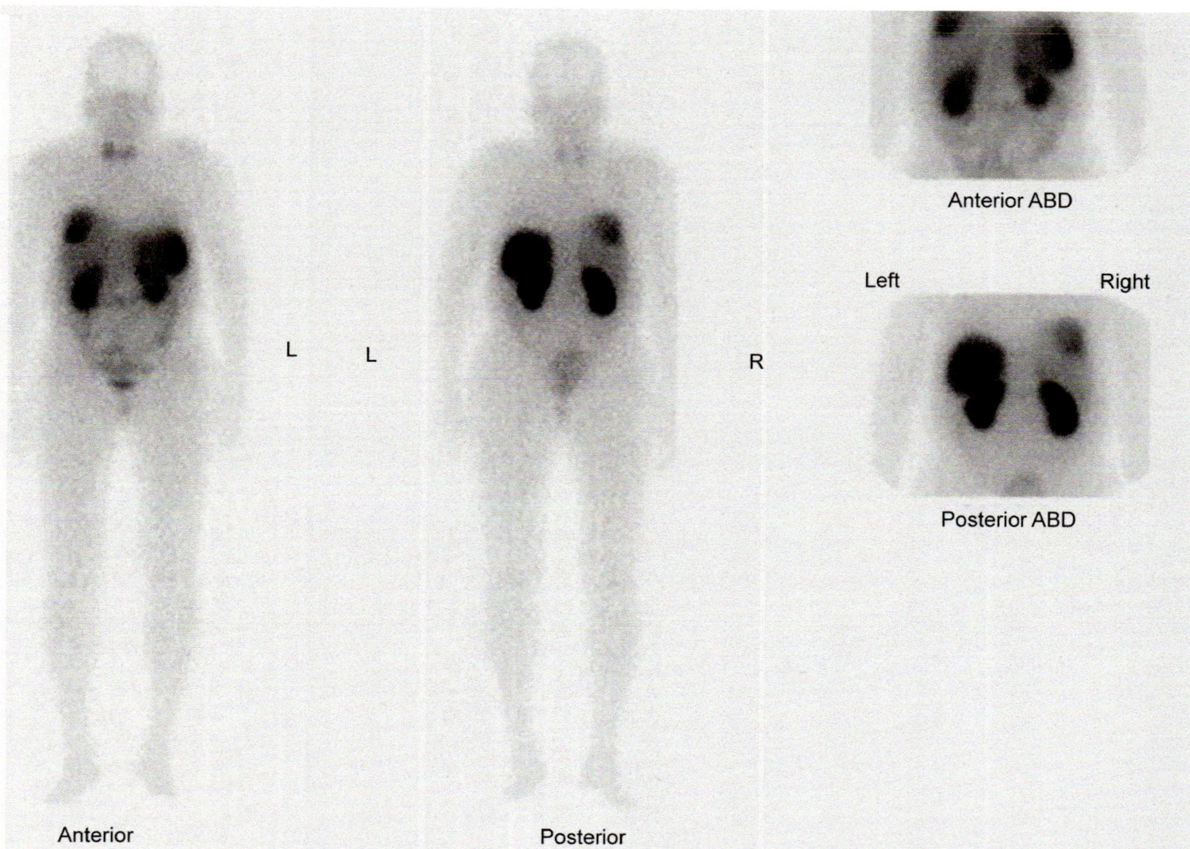

Fig. 1: Whole body In-111 octreotide scan demonstrates abnormal uptake in the hepatic dome consistent with metastasis.

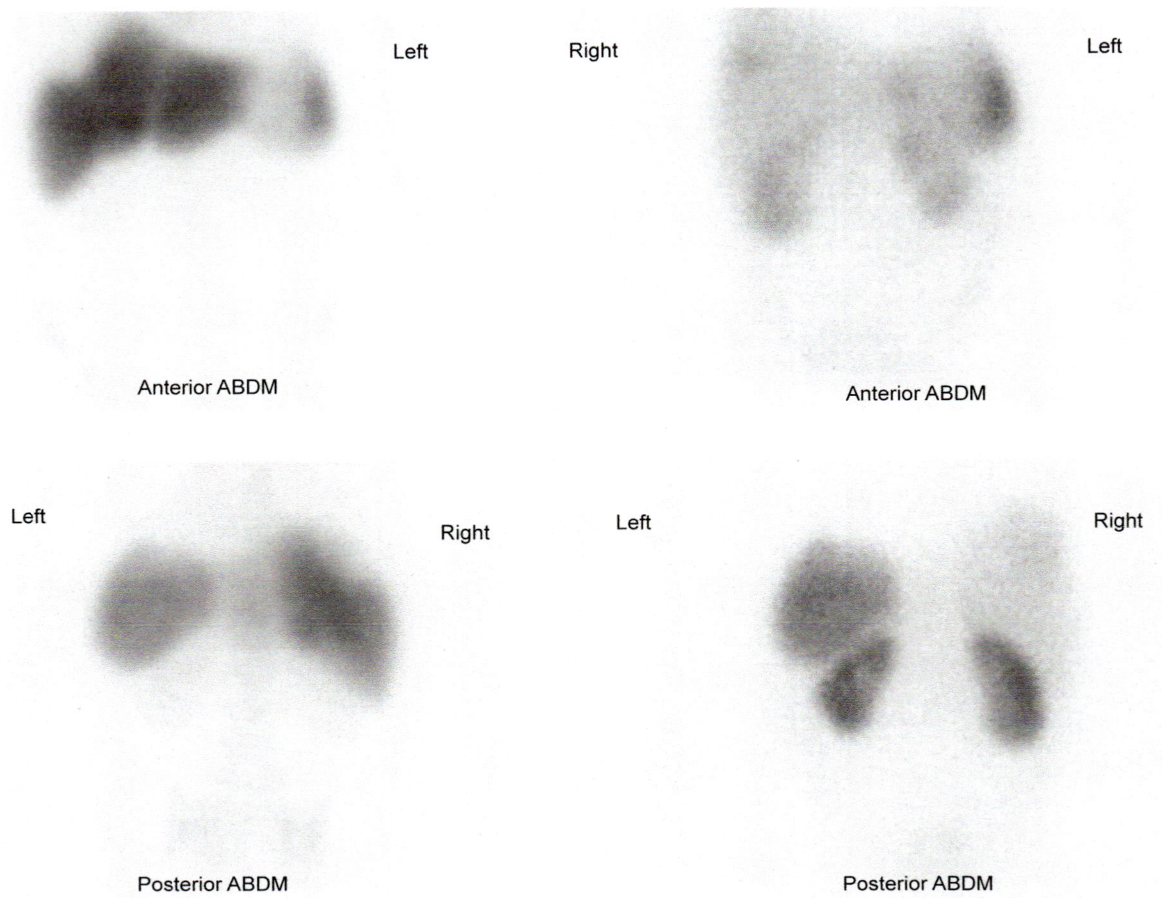

Fig. 2: Tc -99m Sulfur colloid scan reveals photopenic defects in the right hepatic dome, corresponding to the metastatic lesion seen on In-111 Octreotide scan, representing nonfunctioning liver tissue.

REFERENCE

1. Pepe G, Moncayo R, Bombardieri E, et al. Somatostatin receptor SPECT. Eur J Nucl Med Mol Imaging. 2012;39 Suppl 1:S41-51.

CASE 55: ASSESSMENT OF MULTIGATED EQUILIBRIUM ANGIOCARDIOGRAPHY (MUGA) SCAN ARTIFACTS

Brief History

A 53-year-old male with newly diagnosed lymphoma undergoes baseline cardiac evaluation on MUGA scan.

Findings

Initial MUGA scan demonstrates background region of interest (ROI) drawn over free pertechnetate in the stomach which artificially elevates the LVEF. After correcting the background ROI, the EF returns to normal.

Main Teaching Point

- Serial MUGA scan is a gold standard noninvasive evaluation of cardiac function. The combination of MUGA and echocardiography are routinely used to assess LVEF during chemotherapy. Accurate calculation of LVEF is heavily dependent on the ROI over the correct background level activity. ROIs drawn over the region with activity higher than true background artificially elevates the LVEF. Calculation of LVEF is also limited in the setting of cardiac arrhythmias.

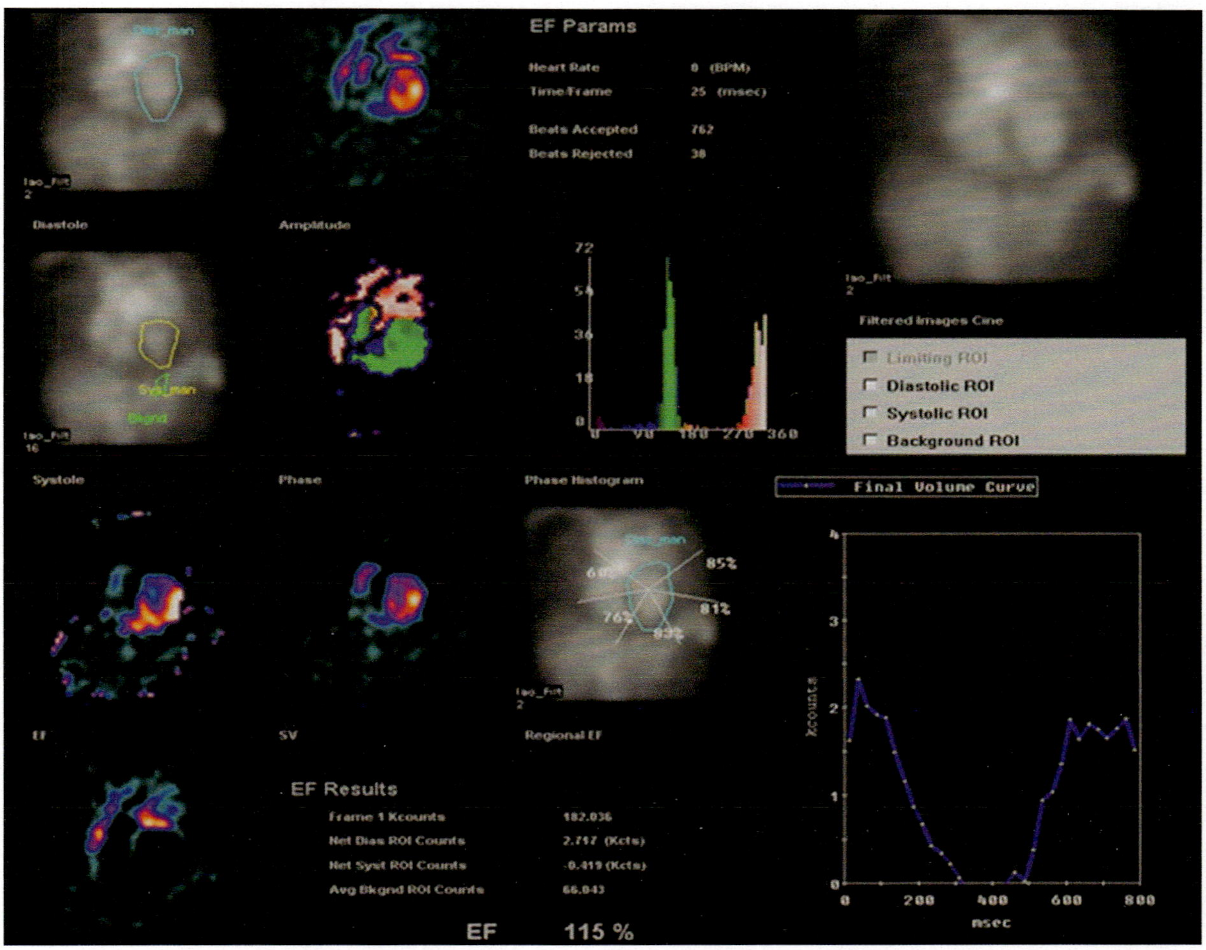

Fig. 1: Multigated cardiac blood pool study obtained following intravenous administration of Tc-99m labeled RBC demonstrates left ventricular ejection fraction of 115%. Images demonstrate that background region of interest (ROI) is drawn over free pertechnetate in the stomach which artificially elevates the LVEF.

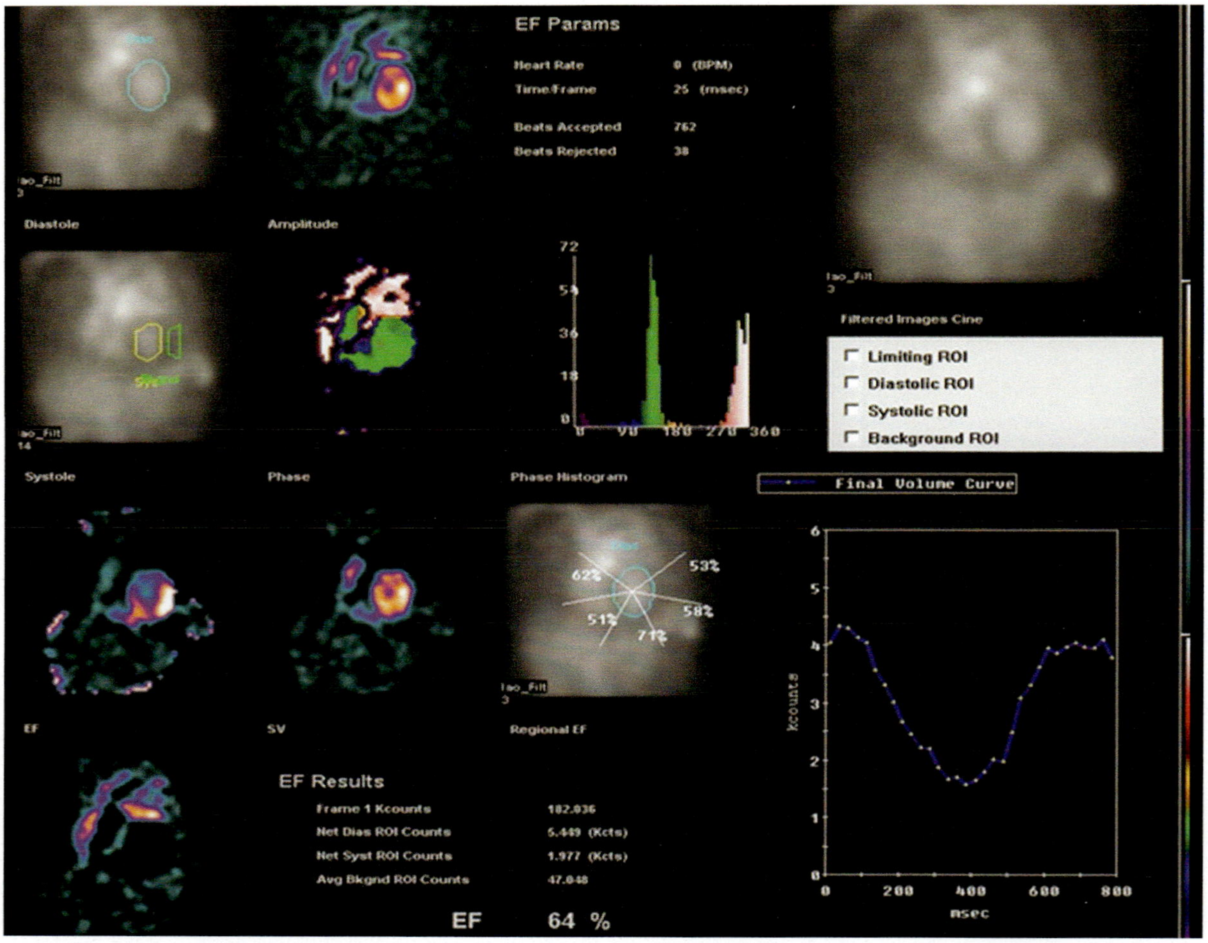

Fig. 2: Multigated cardiac blood pool study obtained following intravenous administration of Tc-99m labeled RBC: After correcting the background ROI, the EF returns to normal.

REFERENCE

1. de Geus-Oei LF, Mavinkurve-Groothuis AM, Bellersen L, et al. Scintigraphic techniques for early detection of cancer treatment-induced cardiotoxicity. J Nucl Med Technol. 2013;41(3):170-81.

Section 2

Nuclear Cardiology

E Gordon DePuey, Munir Ghesani

Introductory Cases

CASE 1: NORMAL FEMALE

In perfusion (A) images tracer distribution is homogeneous throughout the myocardium in vertical long-axis, horizontal long-axis, and short-axis tomograms; in polar maps, and in three-dimensional surface-rendered maps. Note that anterior count density is very slightly less than that of the inferior wall due to photon attenuation by the patient's overlying left breast. End-diastolic and end-systolic tomographic functional images (B) demonstrate normal regional left ventricular function. Left ventricular ejection fraction is 56% (normal = >50%) (Figs. 1A and B).

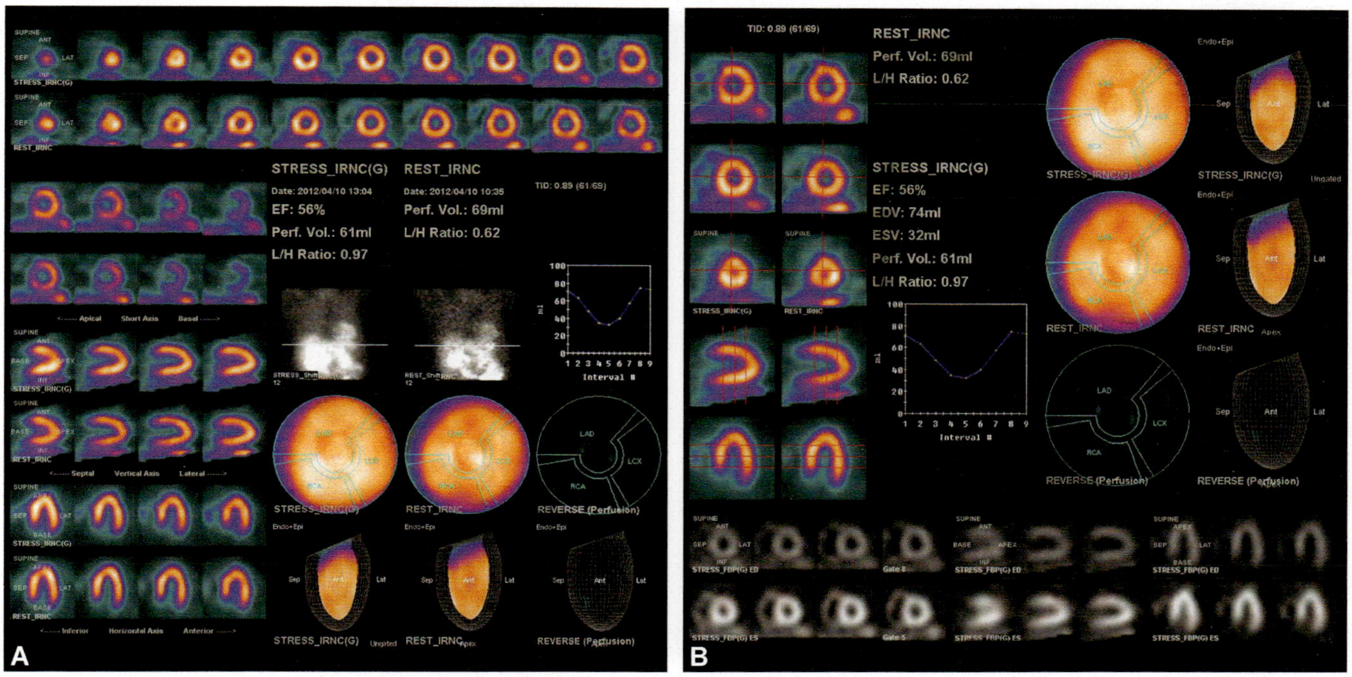

Figs. 1A and B: A 55-year-old female with coronary risk factors and atypical angina.
Imaging protocol: Rest/stress technetium-99m sestamibi.
Stress modality: Treadmill exercise. No chest pain and no ST segment changes.

CASE 2: NORMAL MALE; NONVISUALIZATION OF GALLBLADDER (GB) DUE TO PRIOR CHOLECYSTECTOMY

In perfusion (A) images tracer distribution is homogeneous throughout the myocardium in vertical long-axis, horizontal long-axis, and short-axis tomograms; in polar maps, and in three-dimensional surface-rendered maps. Note that inferior count density is slightly less than that of the anterior wall due to photon attenuation by the patient's left hemidiaphragm which is not counterbalanced by anterior breast attenuation. End-diastolic and end-systolic tomographic functional images (B) demonstrate normal regional left ventricular function. Left ventricular ejection fraction is 55%.

Incidentally noted in both the stress and rest planar projection images (A) is absent tracer concentration in the GB, the due to prior cholecystectomy (Figs. 1A and B).

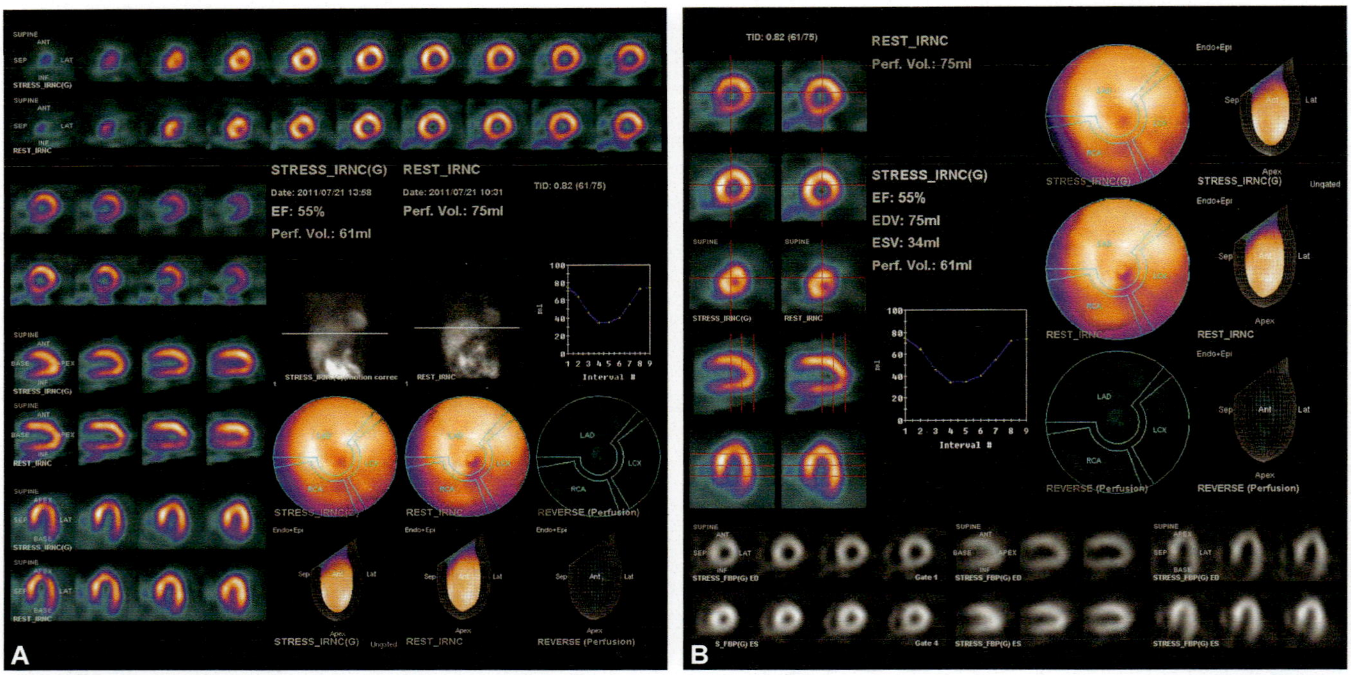

Figs. 1A and B: A 65-year-old male with coronary risk factors and atypical angina.
Imaging protocol: Rest/stress technetium-99m sestamibi.
Stress modality: Treadmill exercise. No chest pain and no ST segment changes.

CASE 3: INADEQUATE RESTING TETROFOSMIN TAG

In stress perfusion (A) images tracer distribution is homogeneous throughout the myocardium in vertical long-axis, horizontal-long axis, and short-axis tomograms; in polar maps, and in three-dimensional surface-rendered maps. However, in the resting images the myocardium is barely visualized due to poor myocardial radiotracer uptake and markedly increased background tracer concentration. This is due to inadequate tagging of the resting technetium-99m (Tc-99m) tetrofosmin dose. Normal tagging efficiency is greater than 90%, preferably greater than 95%. In this case, tagging efficiency was only 40%. End-diastolic and end-systolic post-stress tomographic functional images (B) demonstrate normal regional left ventricular function. Left ventricular ejection fraction is calculated to be 87%. Of note, due to limited resolution of the ventricular cavity in patients with small hearts, end-systolic volume may be significantly underestimated, and therefore left ventricular ejection fraction may be overestimated. Therefore, in general practice left ventricular ejection fractions greater than 70% are only reported as "greater than 70%" (Figs. 1A and B).

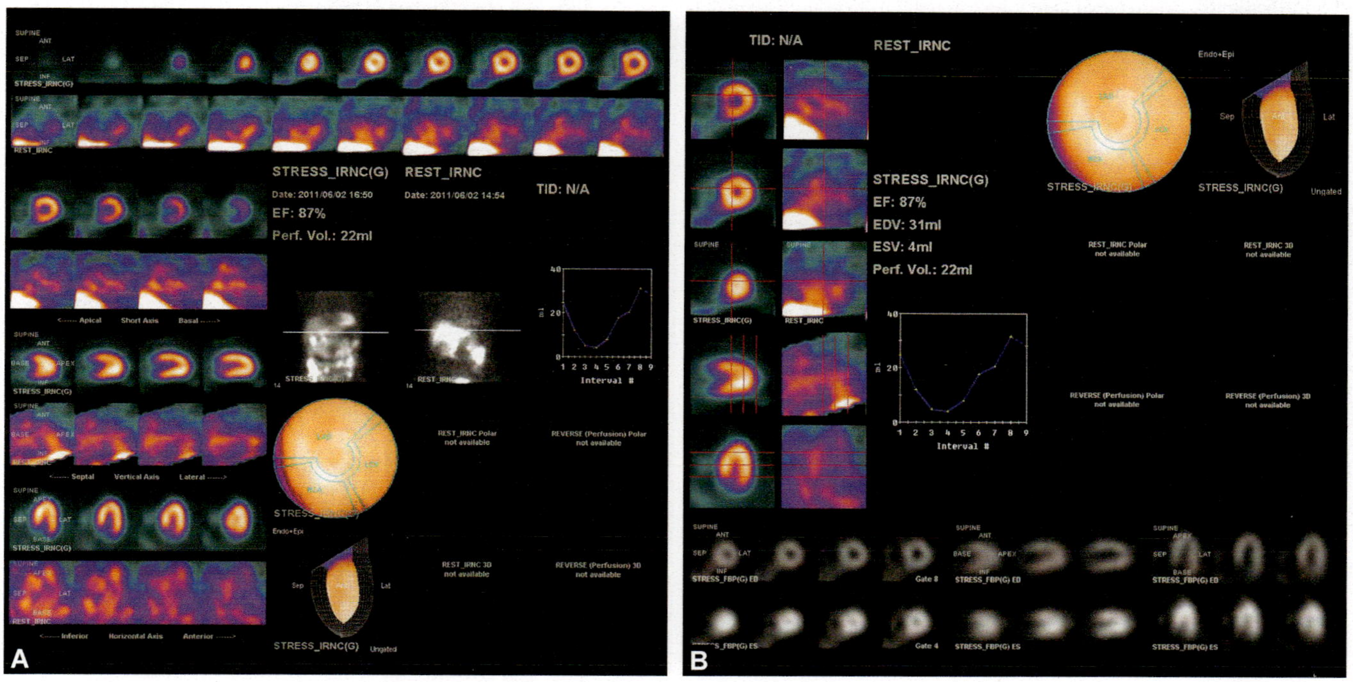

Figs. 1A and B: A 60-year-old female with coronary risk factors and atypical angina.
Imaging protocol: Rest technetium-99m tetrofosmin/stress technetium-99m sestamibi.
Stress modality: Dipyridamole. No chest pain and no ST segment changes.

CASE 4: SHORT SEPTUM

In the horizontal long-axis perfusion tomograms (A) the septum appears short, and there is absent tracer concentration in the basal one-third of the septum. This is due to a long membranous septum and consequently short muscular septum, a common normal variant. In the basal short axis slices, there is a corresponding absence of tracer concentration in the septum. It is important that this defect is not mistaken for a septal infarct. Of note, and infarct involving the base of the septum is unusual since that region of myocardium usually has a dual blood supply, receiving perfusion from both the left anterior descending (LAD) and right coronary artery (RCA). Moreover, if the stress and rest short-axis slices are not precisely aligned, the basal septal defect may appear partially reversible and may be misconstrued as an ischemic abnormality. In the gated tomograms (B) septal wall motion and wall thickening are normal (Figs. 1A and B).

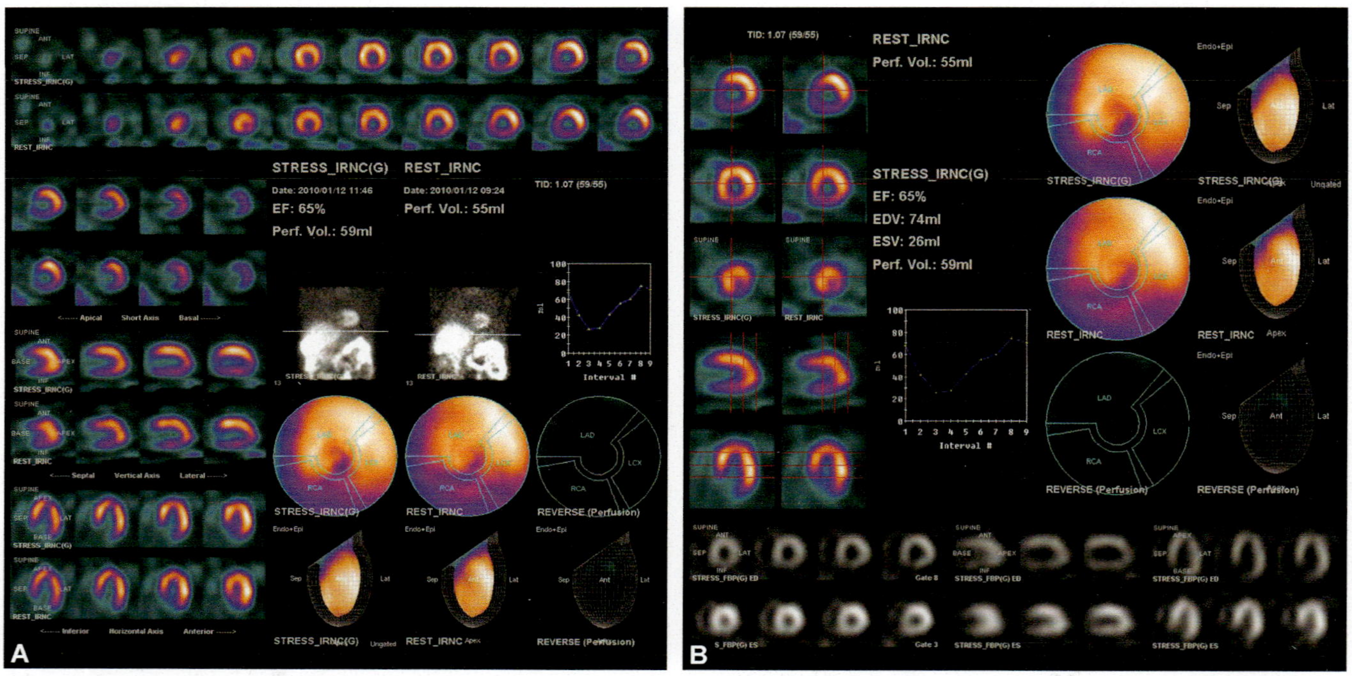

Figs. 1A and B: A 64-year-old female with arrhythmia, coronary artery disease risk factors and atypical angina.
Imaging protocol: Rest technetium-99m tetrofosmin/stress technetium-99m sestamibi.
Stress modality: Dipyridamole. No chest pain and no ST segment changes.

CASE 5: PROMINENT ANTEROSEPTAL RIGHT VENTRICLE INSERTION SITE

In the stress and rest short axis tomograms (A) there is a "cleft-like" perfusion defect in the anteroseptal wall at approximately the 11 o'clock position. This defect is also noted clearly in the stress and rest polar maps and three-dimensional surface-rendered maps. Functional images (B) demonstrate normal wall motion and wall thickening of the entire left ventricular myocardium, including the anteroseptal wall. This small, fixed anteroseptal defect represents a common normal variant associated with the insertion site of the anterior free wall of the right ventricle. Of note, a similar "cleft-like" defect may be observed in the inferoseptal wall at approximately 7 o'clock, associated with the insertion site of the inferior free wall of the right ventricle (Figs. 1A and B).

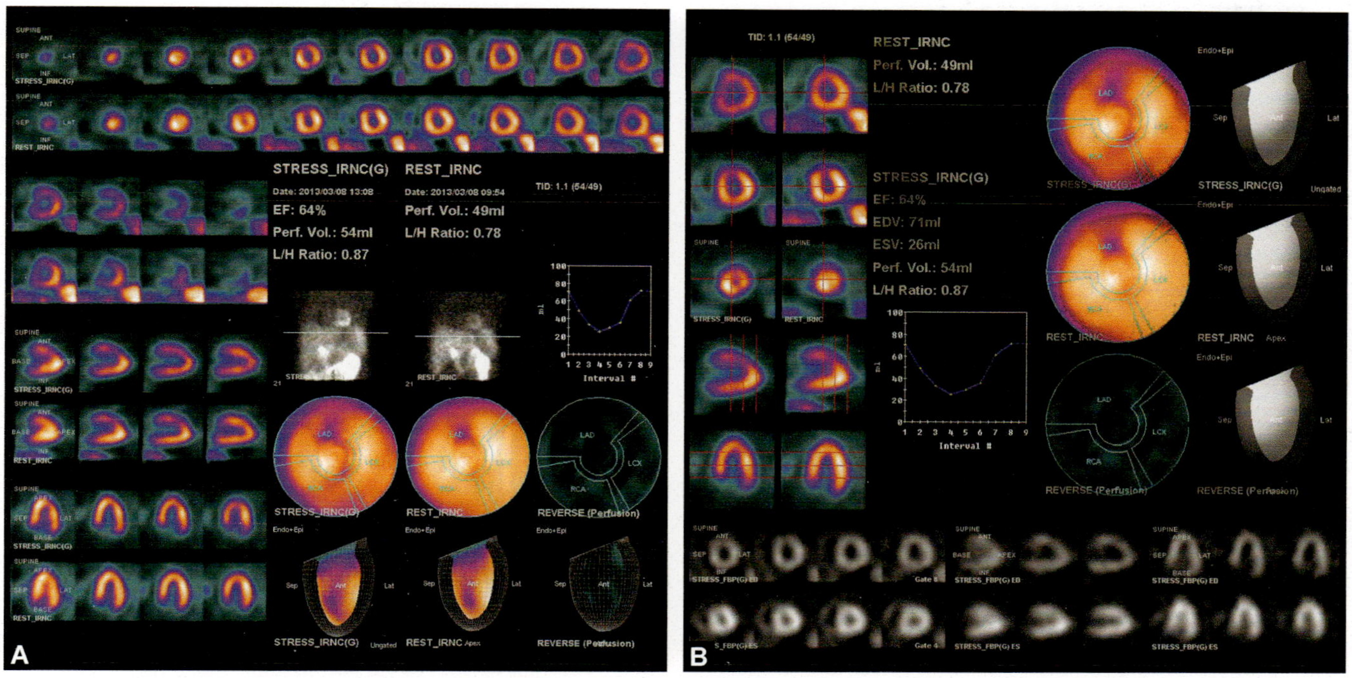

Figs. 1A and B: A 67-year-old female with coronary artery disease risk factors including diabetes and nonanginal chest pain.
Imaging protocol: Rest technetium-99m tetrofosmin/stress technetium-99m sestamibi.
Stress modality: Dipyridamole. No chest pain and no ST segment changes.

CASE 6: APICAL PHYSIOLOGIC THINNING

In both the stress and rest perfusion tomograms (A) there is a small area of moderately decreased tracer concentration at the very apex of the left ventricle. This is also clearly noted in the color maps and three-dimensional surface-rendered maps. Functional images (B) demonstrate normal, vigorous wall motion and thickening of the apex. This finding represents "physiological apical thinning" a normal variant. In gated coronary *computed tomography* angiograms the left ventricular apex is often observed to be just a few millimeters thick. In the *single photon emission computed tomography* (SPECT) images such apical thinning is often not apparent due to blurring of the images secondary to cardiac motion and Compton scatter. In this case example, physiologic apical thinning is more marked than usual (Figs. 1A and B).

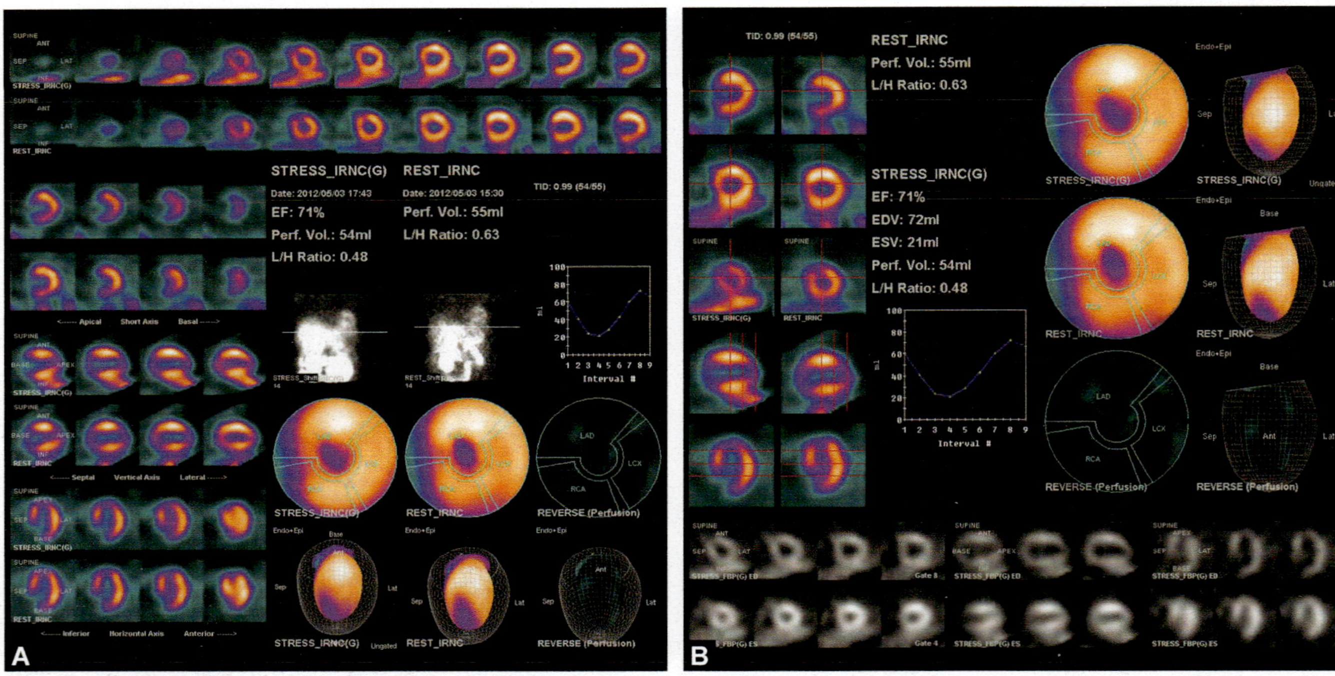

Figs. 1A and B: A 63-year-old female with coronary artery disease risk factors and atypical angina.
Imaging protocol: Rest technetium-99m tetrofosmin/stress technetium-99m sestamibi.
Stress modality: Dipyridamole. No chest pain and no ST segment changes.

CASE 7: MARKED ANTERIOR BREAST ATTENUATION ARTIFACT

In this female patient with a 48 inch chest circumference and DD bra cup perfusion tomograms (A) demonstrate a moderate decrease in tracer concentration in the anterior wall of the left ventricle, best noted in vertical long-axis and short-axis tomograms. However, functional images (B) demonstrate entirely normal anterior wall motion and wall thickening. These findings are secondary to marked photon attenuation by the patient's overlying left breast. Gated imaging is very useful to differentiate fixed defects due to myocardial scarring from those due to attenuation artifact (Figs. 1A and B).

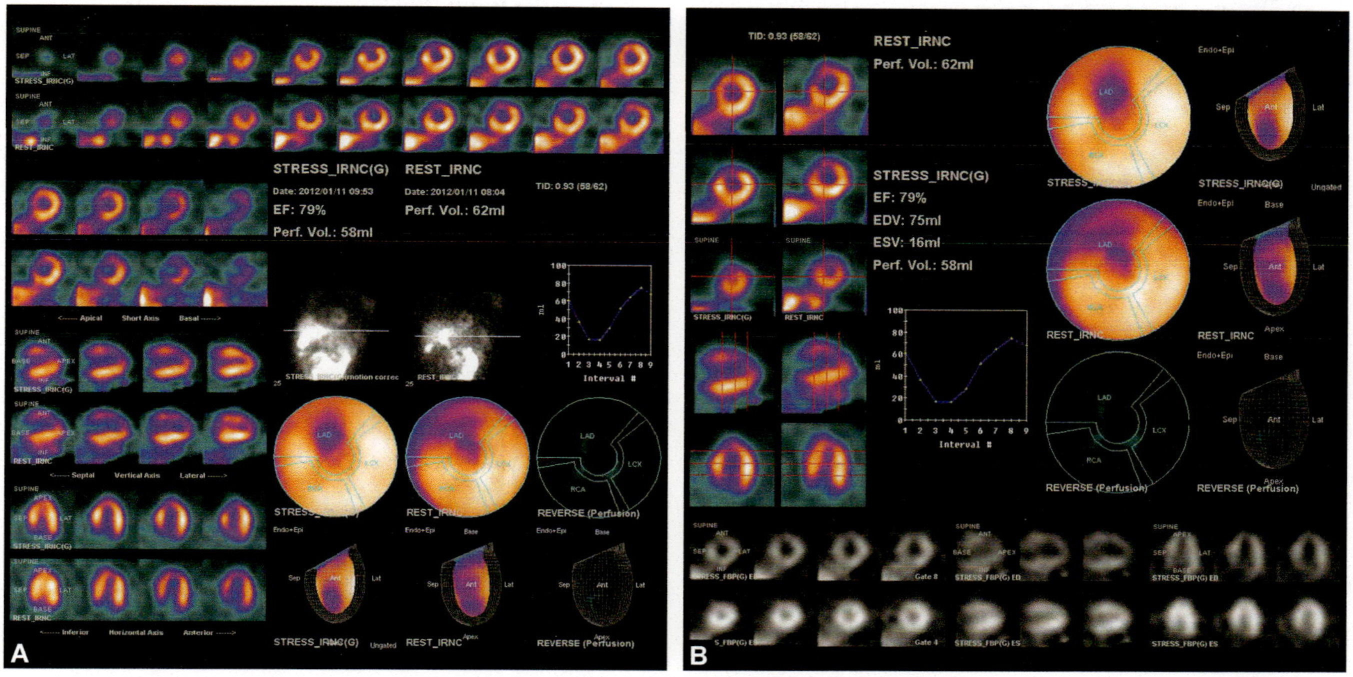

Figs. 1A and B: A 50-year-old obese female with coronary artery disease risk factors and typical angina.
Imaging protocol: Rest technetium-99m tetrofosmin/stress technetium-99m sestamibi. Injected activity was increased to 12 mCi/36 mCi due to the patient's obesity.
Stress modality: Dipyridamole. No chest pain and no ST segment changes.

CASE 8: INFEROLATERAL BREAST ARTIFACT

In this elderly female patient with a 46 inch chest circumference and D bra cup her breasts were very pendulous lying over the anterior abdominal wall when she lay in the supine position for SPECT imaging. Perfusion tomograms (A) demonstrate a moderate decrease in tracer concentration in the inferolateral wall of the left ventricle. However, functional images (B) demonstrate entirely normal inferolateral wall motion and wall thickening. These findings are secondary to marked photon attenuation by the patient's pendulous overlying left breast. Of note, breast position may vary greatly. Therefore, close inspection of planar projection images to determine breast position is critical prior to interpretation of reconstructed tomograms. Also, gated imaging is very useful to differentiate fixed defects due to myocardial scarring from those due to attenuation artifact (Figs. 1A and B).

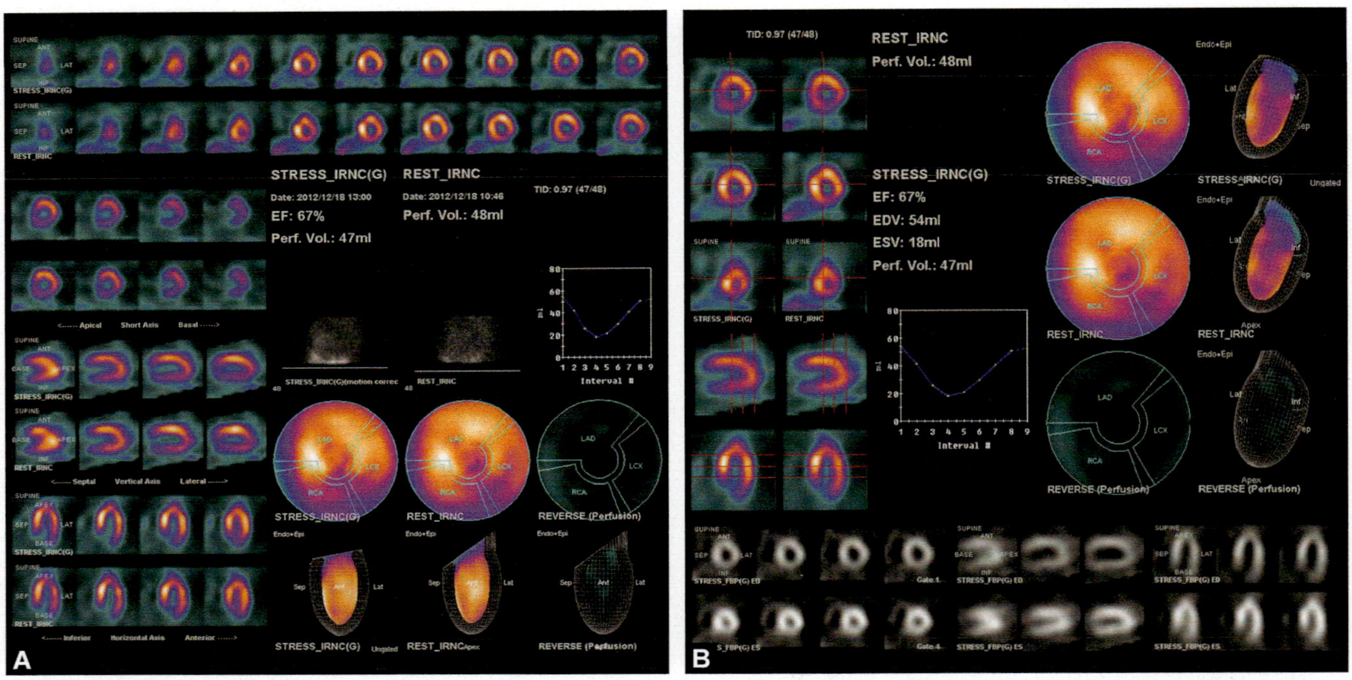

Figs. 1A and B: A 78-year-old female with multiple coronary artery disease risk factors, exertional dyspnea and fatigue, and atypical angina.
Imaging protocol: Rest/stress technetium-99m sestamibi.
Stress modality: Dipyridamole. No chest pain and no ST segment changes.

CASE 9: MODERATE DIAPHRAGMATIC ATTENUATION

Perfusion tomograms (A) demonstrate a moderate decrease in tracer concentration throughout the inferior wall of the left ventricle. Inspection of the stress and rest planar projection images demonstrates elevation of the left hemidiaphragm with a photopenic "shadow" crossing over the inferior wall of the left ventricle with indistinctness of the base of the inferior wall. Of note, the inferior defect appears more marked in the resting tomograms than in the stress tomograms, a finding of "pseudo-reverse-distribution" frequently associated with attenuation artifacts. Functional imaging (B) demonstrates that inferior wall motion and wall thickening are entirely normal, favoring the presence of an attenuation artifact rather than inferior myocardial scarring. Prone imaging is also useful to differentiate inferior attenuation artifacts from true perfusion defects since in the prone position the heart shifts anteriorly and the diaphragm is pushed downward, increasing the distance between the inferior wall of the left ventricle and the left hemidiaphragm (Figs. 1A and B).

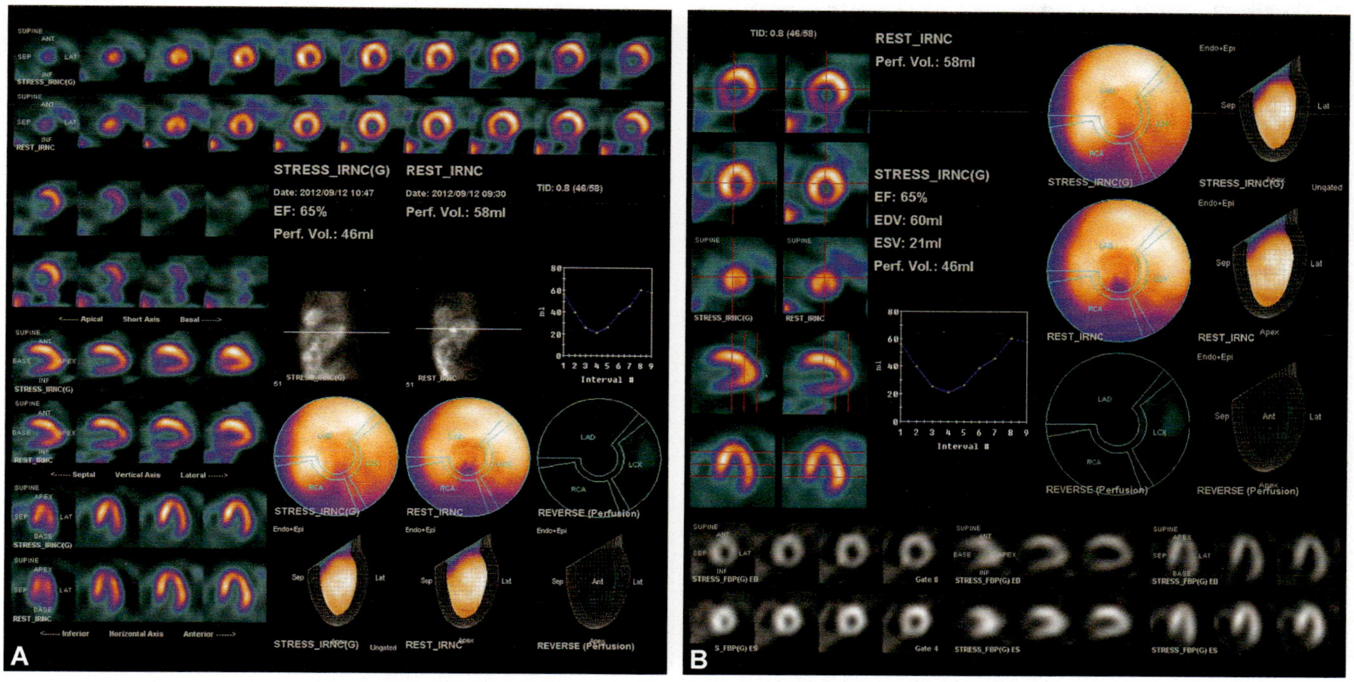

Figs. 1A and B: A 65-year-old obese male with multiple coronary artery disease risk factors and atypical angina.
Imaging protocol: Rest/stress technetium-99m sestamibi.
Stress modality: Dipyridamole. No chest pain and no ST segment changes.

CASE 10: SUBDIAPHRAGMATIC SCATTER

In planar projection images and perfusion tomograms (A) tracer concentration is noted throughout the liver, more marked in the resting images. In the reconstructed resting tomograms, there is a slight increase in inferior wall count density due to Compton scatter from the left lobe of the liver. Because images are normalized to the most intense area of the myocardium, in this case the inferior wall, there is a resulting mild decrease in tracer concentration in the contralateral anterior wall. To minimize radiotracer concentration in the liver, adequate time should be allotted between radiotracer injection and SPECT acquisition to allow for tracer to clear from the liver. In general for the Tc-99m tracers SPECT acquisition should be delayed for 45 minutes following resting radiotracer injection, 45 minutes following radiotracer injection with pharmacologic vasodilatation, and 20–30 minutes following radiotracer injection with treadmill exercise stress. Functional images (B) clearly demonstrate normal ventricular function despite Compton scatter into the inferior wall (Figs. 1A and B).

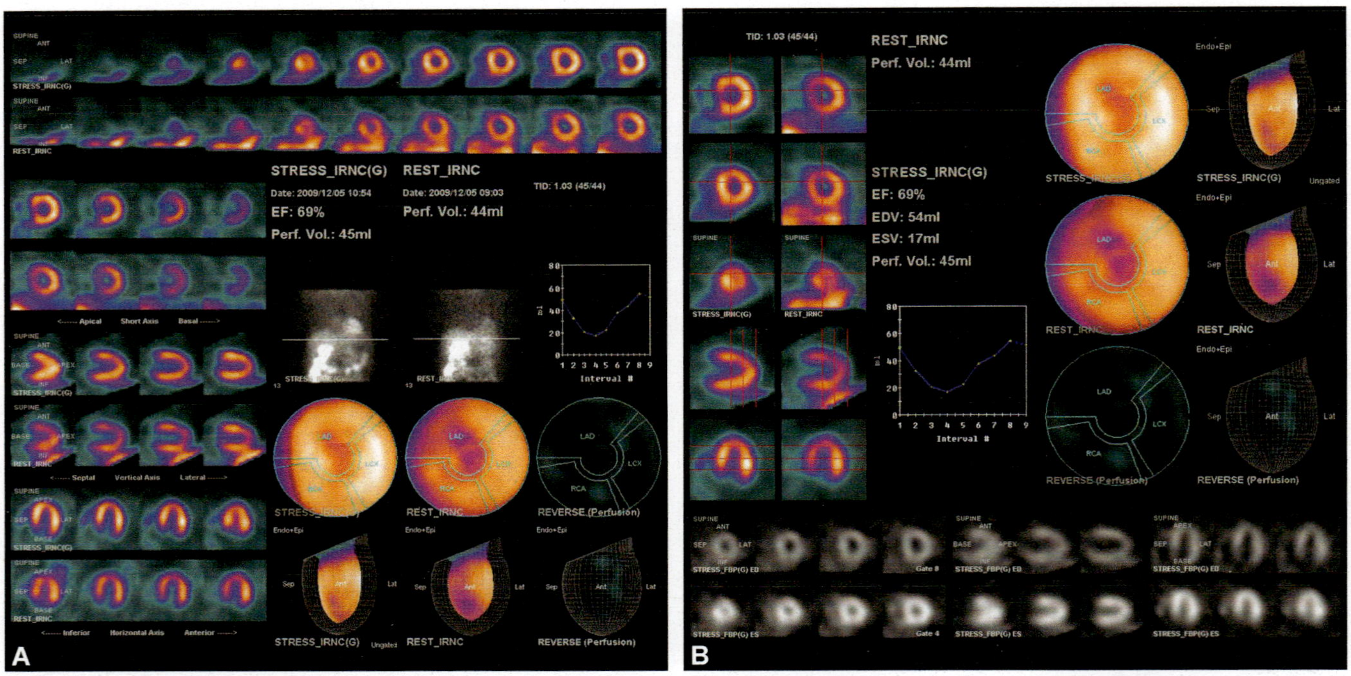

Figs. 1A and B: A 69-year-old male with multiple coronary artery disease risk factors including diabetes and atypical angina.
Imaging protocol: Rest/stress technetium-99m sestamibi.
Stress modality: Regadenoson. No chest pain and no ST segment changes.

CASE 11: SEVERE INFEROLATERAL SCAR; LEFT VENTRICULAR EJECTION FRACTION (LVEF) = 32%

Perfusion tomograms (A) demonstrate a moderately extensive-to-extensive, severe decrease in tracer concentration in the inferolateral wall of the left ventricle. There is no evidence of defect reversibility. Functional imaging (B) demonstrates inferolateral akinesis and absent thickening. The left ventricle is mildly dilated (end-diastolic volume = 124 cc, end-systolic volume = 87 cc), and left ventricular ejection fraction = 30%. These findings are consistent with marked inferolateral myocardial scarring. Absent wall motion and wall thickening of the inferolateral wall would not be consistent with a diaphragmatic attenuation artifact. The moderate decrease in left ventricular ejection fraction is associated with compromised patient prognosis (Figs. 1A and B).

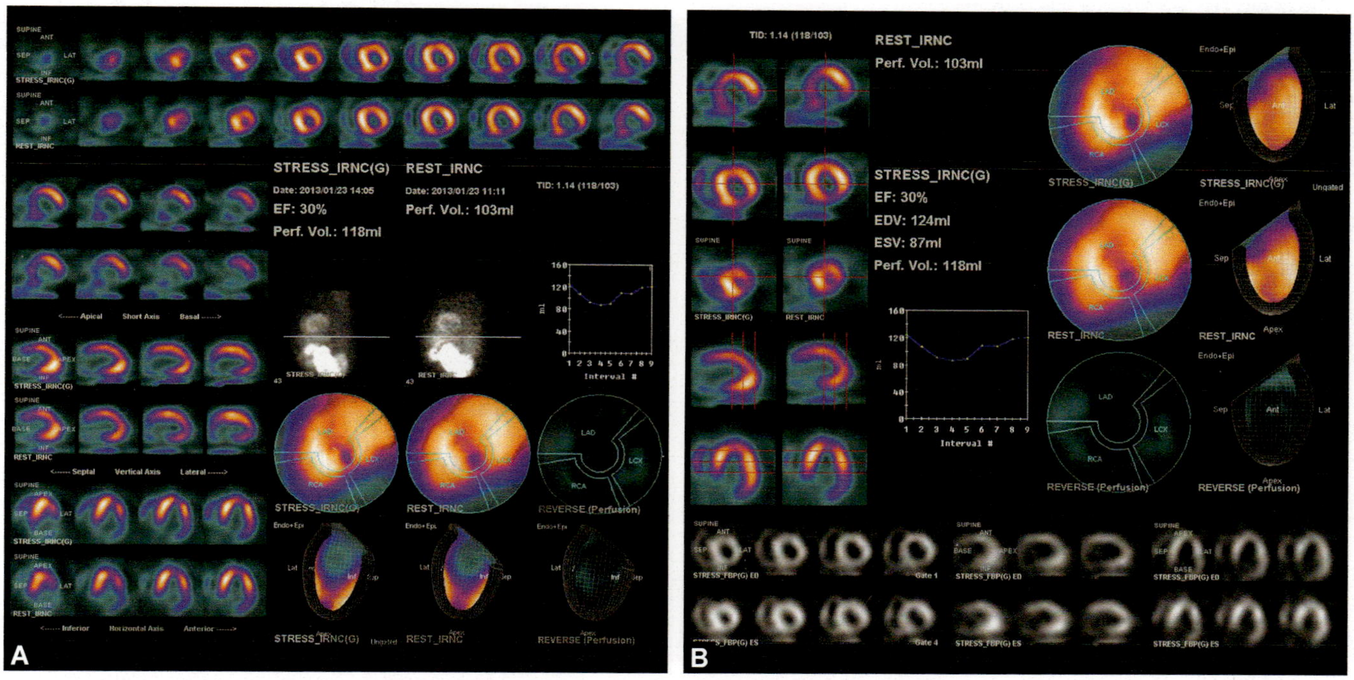

Figs. 1A and B: A 71-year-old man with prior myocardial infarction and exertional fatigue and dyspnea.
Imaging protocol: Rest technetium-99m tetrofosmin/stress technetium-99m sestamibi.
Stress modality: Regadenoson. The resting electrocardiogram demonstrated inferior Q waves. During pharmacologic stress there was no chest pain and no ST segment changes.

CASE 12: SCAR BASAL HALF INFERIOR WALL

Perfusion tomograms (A) demonstrate a marked decrease in tracer concentration in the basal one-third of the inferior wall of the left ventricle. Unlike the tapering of the inferior wall that is frequently noted in patients with photon attenuation by the left hemidiaphragm, in this case there is an abrupt absence of radiotracer concentration in the basal inferior wall. Functional images (B) demonstrate absent wall thickening of the basal third of the inferior wall. Due to the very marked decrease in tracer concentration in this region, it is not possible to accurately assess wall motion. Left ventricular volume is normal (end diastolic volume = 68 cc, end-systolic volume equals 25 cc), and left ventricular ejection fraction is normal (64%). In this patient, the absence of stress-induced ischemia outside of the infarct territory and preservation of normal left ventricular volume and systolic function are associated with a good prognosis (Figs. 1A and B).

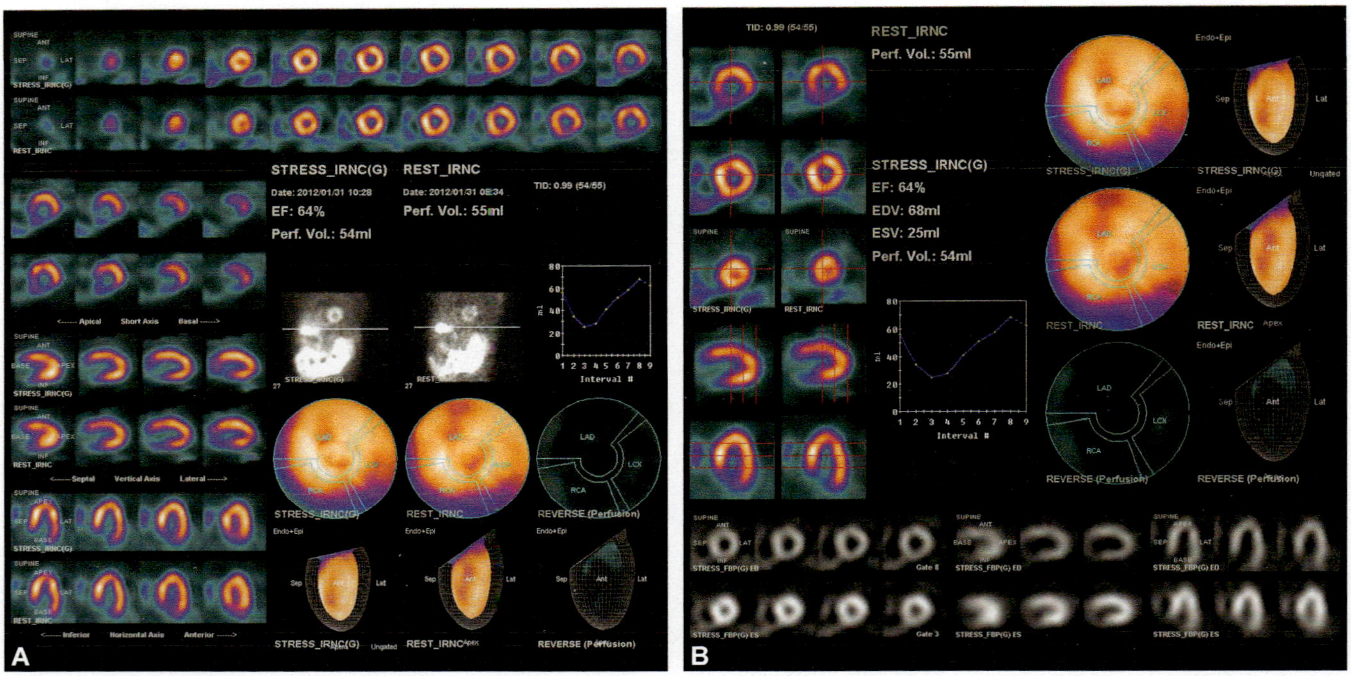

Figs. 1A and B: A 50-year-old man with a history of prior myocardial infarction and atypical angina.

Imaging protocol: Rest technetium-99m tetrofosmin/stress technetium-99m sestamibi.

Stress modality: Regadenoson. The resting electrocardiogram demonstrated nonspecific ST-T wave abnormalities. During pharmacologic stress there was no chest pain and no ST segment changes.

CASE 13: INFEROAPICAL SCAR; LVEF = 50%

Perfusion images (A) demonstrate a moderately extensive, severe decrease in tracer concentration in the inferoapical wall of the left ventricle. There is no evidence of defect reversibility in the resting images. Functional images (B) demonstrate inferoapical akinesis and absent wall thickening. Left ventricular volume is normal, but left ventricular ejection fraction is borderline-low (50%). These findings are consistent with a localized area of inferoapical myocardial scarring. It is important to differentiate this finding from "physiologic apical thinning". With the latter the defect is usually localized to the very apex of the left ventricle, and there is always normal left ventricular regional apical wall motion and wall thickening (Figs. 1A and B).

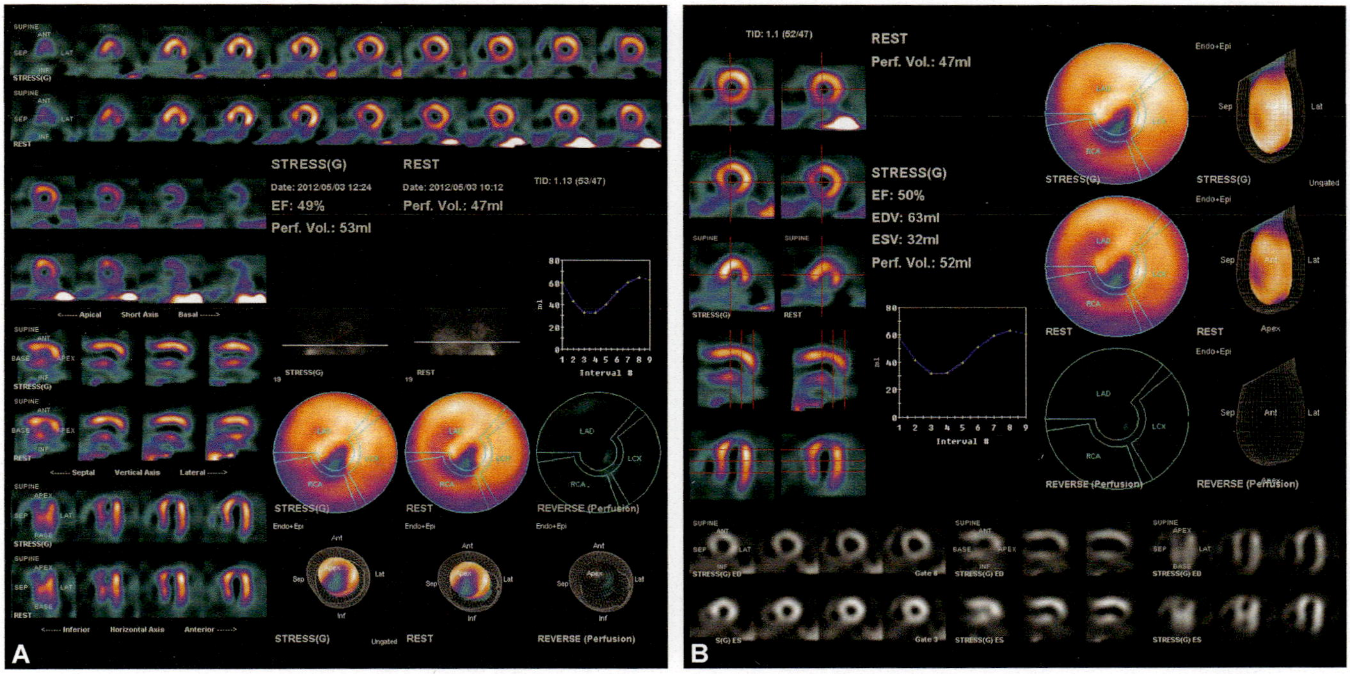

Figs. 1A and B: A 62-year-old man with a history of prior myocardial infarction and exertional dyspnea and fatigue.

Imaging protocol: Rest technetium-99m tetrofosmin/stress technetium-99m sestamibi.

Stress modality: Regadenoson. The resting electrocardiogram demonstrated Q waves in the lateral precordial leads. During pharmacologic stress there was no chest pain and no ST segment changes.

CASE 14: LAD ISCHEMIA

Perfusion images (A) demonstrate a moderately extensive, severe decrease in tracer concentration in the apex and contiguous distal anteroseptal wall of the left ventricle. In resting images the stress perfusion abnormality is completely reversible. These findings are consistent with stress-induced ischemia. Functional images (B) demonstrate borderline left ventricular dilatation (end-diastolic volume = 109 cc, end-systolic volume = 53 cc) and a borderline-low left ventricular ejection fraction (51%). Left ventricular regional wall motion is normal. Note that since post-stress SPECT is acquired 30–45 minutes following exercise or pharmacologic stress, stress-induced regional wall motion abnormalities generally have resolved by the time of SPECT imaging acquisition (Figs. 1A and B).

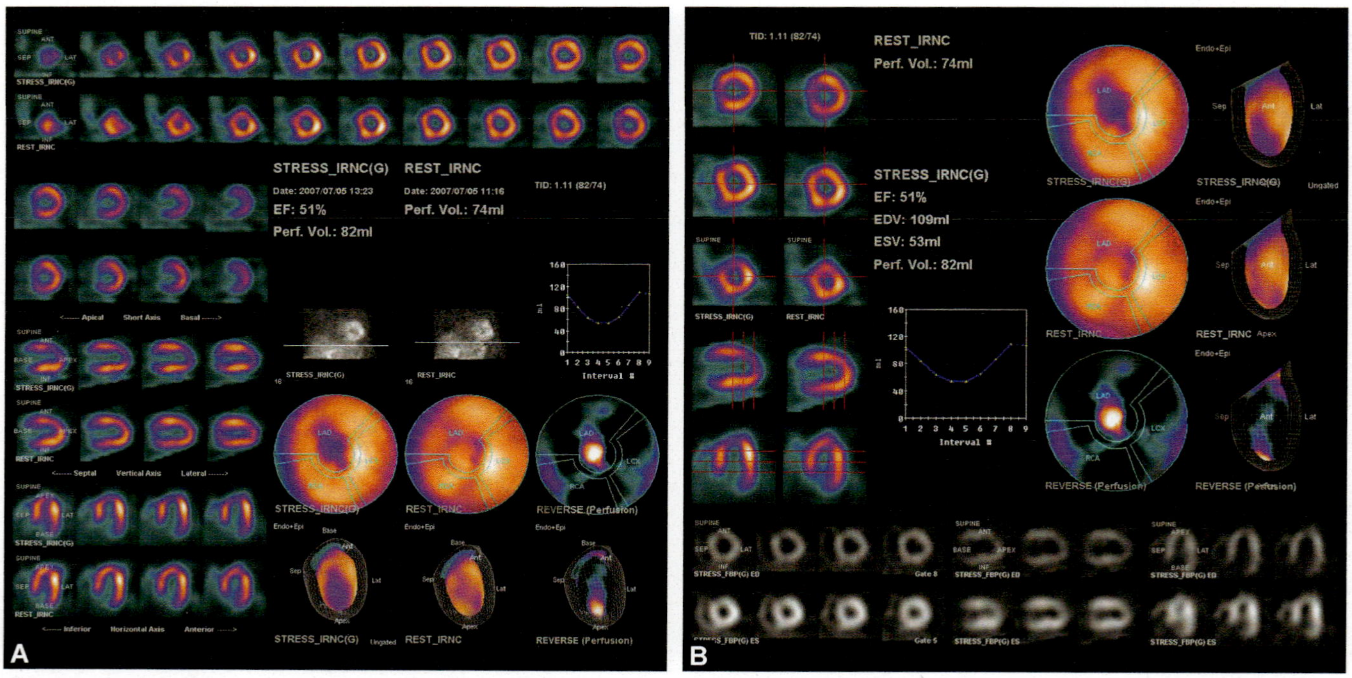

Figs. 1A and B: A 44-year-old man with coronary artery disease risk factors and typical angina.
Imaging protocol: Rest/stress technetium-99m sestamibi.
Stress modality: Dipyridamole. No chest pain and no ST segment changes.

CASE 15: MARKED INFEROAPICAL ISCHEMIA

Perfusion images (A) demonstrate an extensive, moderately severe decrease in tracer concentration throughout the inferior wall of the left ventricle, more marked in the distal one-third of the inferior wall/inferoapical region. In resting images, the stress perfusion abnormality is reversible, except for a mild residual abnormality in the distal inferior wall inferoapical region. These findings are consistent with stress-induced ischemia. The residual resting abnormality in the distal inferior wall to be consistent with underlying scar or resting ischemia. Functional images (B) demonstrate normal left ventricular volume and ejection fraction (62%) and normal regional function. Normal wall motion and wall thickening of the inferoapical wall would perhaps favor resting ischemia rather than scar as a cause of the residual resting perfusion abnormality in that region (Figs. 1A and B).

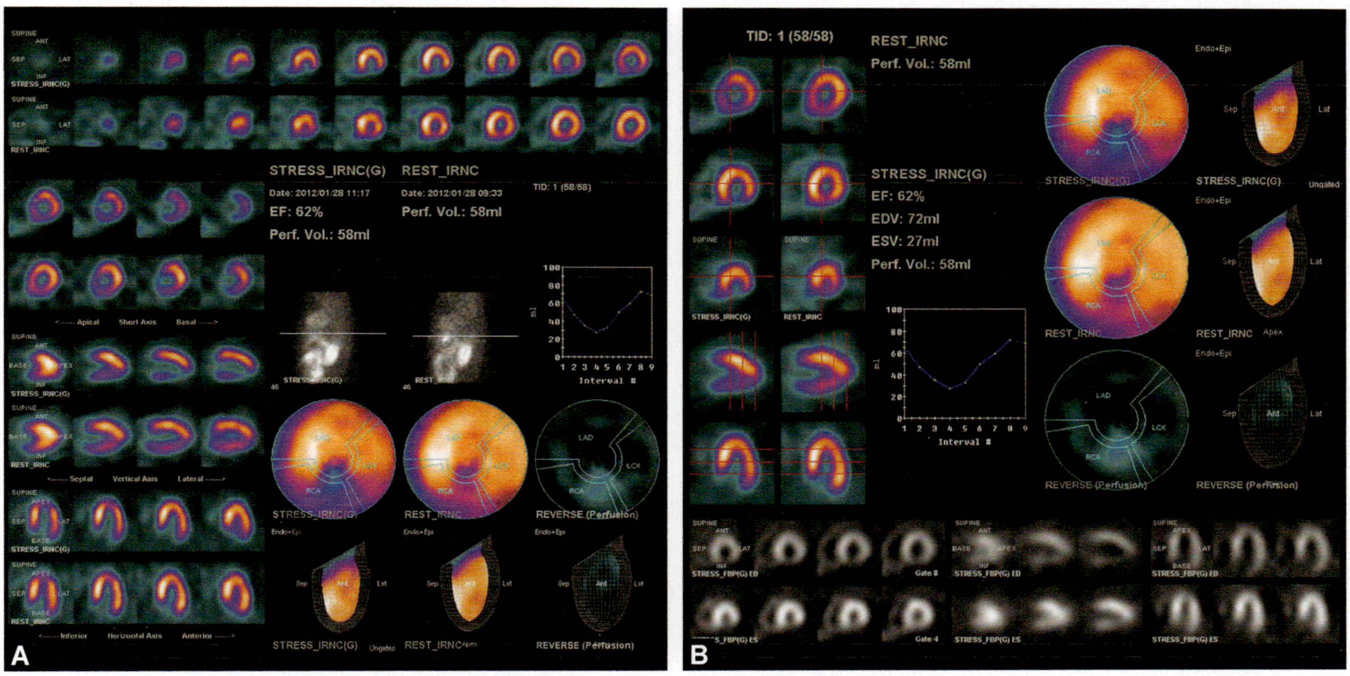

Figs. 1A and B: An 80-year-old man with coronary artery disease risk factors and atypical angina.
Imaging protocol: Rest/stress technetium-99m sestamibi.
Stress modality: Dipyridamole. No chest pain; 1 mm ST segment depression in leads II and III.

CASE 16: INCREASED SEPTAL UPTAKE DUE TO LEFT VENTRICULAR HYPERTROPHY (LVH) (S/P AVR)

This patient underwent myocardial perfusion imaging several years following aortic valve replacement for aortic stenosis. In both the stress and rest perfusion tomograms (A) there is a mild/moderate relative increase in tracer concentration in the septum, a finding frequently observed in hypertensive patients and in those with left ventricular hypertrophy. This patient had left ventricular hypertrophy, confirmed echocardiographically, due to prior aortic stenosis. Otherwise, tracer distribution is normal. Gated tomographic images (B) demonstrate normal left ventricular volume (end-diastolic volume = 55 cc, end-systolic volume = 24 cc) and a low-normal ejection fraction (54%). Note that it is often difficult to interpret SPECT myocardial perfusion images in patients with increased septal radiotracer concentration due to left ventricular hypertrophy. Images are normalized to the "hot" septum, giving the impression of decreased radiotracer concentration throughout the remainder of the left ventricular myocardium. However, normal left ventricular volume and preserved regional wall motion of the anterior, lateral and inferior walls suggests that myocardial scarring as a cause of relatively decreased radiotracer concentration in these segments would be unlikely (Figs. 1A and B).

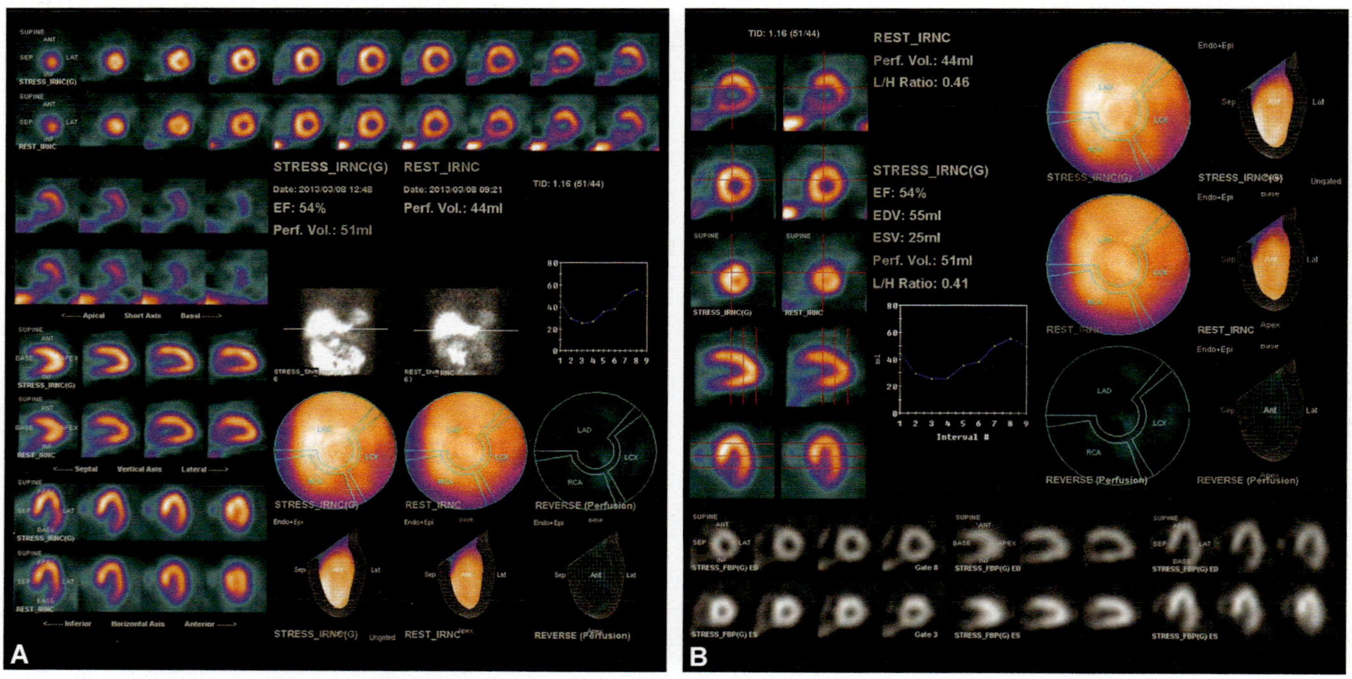

Figs. 1A and B: A 63-year-old man status postaortic valve replacement with atypical chest pain and exertional dyspnea.
Imaging protocol: Rest/stress technetium-99m sestamibi.
Stress modality: Treadmill exercise. The resting electrocardiogram demonstrated LVH. During exercise there were 2 mm of ST segment depression. The patient experienced no chest pain.

CASE 17: HYPERTROPHIC CARDIOMYOPATHY

This patient had a long-standing history of hypertension and several episodes of congestive heart failure. Stress and rest perfusion images (A) demonstrate normal perfusion distribution. The myocardium appears diffusely thickened. In planar projection images myocardial thickening is also apparent, and the myocardial-to-background ratio is increased. All of these findings are suggestive of increased myocardial mass/myocardial hypertrophy. Functional images (B) demonstrate marked left ventricular dilatation (end-diastolic volume = 244 cc, end-systolic volume = 160 cc), and left ventricular ejection fraction is moderately decreased (34%). These combined findings are most consistent with a nonischemic, hypertensive cardiomyopathy (Figs. 1A and B).

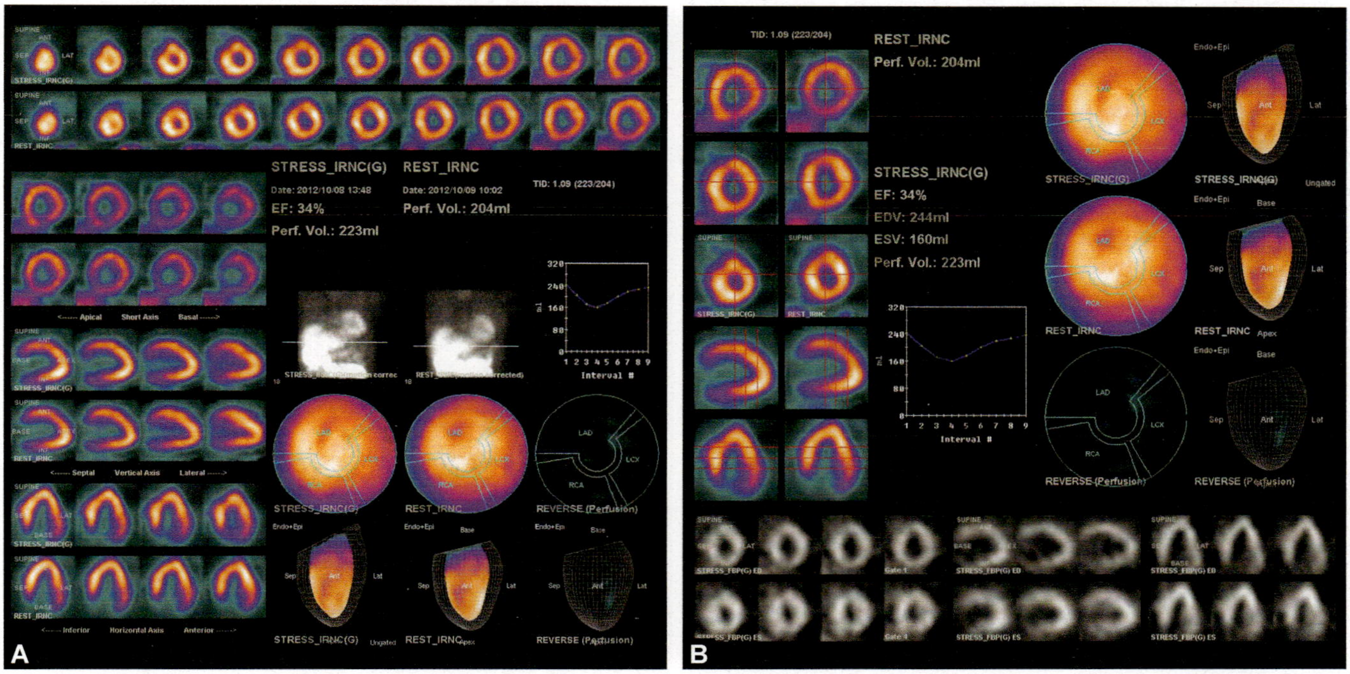

Figs. 1A and B: A 73-year-old man with coronary artery disease risk factors including long-standing hypertension with exertional dyspnea and atypical chest pain.

Imaging protocol: Rest technetium-99m tetrofosmin/stress technetium-99m sestamibi.

Stress modality: Regadenoson. The resting electrocardiogram demonstrated LVH and nonspecific ST-T wave abnormalities. During pharmacologic stress there was no chest pain and no additional ST segment changes.

CASE 18: REST/DELAYED THALLIUM; INFERIOR RESTING ISCHEMIA

A rest/stress Tc-99m sestamibi myocardial perfusion scan performed previously had demonstrated a fixed inferior myocardial perfusion defect, consistent with either myocardial scarring or resting ischemia of viable, jeopardized myocardium. Therefore, a rest/delayed thallium-201 scan was performed. The patient received an intravenous dose of 4.0 mCi thallium-201 at rest. SPECT imaging was performed 10 minutes thereafter and at a 4 hour delayed interval. The immediate and delayed perfusion images (A) demonstrate an extensive, moderately severe decrease in tracer concentration in the inferior wall in the immediate images, which is completely reversible in the delayed images. Polar plots (B) also demonstrate the reversible inferior perfusion defect. These findings are consistent with resting ischemia of viable, jeopardized myocardium and do not favor myocardial scarring. Initial thallium-201 uptake is proportional to myocardial blood flow, which may be decreased with either myocardial scarring or resting ischemia. In delayed images, there will be thallium-201 redistribution into viable myocardium but not into scar (Figs. 1A and B).

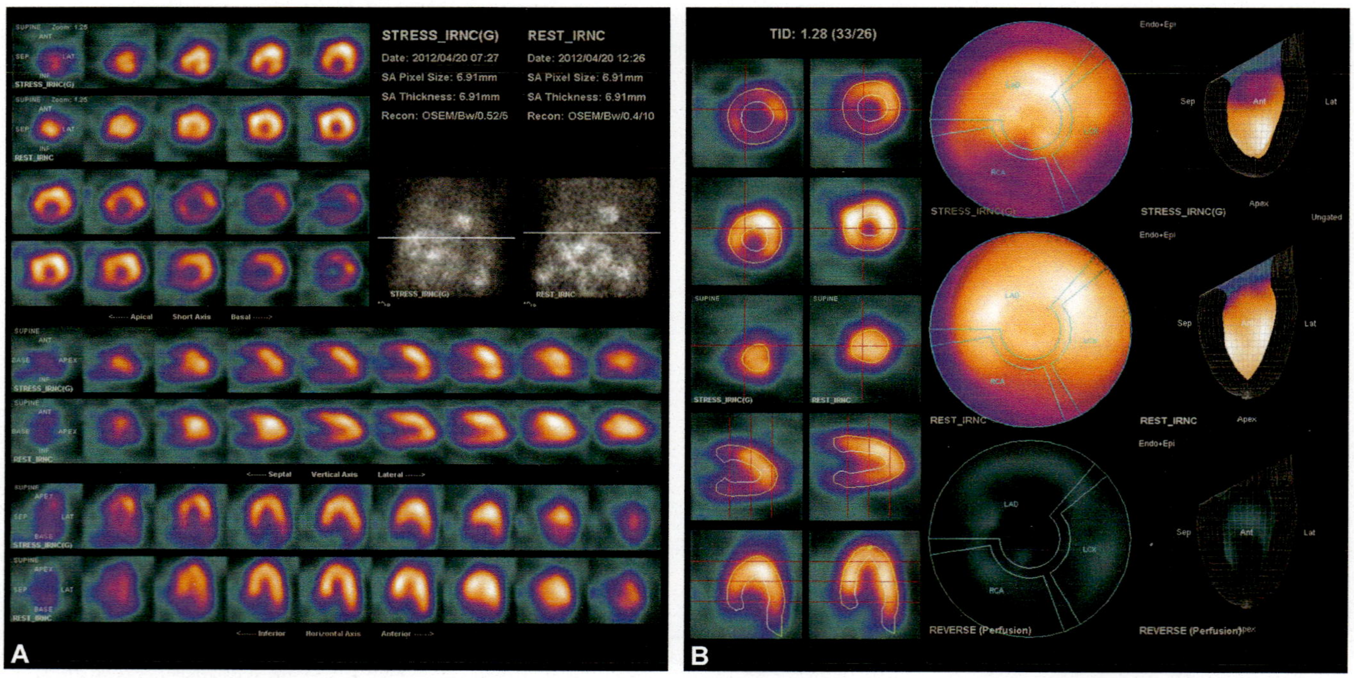

Figs. 1A and B: A 75-year-old man with coronary artery disease risk factors and exertional chest pain. The resting electrocardiogram demonstrated new ST segment abnormalities. A prior rest/stress technetium-99m sestamibi myocardial perfusion scan had demonstrated a fixed inferior myocardial perfusion defect.

Imaging protocol: Rest/4-hour delayed thallium-201 SPECT.

CASE 19: REST/DELAYED THALLIUM; SCAR WITHOUT ISCHEMIA

This patient presented with a history of prior myocardial infarction and acutely worsening congestive heart failure. The resting electrocardiogram demonstrated new ST-T wave abnormalities. There was a clinical concern of resting ischemia of viable, jeopardized myocardium as a cause of the patient's worsening heart failure. Therefore, a rest/delayed thallium-201 scan was performed. The patient received an intravenous dose of 4.0 mCi thallium-201 at rest. SPECT imaging was performed 10 minutes thereafter and at a 4-hour delayed interval. The immediate and delayed perfusion images (A) demonstrate an extensive, severe decrease in tracer concentration in the left ventricular apex and adjacent anteroapical region and inferior wall. There is no evidence of defect reversibility in delayed images. These findings are consistent with myocardial scarring with no evidence of resting ischemia of viable, jeopardized myocardium. The lung/heart (L/H) ratio, determined by placing regions of interest over the mid right lung and the brightest area of myocardium, is increased in anterior planar projection images (B) (immediate = 1.09, delayed = 0.61), consistent with poor left ventricular function (Figs. 1A and B).

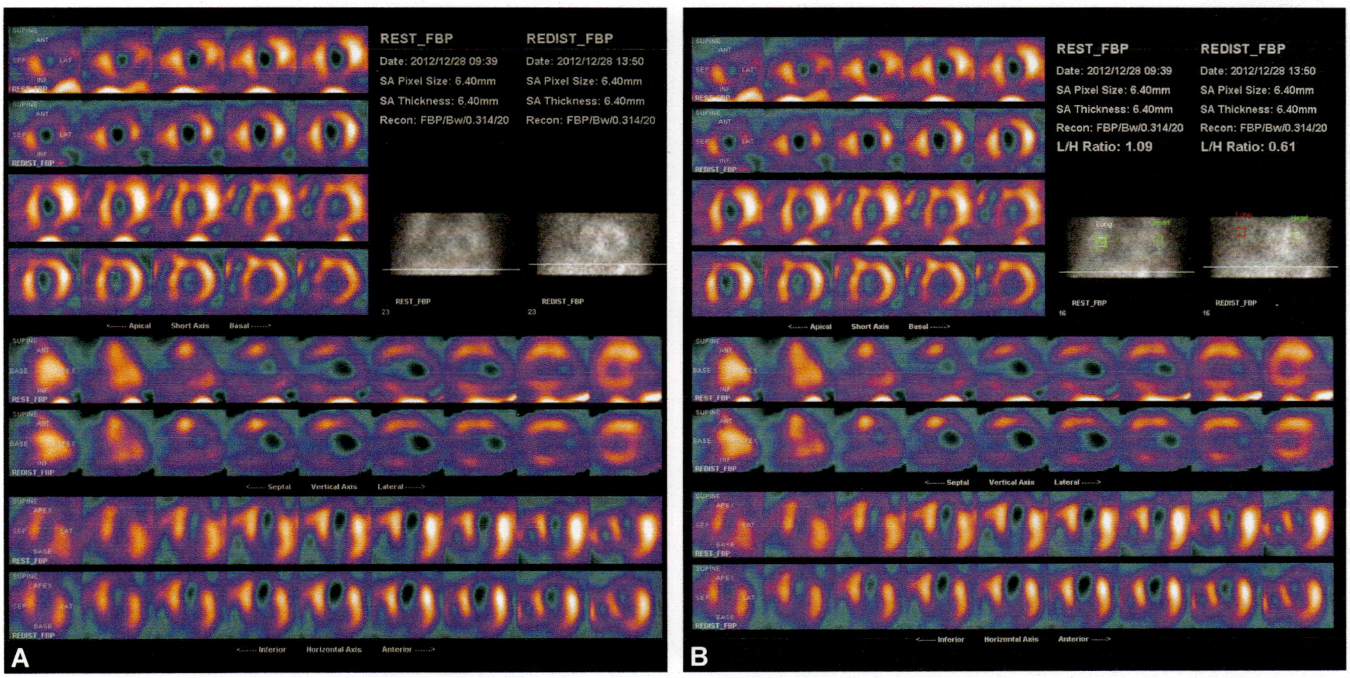

Figs. 1A and B: A 73-year-old female with a history of prior myocardial infarction and acutely worsening congestive heart failure.
Imaging protocol: Rest/4-hour delayed thallium-201 SPECT.

CASE 20: MUGA, DECLINE IN LVEF POSTCHEMOTHERAPY

In this patient with breast cancer undergoing doxorubicin chemotherapy, equilibrium radionuclide ventriculography (MUGA) was performed prior to institution of chemotherapy (A), and after the patient had received 300 mg/m^2 of doxorubicin (B). The initial left ventricular ejection fraction was normal (74%) and decreased significantly to 44% following chemotherapy, consistent with doxorubicin cardiotoxicity. If the baseline left ventricular ejection fraction is greater than 50%, a decrease in ejection fraction by 10 ejection fraction points to an absolute value of less than 50% is consistent with cardiotoxicity. If the baseline left ventricular ejection fraction (LVEF) is less than 50%, a decrease by 10 ejection fraction points or a value of less than 30% is consistent with cardiotoxicity. If cardiotoxicity is demonstrated, the patient should be given a "holiday" from chemotherapy and a repeat MUGA scan should be performed to determine if the LVEF has recovered prior to administration of additional chemotherapy. Prior to each subsequent chemotherapy dose, a repeat MUGA scan should be performed to determine if cardiotoxicity has recurred (Figs. 1A and B).

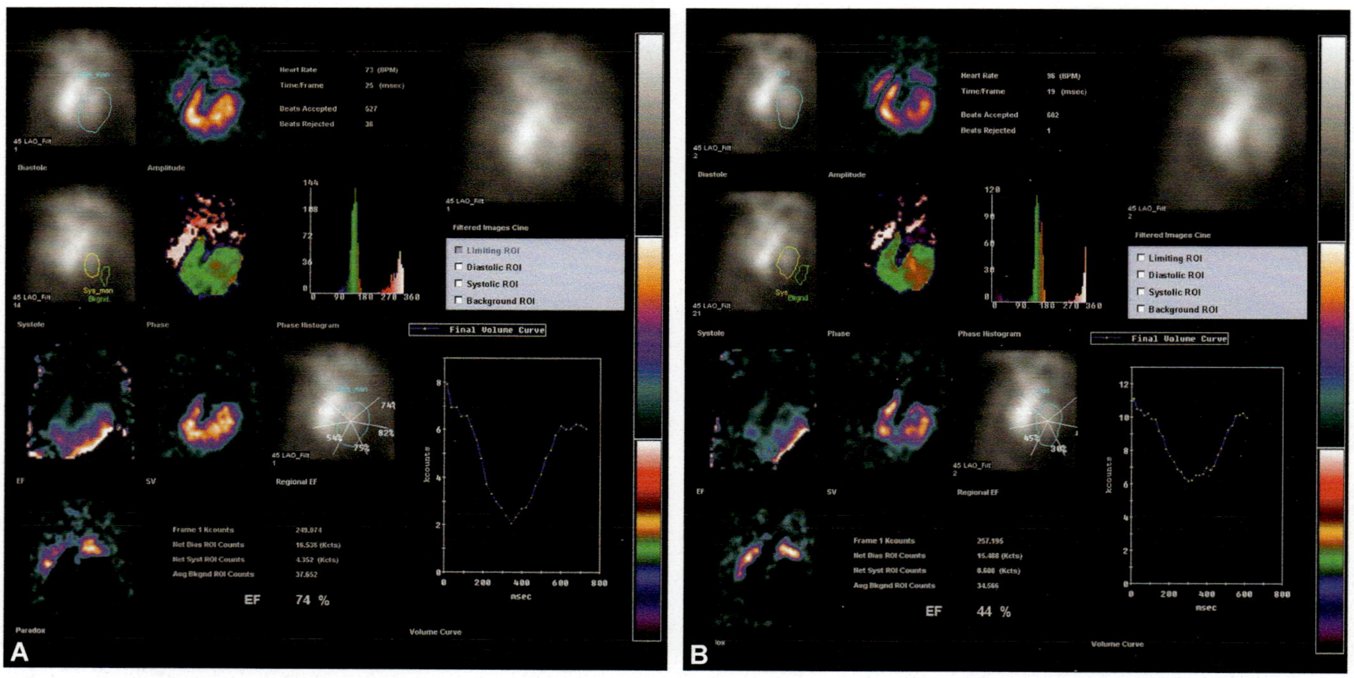

Figs. 1A and B: A 48-year-old asymptomatic female with breast cancer undergoing doxorubicin chemotherapy.
Imaging protocol: Equilibrium radionuclide ventriculography with in vitro technetium-99m labeled red blood cells.

Intermediate Cases

CASE 1: ANTERIOR, APICAL, AND INFERIOR SCAR

Perfusion images (A) demonstrate fixed severe apical, and extensive and moderately severe anteroseptal and inferior perfusion abnormalities. There is no evidence of defect reversibility. Functional images (B) demonstrate akinesis and absent thickening of the apex, and marked hypokinesis and absent thickening of the anteroseptal and inferior walls. The left ventricle is mildly/moderately dilated (end-diastolic volume = 133 cc, end-systolic volume equals 83 cc), and left ventricular ejection fraction is moderately decreased (37%). Although there is no evidence of stressed-induced ischemia, the extent of the perfusion abnormalities in a multivessel distribution (left anterior descending [LAD] and right coronary artery [RCA]) and the moderate decrease in LVEF impart a poor prognosis for this patient (Figs. 1A and B).

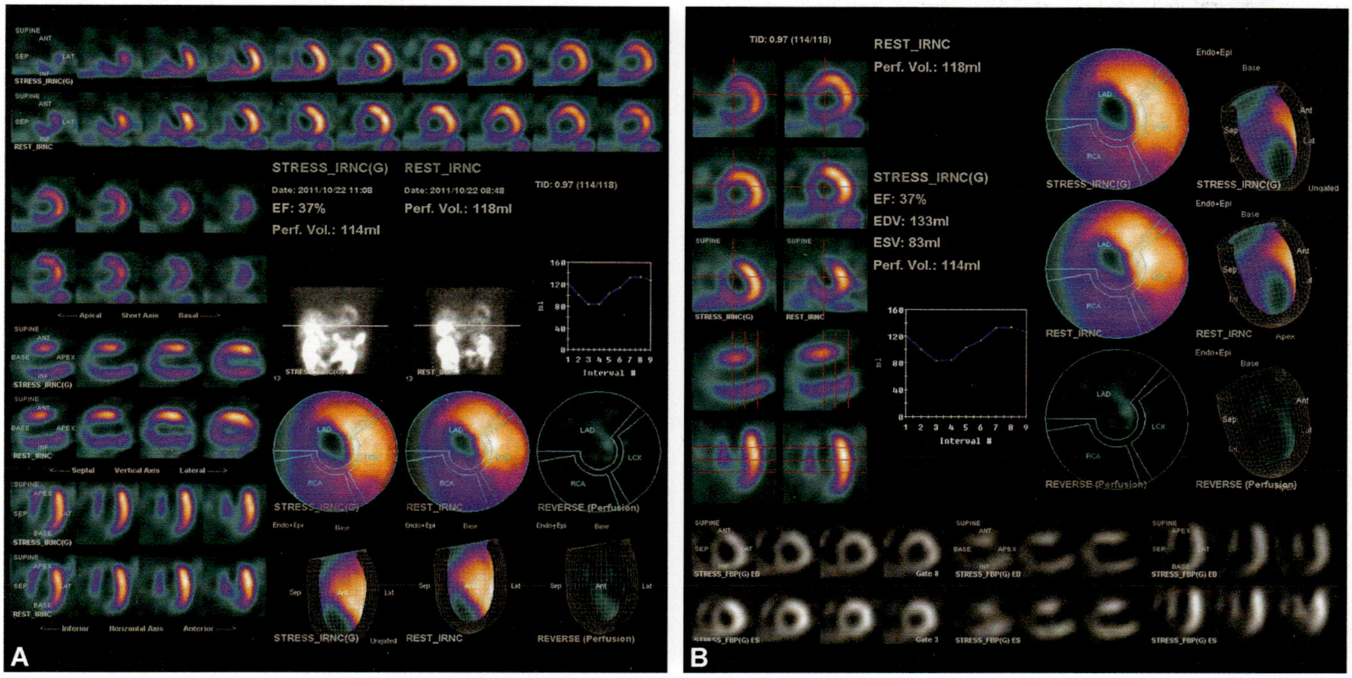

Figs. 1A and B: A 74-year-old male with prior myocardial infarction and exertional dyspnea.
Imaging protocol: Rest/stress technetium-99m sestamibi.
Stress modality: Dipyridamole. The resting electrocardiogram demonstrated Q waves in the precordial leads. The patient experienced no chest pain and no ST segment changes during pharmacologic stress.

CASE 2: D1 AND LCX ISCHEMIA

Stress perfusion images (A) demonstrate an extensive, moderately severe decrease in tracer concentration throughout the lateral wall of the left ventricle in the distribution of the left circumflex coronary artery, and a moderately extensive, mild decrease in concentration in the basal portion of the anterior wall, characteristic of the distribution of the first diagonal territory. It is important to note that the perfusion abnormality extends beyond the normal distribution of the left circumflex coronary artery into the diagonal territory and is therefore consistent with multivessel disease. In resting images, these perfusion abnormalities are completely reversible. Functional images (B) demonstrate normal left ventricular volume and regional function. Left ventricular ejection fraction is normal (63%). Multivessel ischemia is associated with a higher risk of subsequent cardiac events than single-vessel disease and is therefore important to recognize with myocardial perfusion SPECT (Figs. 1A and B).

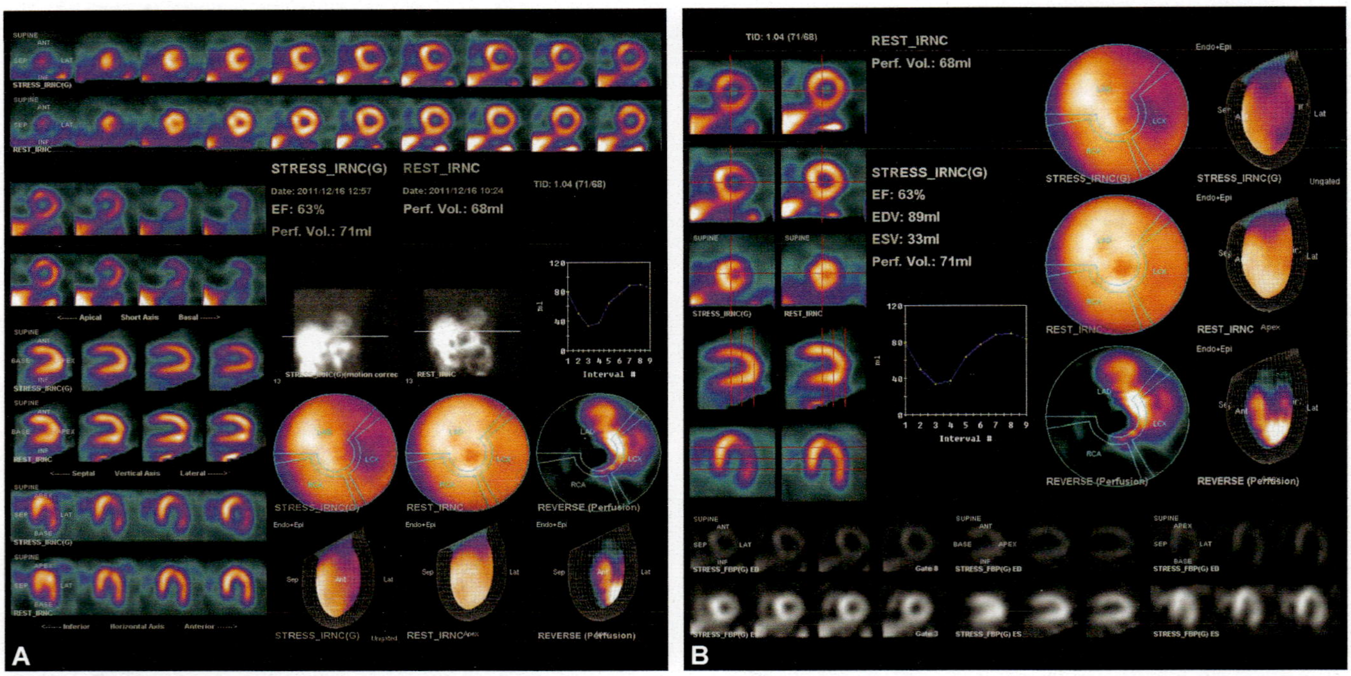

Figs. 1A and B: A 55-year-old male with typical angina.
Imaging protocol: Rest/stress technetium-99m sestamibi.
Stress modality: Treadmill exercise. No chest pain but 2 mm ST segment depression in leads II and III during exercise.

CASE 3: APICAL AND INFEROLATERAL ISCHEMIA; MULTIVESSEL DISEASE

Stress perfusion images (A) demonstrate a severe apical perfusion abnormality and a moderately extensive, moderately severe abnormality in the basal half of the inferior wall. These perfusion abnormalities are in distinctly separate vascular territories, thus consistent with multivessel disease. In resting images, these perfusion abnormalities are completely reversible. Functional images (B) demonstrate normal left ventricular volume and regional function. Left ventricular ejection fraction is normal (71%). Multivessel ischemia is associated with a higher risk of subsequent cardiac events than single-vessel disease and is therefore important to recognize with myocardial perfusion SPECT (Figs. 1A and B).

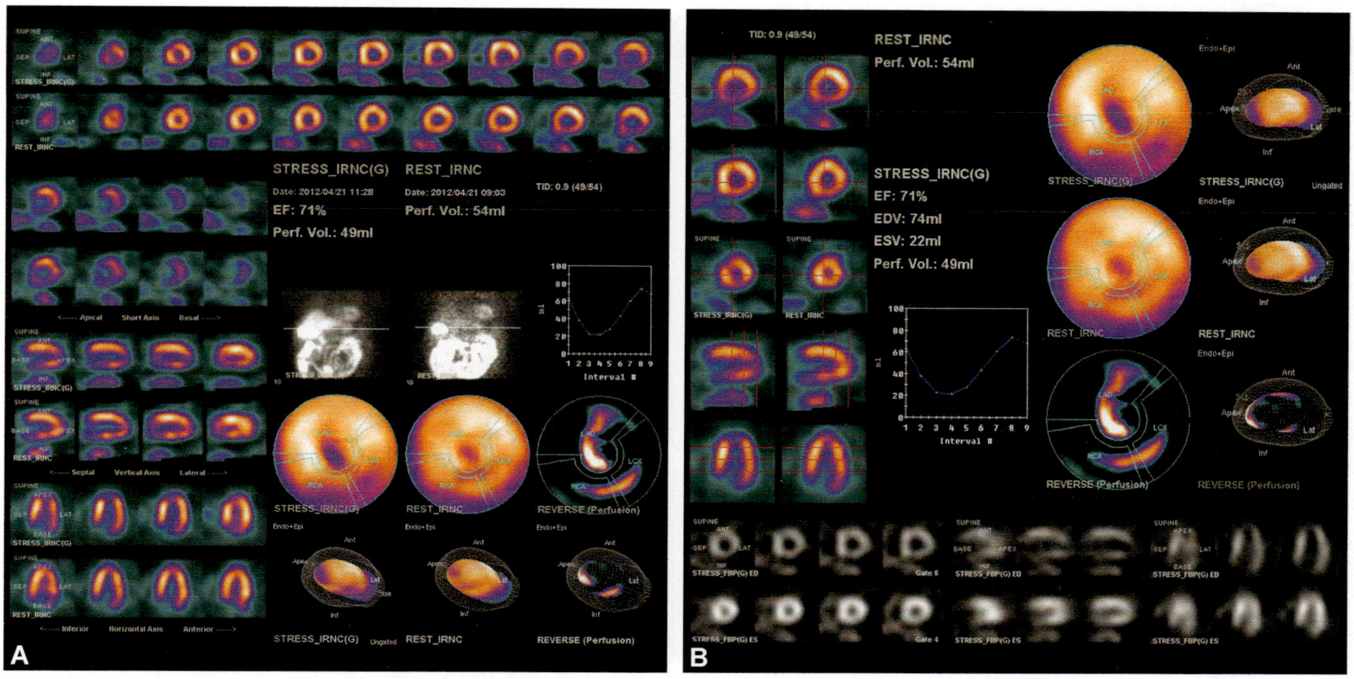

Figs. 1A and B: A 67-year-old male with exertional dyspnea and fatigue.
Imaging protocol: Rest/stress technetium-99m sestamibi.
Stress modality: Treadmill exercise. No chest pain and no ST segment changes during exercise.

CASE 4: LAD AND RCA ISCHEMIA; TRANSIENT ISCHEMIC DILATATION (TID)

Stress perfusion images (A) demonstrate a severe apical perfusion abnormality, a moderately extensive, moderately severe abnormality in contiguous distal anterolateral wall, and an extensive, moderately severe abnormality involving the entire inferior wall. These perfusion abnormalities involve the LAD and RCA vascular territories, respectively, and therefore are consistent with multivessel disease. In resting images, these perfusion abnormalities are completely reversible. The left ventricular cavity is noted to be mildly larger at stress than at rest (mild TID), consistent with stress-induced subendocardial ischemia. Of note, the automatically calculated TID ratio is 1.1 (abnormal = >1.12); however, visually the degree of TID appears greater. Functional images (B) demonstrate moderate left ventricular dilatation (end-diastolic volume = 152 cc, end-systolic volume = 95 cc). Left ventricular ejection fraction moderately decreased (38%). In this patient multivessel ischemia, TID, increased left ventricular volume, and moderately decreased LVEF are all associated with a higher risk of subsequent cardiac events (Figs. 1A and B).

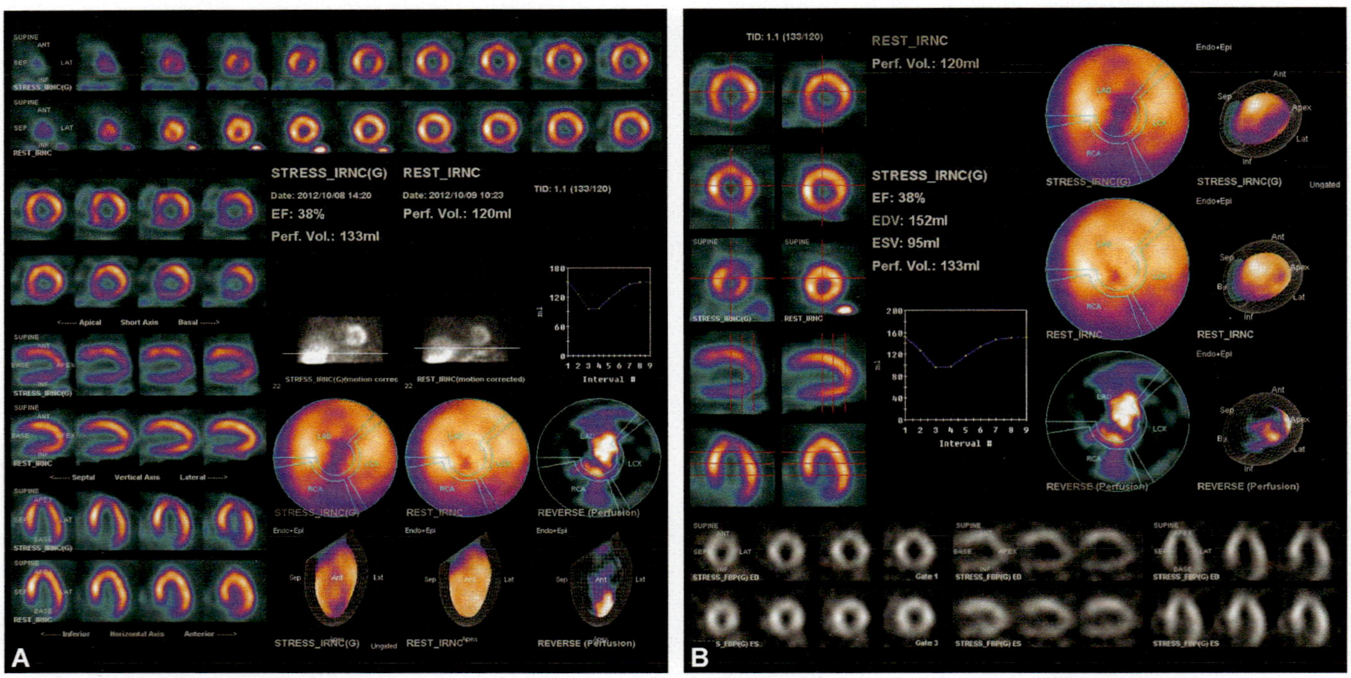

Figs. 1A and B: A 57-year-old female with multiple coronary artery disease risk factors and atypical angina.
Imaging protocol: Rest technetium-99m tetrofosmin/stress technetium-99m sestamibi.
Stress modality: Regadenoson. The patient experienced no chest pain during pharmacologic stress. There was 1 mm of horizontal ST segment depression in V2 and V3.

CASE 5: ANTERIOR AND INFEROLATERAL ISCHEMIA; TID, CONSISTENT WITH MULTIVESSEL DISEASE

Stress perfusion images (A) demonstrate a small-to-moderately extensive anterior perfusion abnormality, and a moderately extensive, severe inferior abnormality. These perfusion abnormalities involve the LAD and RCA vascular territories, respectively, and therefore are consistent with multivessel disease in the LAD and RCA territories. In resting images, these perfusion abnormalities are completely reversible. The left ventricular cavity is noted to be mildly/moderately larger at stress than at rest (mild transient ischemic dilatation or TID), consistent with stress-induced subendocardial ischemia. The calculated TID ratio is 1.26 (abnormal = >1.12). Of note, although TID is often associated with multivessel stress-induced ischemia, it may be present with extensive or severe single-vessel ischemia. Functional images (B) demonstrate normal left ventricular volume and ejection fraction (73%). In this patient multivessel ischemia and TID are associated with a higher risk of subsequent cardiac events (Figs. 1A and B).

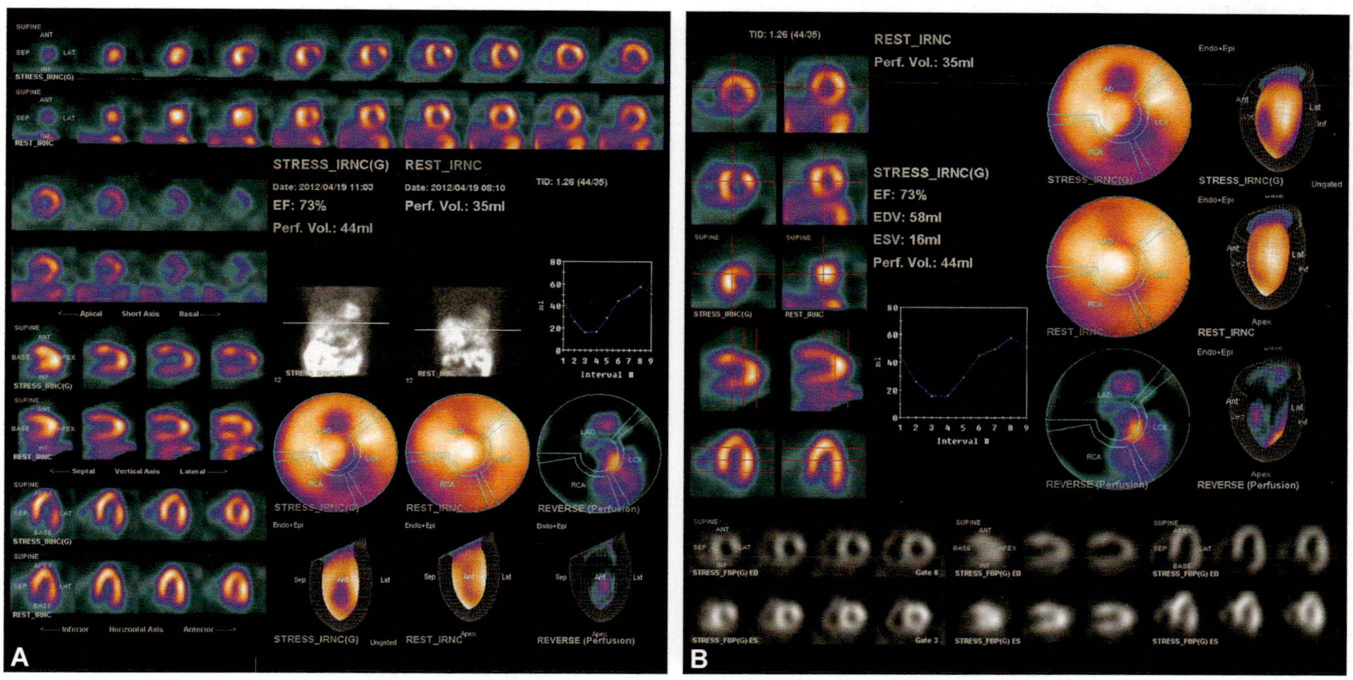

Figs. 1A and B: A 72-year-old male with coronary artery disease risk factors exertional dyspnea, and atypical angina.
Imaging protocol: Rest/stress technetium-99m sestamibi.
Stress modality: Treadmill exercise. No chest pain and 1 mm ST segment upsloping depression in leads II, III, and aVF during exercise.

CASE 6: APICAL ISCHEMIA AND BASAL INFERIOR ISCHEMIA

Stress perfusion images (A) demonstrate a small, severe apical perfusion abnormality, and a small, severe perfusion abnormality involving the basal one-third of the inferior wall. These perfusion abnormalities involve the LAD and RCA vascular territories, respectively, and therefore are consistent with multivessel disease. In resting images, these perfusion abnormalities are completely reversible. There is no evidence of TID. Functional images (B) demonstrate normal resting left ventricular volume and ejection fraction (>70%). Of note, the stress perfusion abnormalities alone could be interpreted as physiologic apical thinning and diaphragmatic attenuation of the base of the inferior wall. However, their complete reversibility in resting perfusion images is consistent with multivessel ischemia rather than normal variants (Figs. 1A and B).

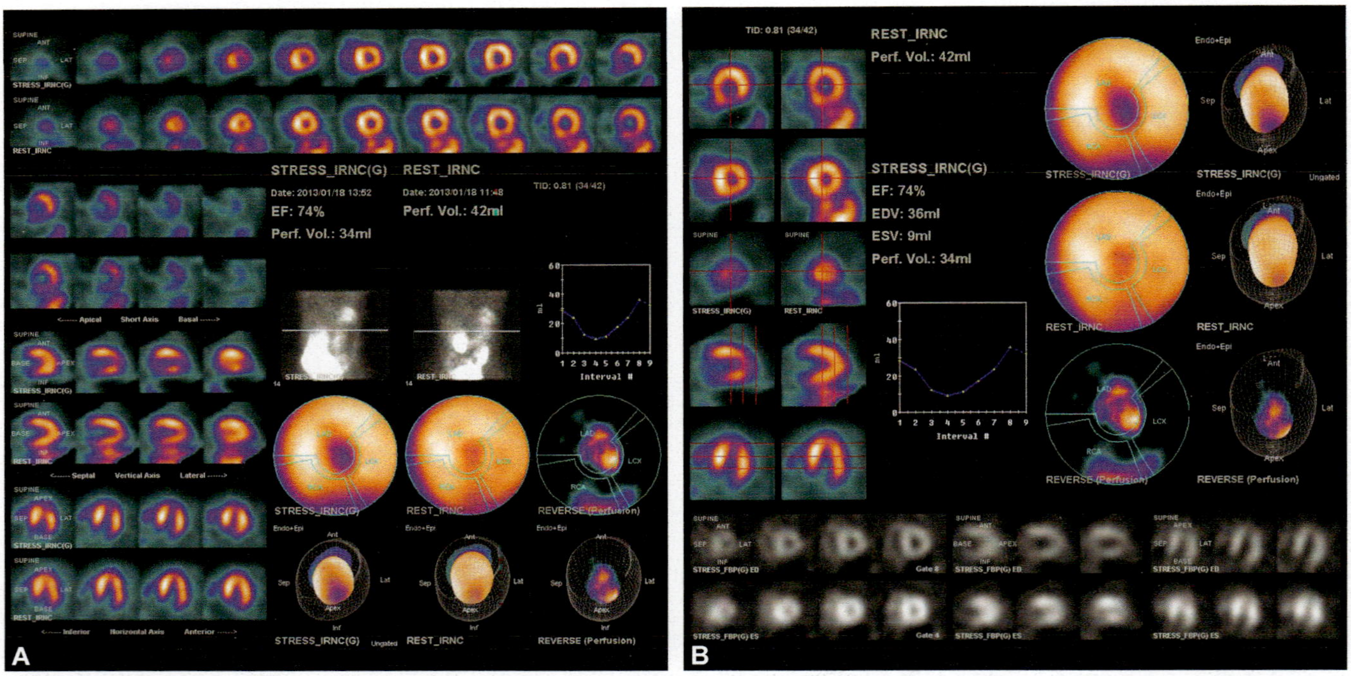

Figs. 1A and B: A 55-year-old male with coronary artery disease risk factors including diabetes and nonanginal chest pain.
Imaging protocol: Rest/stress technetium-99m sestamibi.
Stress modality: Regadenoson. No chest pain and no ST segment changes during exercise.

CASE 7: EXTENSIVE LATERAL SCAR WITH MODERATE PERI-INFARCT ISCHEMIA AT ANTEROLATERAL BORDER; MILD TID

Stress perfusion images (A) demonstrate extensive and severe decrease in tracer concentration throughout the lateral wall of the left ventricle. In resting images, there is slight reversibility of the stress defect at its anterolateral border, consistent with peri-infarct ischemia. Left ventricular cavity is slightly larger at stress than at rest (mild TID). The TID ratio is 1.14 (normal = <1.12). Functional images (B) demonstrate marked left ventricular dilatation (end-diastolicvolume=220cc,end-systolicvolume=188cc), and the left ventricular ejection fraction is markedly decreased (14%). Of note, it is important to recognize peri-infarct ischemia since it is associated with an increased risk of subsequent cardiac events, including myocardial infarction, worsening heart failure and arrhythmias (Figs. 1A and B).

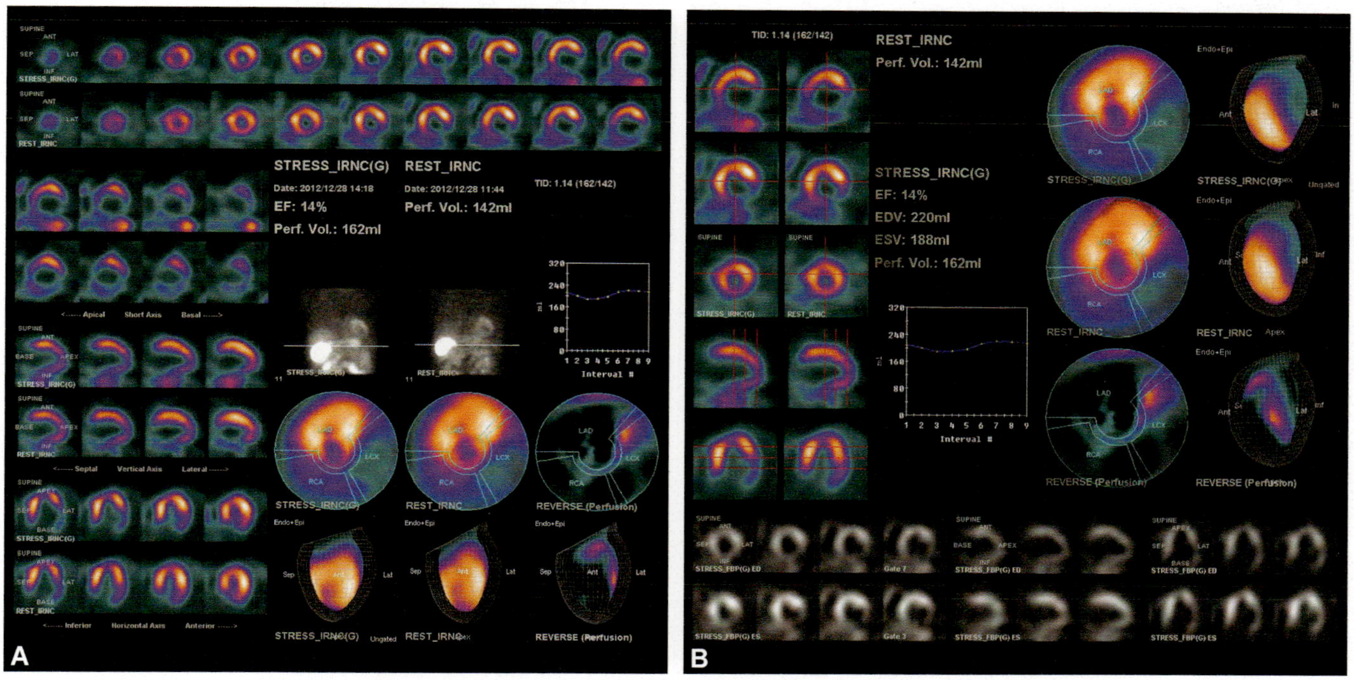

Figs. 1A and B: A 74-year-old male with a history of prior myocardial infarction, exertional dyspnea and atypical angina.
Imaging protocol: Rest/stress technetium-99m sestamibi.
Stress modality: Regadenoson. No chest pain and no ST segment changes during exercise.

CASE 8: ANTERIOR ISCHEMIA; LATERAL SCAR + ISCHEMIA

Stress perfusion images (A) demonstrate a marked and extensive decrease in the lateral wall of the left ventricle, and a moderately extensive, mild-to-moderately severe decrease in tracer concentration in the anterior wall. In resting images, there is reversibility at the anterolateral and inferolateral borders of the stress lateral wall perfusion defect, and there is complete reversibility of the anterior stress defect. These findings are consistent with lateral wall scarring with moderate stress-induced peri-infarct ischemia and also stress-induced anterior ischemia. Functional images (B) demonstrate normal left ventricular volume and ejection fraction (54%) (Figs. 1A and B).

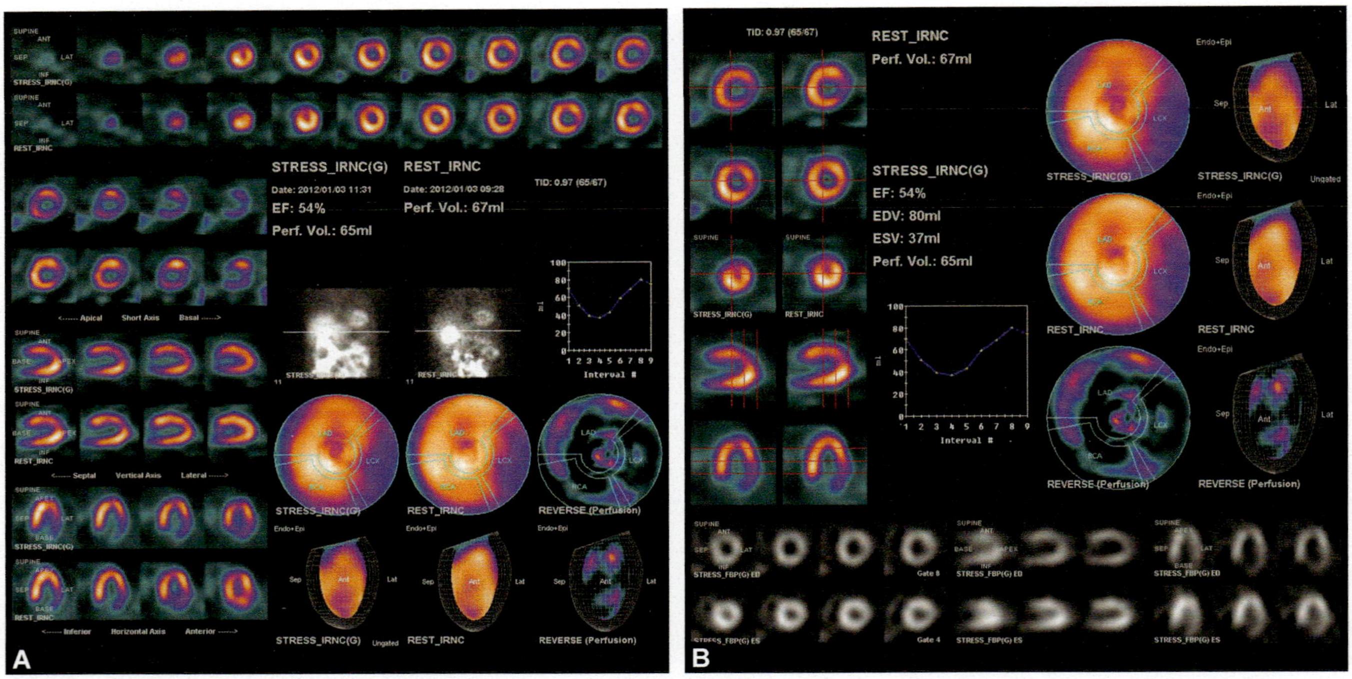

Figs. 1A and B: An 84-year-old female with a history of prior myocardial infarction, exertional dyspnea and atypical angina.
Imaging protocol: Rest technetium-99m tetrofosmin/stress technetium-99m sestamibi.
Stress modality: Regadenoson. The resting electrocardiogram demonstrated Q waves in leads II and III. There was 1 mm of horizontal ST segment depression in the lateral precordial leads during exercise.

CASE 9: ANTERIOR ISCHEMIA WITH MARKED POST-STRESS STUNNING

Stress perfusion images (A) demonstrate a moderately extensive, moderately-to-markedly severe decrease in tracer concentration in the distal half of the anterior wall, and apex of the left ventricle. In resting images, there is a small residual apical defect, but the anterior defect is completely reversible. Post-stress functional images (B) demonstrate moderate anterior hypokinesis despite reversibility of the stress perfusion defect. The left ventricle is mildly dilated (end-diastolic volume = 127 cc, end-systolic volume = 63 cc), and left ventricular ejection fraction is low-normal (51%). Of note, since post-stress perfusion imaging is performed approximately 30–45 minutes following the termination of exercise or pharmacologic stress, stress-induced functional abnormalities generally will have resolved by the time of SPECT image acquisition. However, in this case anterior hypokinesis persists, consistent with "post-stress stunning". Post-stress stunning is generally associated with severe stress-induced ischemia (Figs. 1A and B).

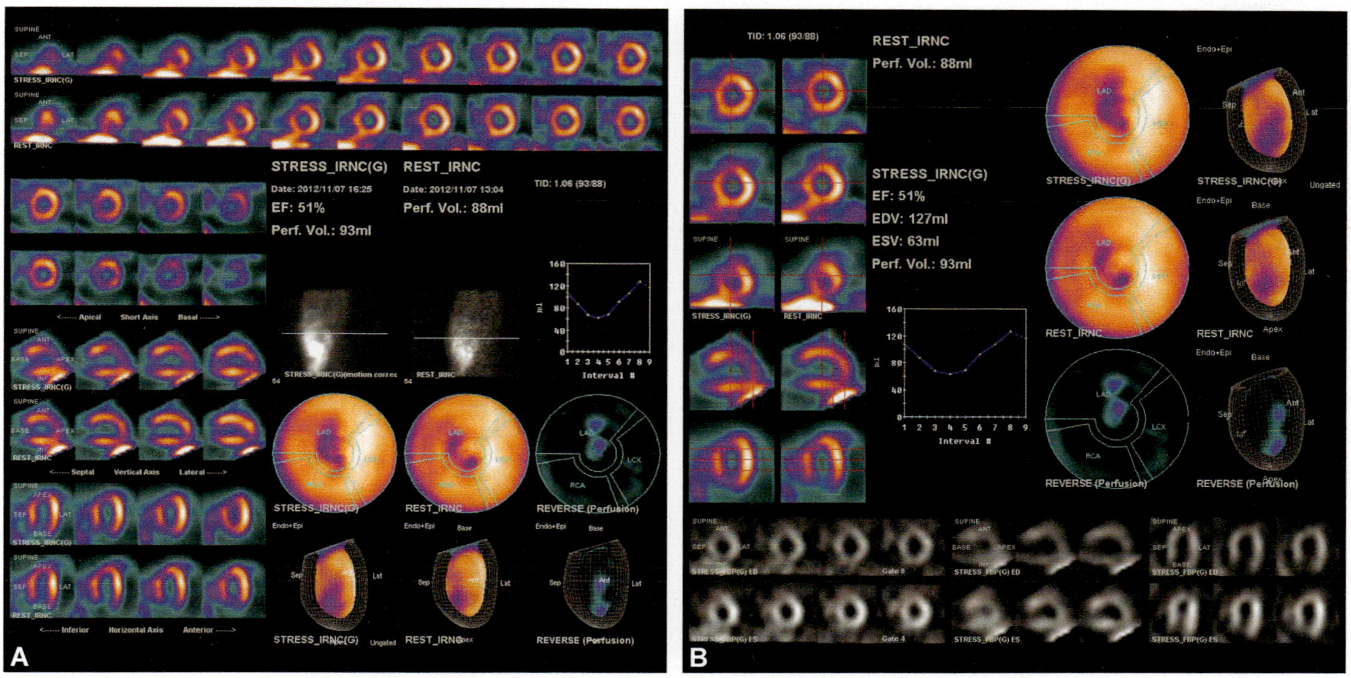

Figs. 1A and B: A 58-year-old male with multiple coronary artery disease risk factors including diabetes and atypical angina.
Imaging protocol: Rest technetium-99m tetrofosmin/stress technetium-99m sestamibi.
Stress modality: Treadmill exercise. During exercise the patient became hypotensive but developed no chest pain, and there were no ST segment changes.

CASE 10: LEFT VENTRICULAR ANEURYSM WITH SLIGHT PERI-INFARCT ISCHEMIA

Perfusion images (A) demonstrate a severe and extensive defect involving the anterior wall and apex of the left ventricle. The perfusion defect is slightly less extensive in resting images, consistent with mild peri-infarct ischemia. The peri-infarct ischemia is best appreciated in the polar maps. Functional images (B) demonstrate akinesis and absent thickening of the extensive anterior/apical perfusion abnormality. The left ventricle is markedly dilated (end-diastolic volume = 219 cc, end-systolic volume = 157 cc), and left ventricular ejection fraction is markedly decreased (28%). Inspection of the configuration of the left ventricular cavity demonstrates diastolic bulging. This finding is best appreciated in the three-dimensional surface-rendered images. There is relatively preserved contraction of the basal segments of the left ventricle. These findings are consistent with a left ventricular aneurysm (Figs. 1A and B).

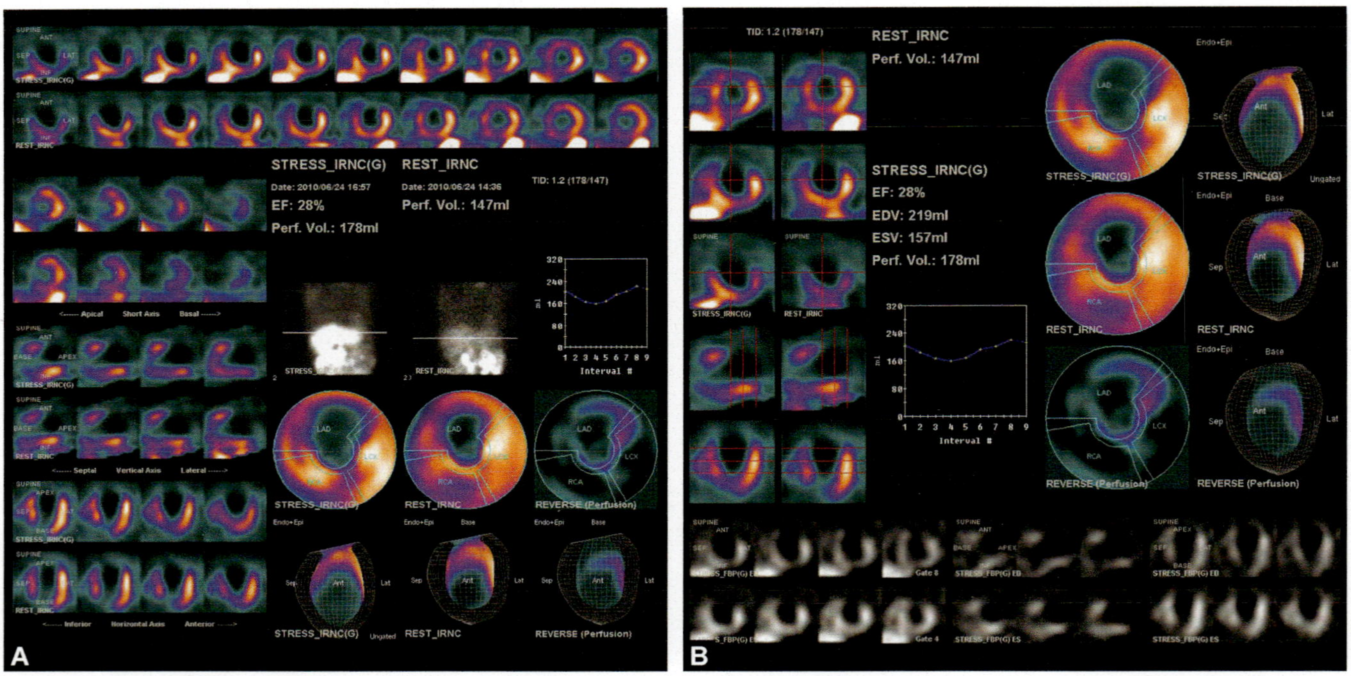

Figs. 1A and B: A 70-year-old male with prior myocardial infarction and exertional dyspnea.
Imaging protocol: Rest/stress technetium-99m sestamibi.
Stress modality: Regadenoson. The resting electrocardiogram demonstrated mild ST segment elevation in the anterior precordial leads the patient developed no chest pain. There was slight further ST segment elevation during pharmacologic stress.

CASE 11: PULMONARY HYPERTENSION WITH RIGHT VENTRICULAR (RV) HYPERTROPHY AND HYPOKINESIS (REST ONLY)

Resting perfusion images demonstrate an enlarged RV cavity and relatively increased radiotracer concentration in the RV myocardium, consistent with RV hypertrophy. Left ventricular myocardial perfusion and volume are normal. The right ventricle is best visualized in functional end-diastolic/end-systolic gated tomograms, displayed in black and white. These findings may be associated with pulmonary hypertension, valvular heart disease, or congenital heart disease. This patient had pulmonary hypertension due to chronic obstructive lung disease (Fig. 1).

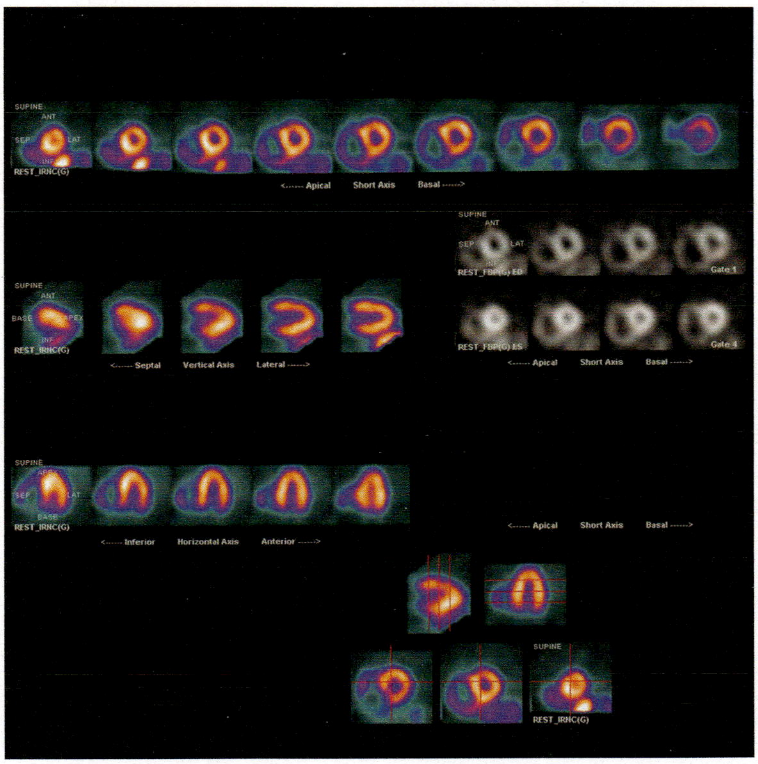

Fig. 1: A 61-year-old male with a history of chronic obstructive pulmonary disease, exertional dyspnea and atypical angina.
Imaging protocol: Rest/stress technetium-99m sestamibi.
Stress modality: Regadenoson. The patient developed dyspnea during pharmacologic stress, which was promptly relieved following the intravenous administration of 50 mg of aminophylline. There were no ST segment changes during pharmacologic stress.

CASE 12: PERMANENT PACEMAKER WITH APICAL FIXED DEFECT AND DYSKINESIS

Perfusion images (A) demonstrate a small area of mildly decreased tracer concentration in the apex of the left ventricle in stress images, which is slightly more marked in resting perfusion images. Otherwise, tracer distribution throughout the left ventricular myocardium is normal. However, functional images (B) demonstrate apical akinesis/mild dyskinesis. Left ventricular volume is normal, but left ventricular ejection fraction is moderately decreased. In this case, the severity of the apical functional abnormality (akinesis/mild dyskinesis) is much greater than that expected from the mild, localized perfusion defect. This patient had a ventricular pacemaker with a lead positioned in the left ventricular apex. Retrograde conduction from the pacemaker lead results in dyssynergic apical wall motion. It is likely that this also prevents maximal filling of the coronary arteries supplying the apex during ventricular diastole, with a resulting perfusion abnormality (Figs. 1A and B).

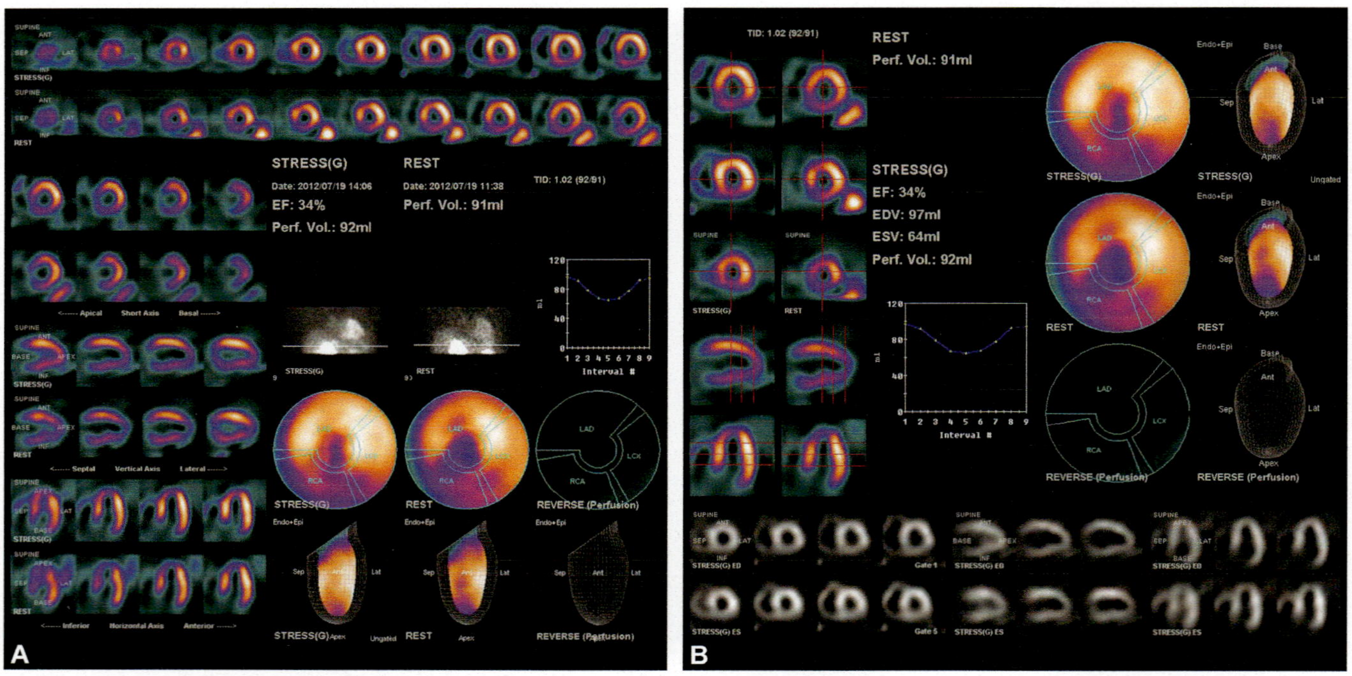

Figs. 1A and B: A 71-year-old female with coronary artery disease risk factors and atypical angina.
Imaging protocol: Rest/stress technetium-99m sestamibi.
Stress modality: Regadenoson. The resting electrocardiogram demonstrated a ventricular paced rhythm. The stress electrocardiogram was uninterpretable due to the paced rhythm. The patient experienced no chest pain during pharmacologic stress.

CASE 13: APICAL HYPERTROPHY

Perfusion images (A) demonstrate a relative increase in tracer concentration in the apex, which appears to be somewhat thickened, in both the stress and rest tomographic images. This is due to apical hypertrophy which may occur in hypertensive patients but may also be an isolated pathophysiologic phenomenon. Due to normalization of images to the most intense area of the myocardium, i.e. the apex, tracer concentration appears relatively decreased in the more basal aspects of the left ventricular myocardium. This is particularly apparent in the polar plots. Of note, the reader must be cautious not to misinterpret perfusion abnormalities in the basal myocardium when images are normalized to the "hot" apex. Functional images (B) demonstrate normal left ventricular wall motion and ejection fraction (66%) (Figs. 1A and B).

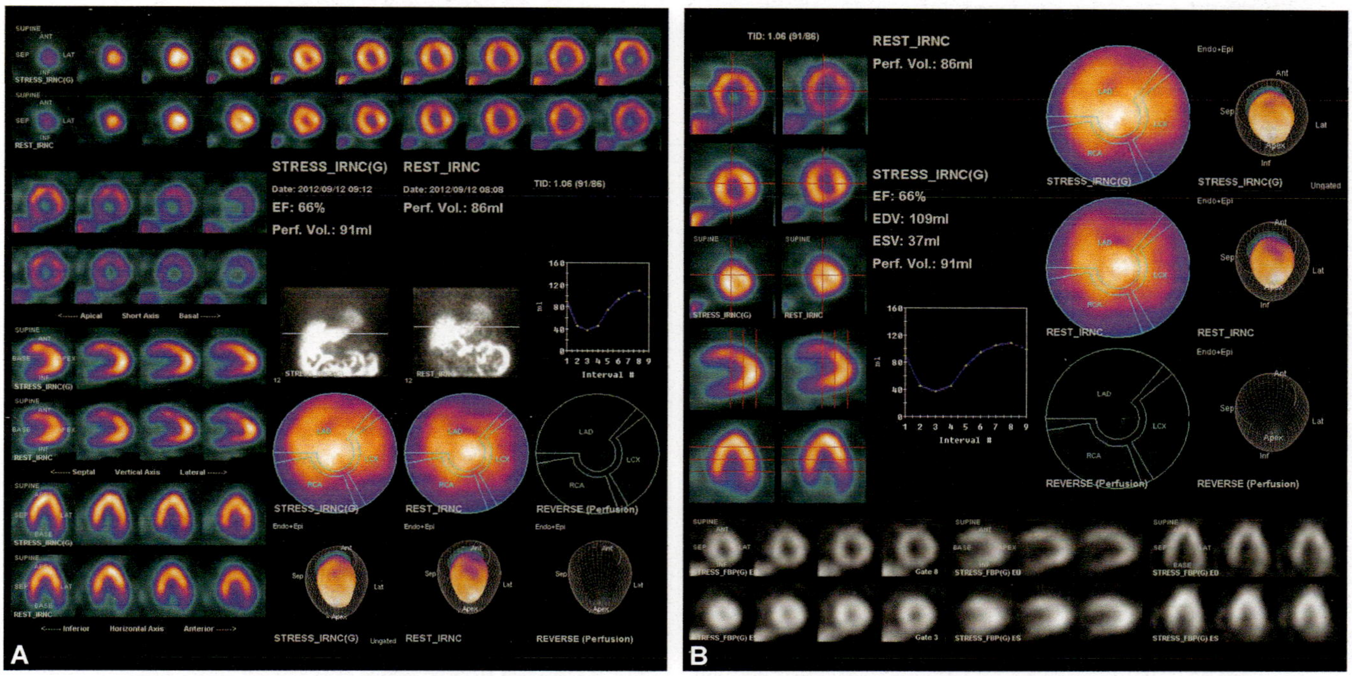

Figs. 1A and B: A 58-year-old male with coronary artery disease risk factors including hypertension and atypical angina.
Imaging protocol: Rest technetium-99m tetrofosmin/stress technetium-99m sestamibi.
Stress modality: Treadmill exercise. There were 2 mm of ST segment depression in leads II, III, aVF, the one, and V2 during exercise. The patient experienced no chest pain.

CASE 14: STATUS POST LEFT MASTECTOMY; NORMAL FEMALE

This patient had undergone a radical left mastectomy several years prior to myocardial perfusion imaging. In stress and rest perfusion tomograms (A) there is a mild/moderate relative decrease in tracer concentration in the inferior wall of the left ventricle. There is no evidence of reversibility of the inferior defect. Of note, no breast shadow is apparent in the planar projection images. Functional images (B) demonstrate normal left ventricular volume and ejection fraction (58%). With normal regional function, the mild/moderate fixed inferior defect is consistent with attenuation artifact rather than myocardial scarring.

Although this perfusion pattern would be considered normal for a man, consistent with photon attenuation by the left hemidiaphragm, in women anterior and inferior count density should be equivalent, or there may be a relative decrease in anterior count density due to attenuation by the overlying left breast. However, in this woman, status post left mastectomy, body habitus is similar to that of a man, so inferior diaphragmatic attenuation, not counterbalanced by anterior breast attenuation, can be anticipated. Therefore, when patient data are compared to gender-matched normal files using quantitative analysis, women having undergone left mastectomy should be analyzed using the normal male file (Figs. 1A and B).

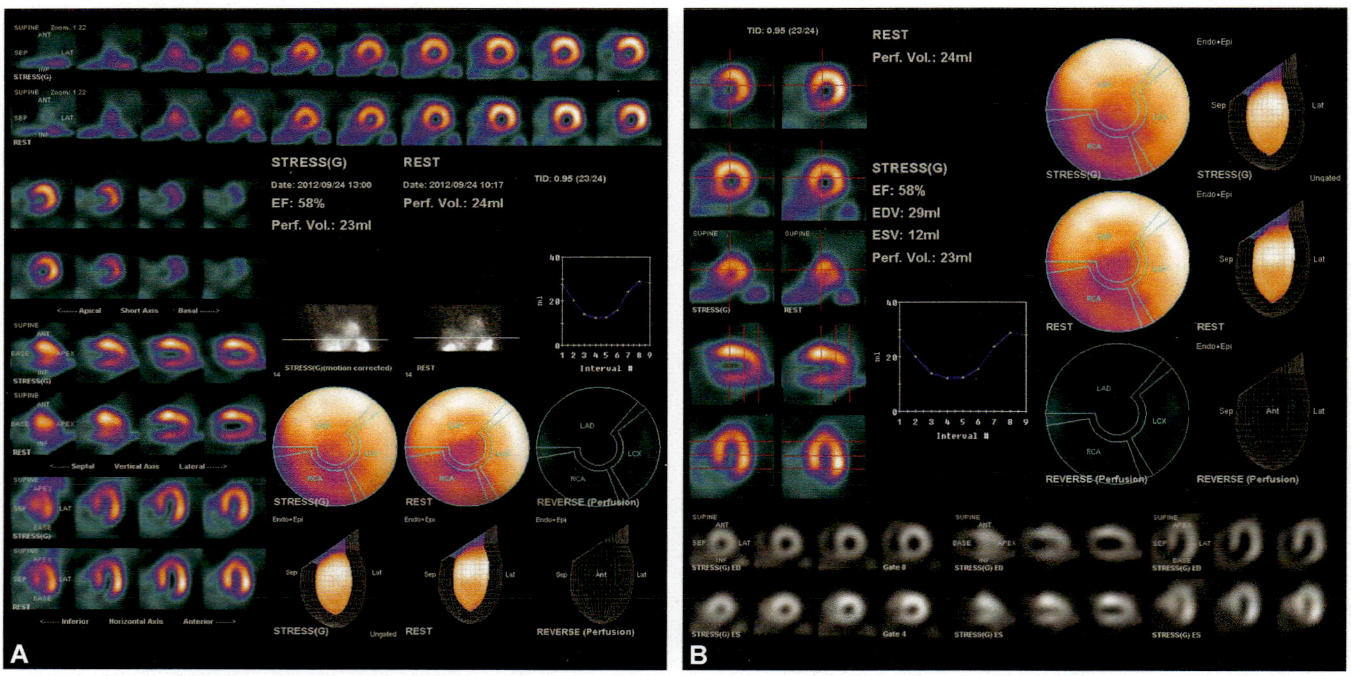

Figs. 1A and B: A 50-year-old female with coronary artery disease risk factors and atypical angina.
Imaging protocol: Rest technetium-99m tetrofosmin/stress technetium-99m sestamibi.
Stress modality: Treadmill exercise. No chest pain and no ST segment abnormalities during exercise.

CASE 15: SHIFTING BREAST ATTENUATION ARTIFACT; ENTIRE SCAN REPEATED

In planar projection images (A) a "shadow" from the patient's large, dense left breast can be observed. In the stress planar images (left) the position of the left breast is anterior and relatively high on the chest wall. In the rest planar images, the breast is positioned somewhat lower, covering a greater proportion of the left ventricle. Stress perfusion tomograms (A) demonstrate a moderate decrease in tracer concentration in the anterior wall, which is much less apparent in the resting tomograms. This finding is particularly evident in the stress and rest polar plots. It is not possible to differentiate a variable anterior attenuation artifact due to the patient's shifting left breast position versus stress-induced anterior ischemia. Functional images (B) demonstrate normal left ventricular wall motion and ejection fraction. There are not at all helpful to differentiate a variable attenuation artifact from stress-induced ischemia since in the post-stress gated images resting left ventricular function will be normal in both instances. Therefore, the perfusion scan was repeated (C) with the technologist assuring that the left breast was in the very same position during the stress and rest SPECT acquisitions. In this repeat study, there is a fixed anterior perfusion defect. Repeat functional images (D) again demonstrate normal wall motion and wall thickening, including that of the anterior wall. These findings present on the repeat study are consistent with breast attenuation artifact.

It is important to assure that breast position is constant during stress and rest SPECT acquisitions. Women should be imaged with their bra off, and the degree of elevation of the left arm over the head should be constant since changing arm position will result in changing breast position. Attenuation correction will also help to avoid breast attenuation artifacts (Figs. 1A to D).

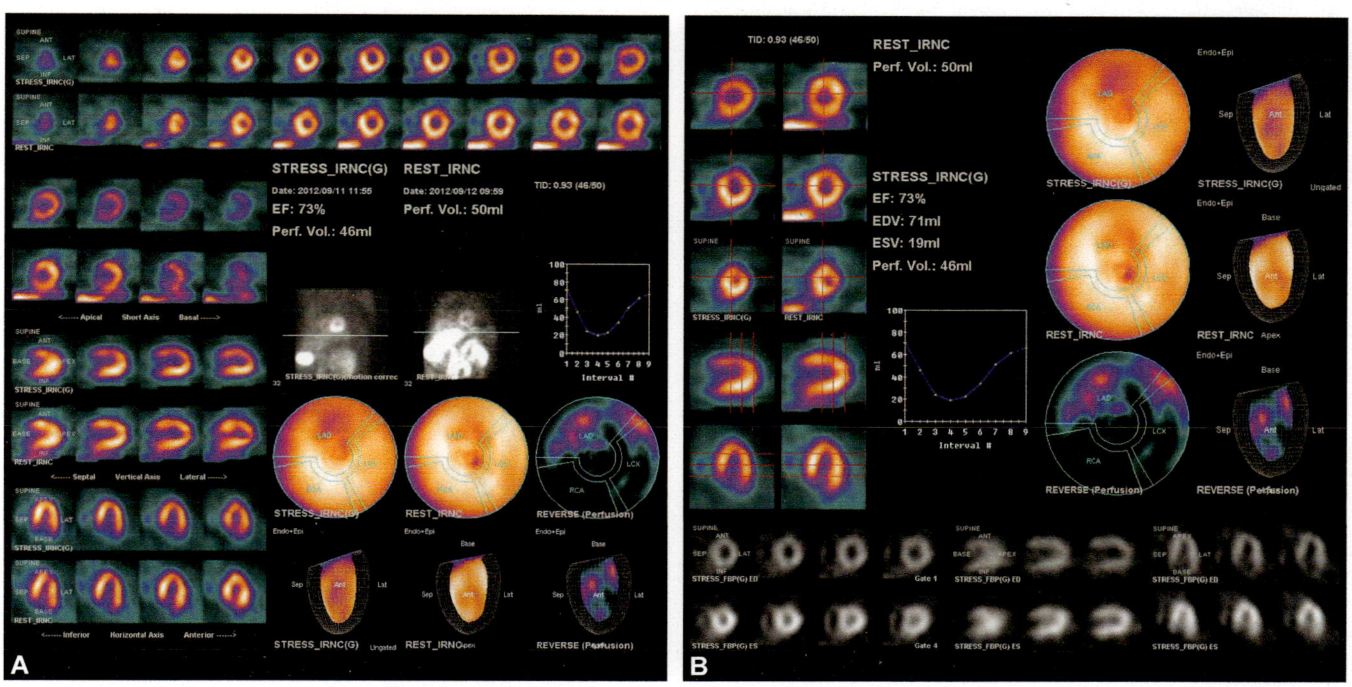

Figs. 1A and B

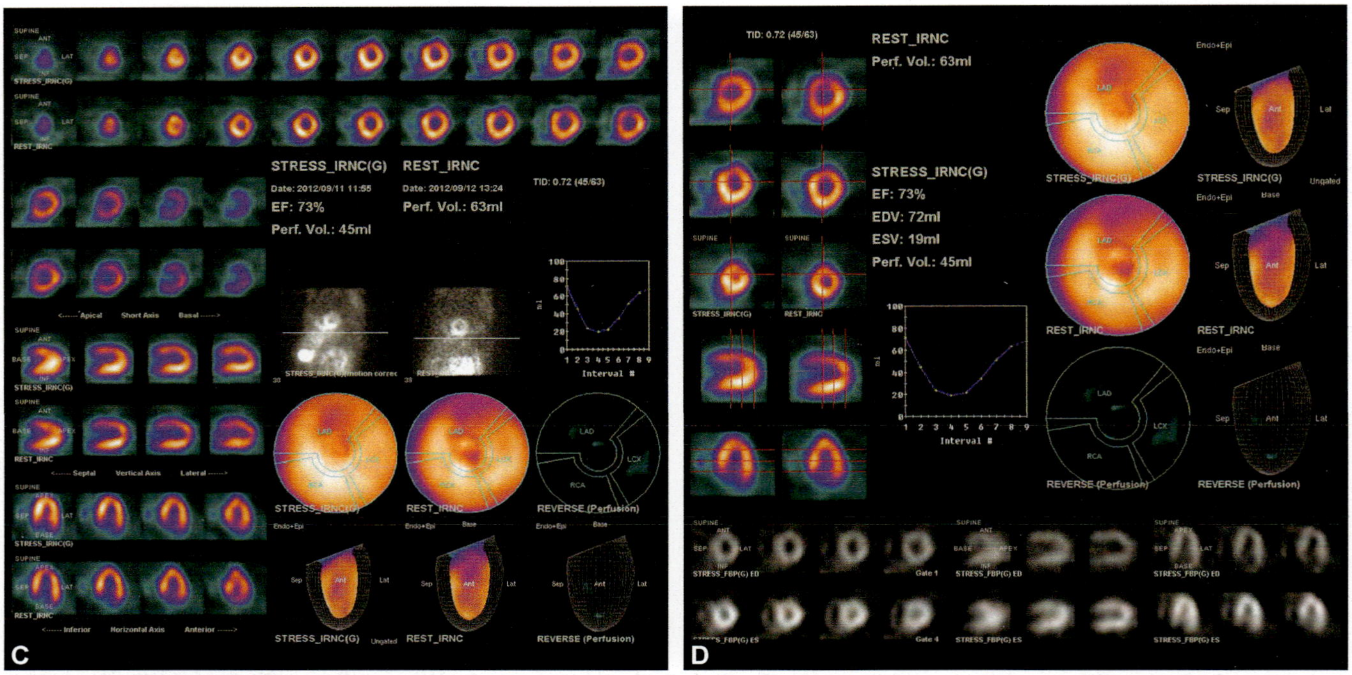

Figs. 1A to D: A 55-year-old obese female with coronary artery disease risk factors and nonanginal chest pain.
Imaging protocol: Rest/stress technetium-99m sestamibi.
Stress modality: Regadenoson. The patient experienced no chest pain during pharmacologic stress. There was 1 mm of ST segment depression in leads II and III.

CASE 16: LEFT BREAST CANCER; ANTERIOR AND LATERAL ISCHEMIA WITH MODERATE TID

Stress perfusion images (A) demonstrate an extensive, moderately severe decrease in tracer concentration throughout the anterior and lateral wall of the left ventricle, which is completely reversible in resting images. There is borderline TID (TID ratio = 1.1). Functional images (B) demonstrate normal left ventricular volume and ejection fraction (71%). These findings are consistent with multivessel coronary artery disease involving the LAD and left circumflex coronary arteries. Incidentally noted in the stress and rest planar projection images (A) is a focus of moderately increased tracer concentration in the left breast. Subsequent mammography demonstrated a left breast cancer. Of note, Tc-99m sestamibi accumulates in neoplasms due to increased mitochondrial density and activity. The interpreting physician should always be attentive to such incidental scan findings (Figs. 1A and B).

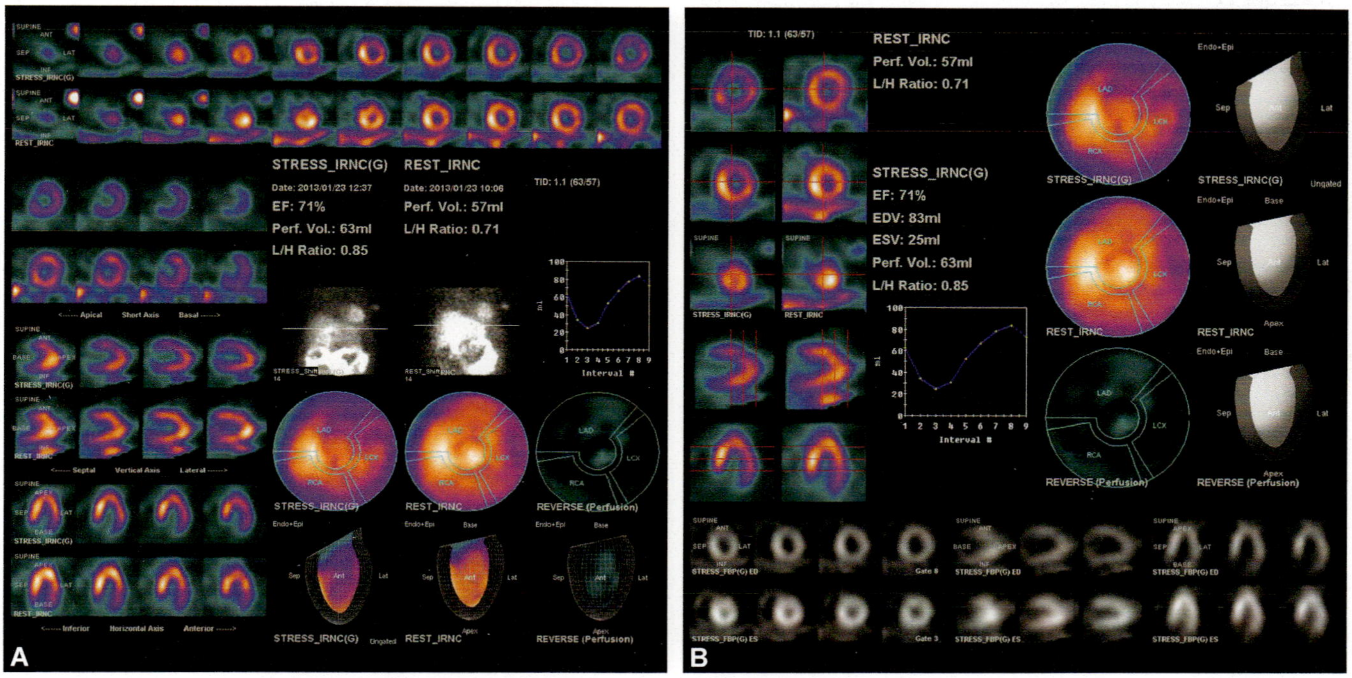

Figs. 1A and B: A 76-year-old female with coronary artery disease risk factors and atypical angina.
Imaging protocol: Rest/stress technetium-99m sestamibi.
Stress modality: Dipyridamole. The patient experienced no chest pain during pharmacologic stress. There was 1 mm of ST segment depression in leads II, III, aVF, and V1–V2.

CASE 17: ABSENT GALLBLADDER STATUS POST CHOLECYSTECTOMY; SPLENOMEGALY (CLL); MILD ISCHEMIA BASAL HALF OF THE ANTERIOR WALL (NO FUNCTIONAL IMAGES)

Stress perfusion tomograms (A) demonstrate a mild decrease in tracer concentration in the anterior wall, which is reversible in resting tomograms. This is consistent with stress-induced ischemia in the territory of the left anterior descending coronary artery. Incidentally noted in anterior stress and rest planar projection images is absent tracer concentration in the gall bladder (GB). This is consistent with the patient's history of prior cholecystectomy. However, this finding may be observed in patients with acute and/or chronic cholecystitis. In planar projections in the steep left anterior oblique projection (B) moderate/marked splenomegaly is noted. This is consistent with the patient's history of chronic lymphocytic leukemia (CLL). Of note, planar projection images should always be inspected carefully for incidental sub diaphragmatic findings such as those described above (Figs. 1A and B).

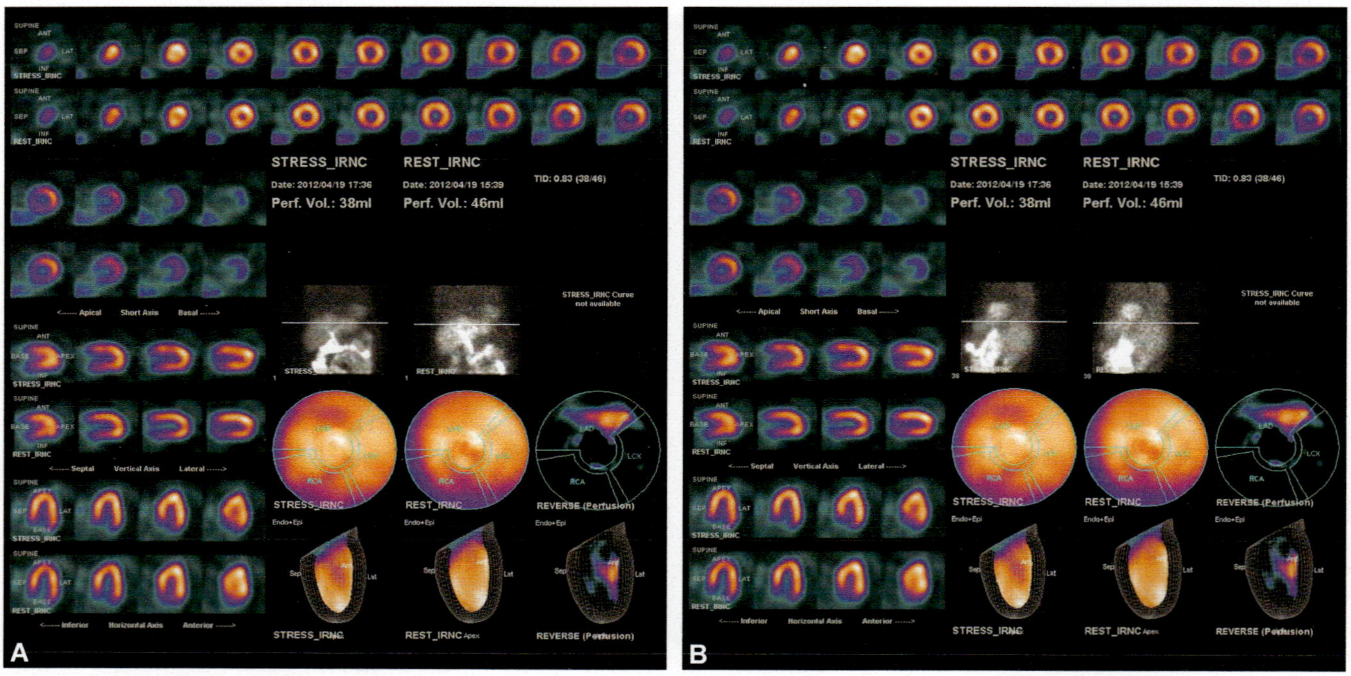

Figs. 1A and B: A 69-year-old female with chronic lymphocytic leukemia, coronary artery disease risk factors, and typical angina.
Imaging protocol: Rest/stress technetium-99m sestamibi.
Stress modality: Regadenoson. The patient experienced no chest pain during pharmacologic stress, and there were no ST segment abnormalities.

CASE 18: UPPER MEDIASTINAL NEOPLASM; NORMAL MYOCARDIAL PERFUSION

Stress and rest perfusion tomograms (A) are normal. Incidentally noted in planar projection images is a large area of intense, irregular focal tracer accumulation in the upper mediastinum. This is noted best in the resting planar projection images where the patient is positioned slightly lower in the camera field-of-view. Functional images (B) demonstrate normal left ventricular volumes and ejection fraction (71%).

Technetium-99m accumulates in the neoplastic tissue due to increased mitochondrial density and activity. The myocardial perfusion scan in this patient with multiple coronary artery disease risk factors was performed as part of preoperative screening prior to resection of the known upper mediastinal neoplasm (Figs. 1A and B).

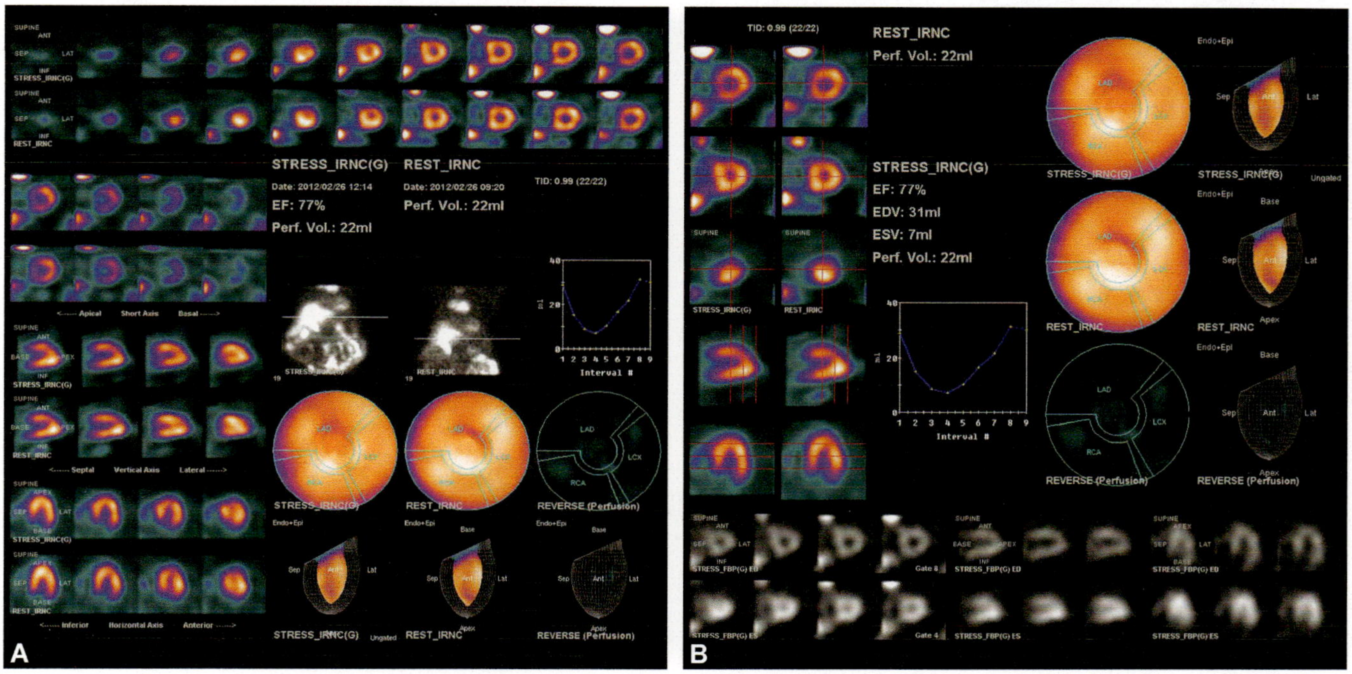

Figs. 1A and B: A 52-year-old female with coronary artery disease risk factors. Preoperative evaluation for resection of an upper mediastinal mass.

Imaging protocol: Rest technetium-99m tetrofosmin/stress technetium-99m sestamibi.

Stress modality: Regadenoson. No chest pain or ST segment abnormalities during pharmacologic stress.

CASE 19: GRANULOMATOUS LUNG DISEASE (REST ONLY); NORMAL MYOCARDIAL PERFUSION

A resting myocardial perfusion scan (A) demonstrates normal myocardial perfusion. In planar projection images, there is moderately/markedly increased radiotracer concentration in the right lower lung field, and mildly and irregularly increased tracer concentration throughout the remainder of both lungs. The L/H count density ratio (B), using a lung region of interest placed over the right lower lung field, is 0.61 (normal = <0.42 for Tc-99m sestamibi). In this patient, increased radiotracer concentration in the lungs is due to granulomatous lung disease. More commonly, homogenously increased lung uptake is noted due to poor left or right ventricular function (Figs. 1A and B).

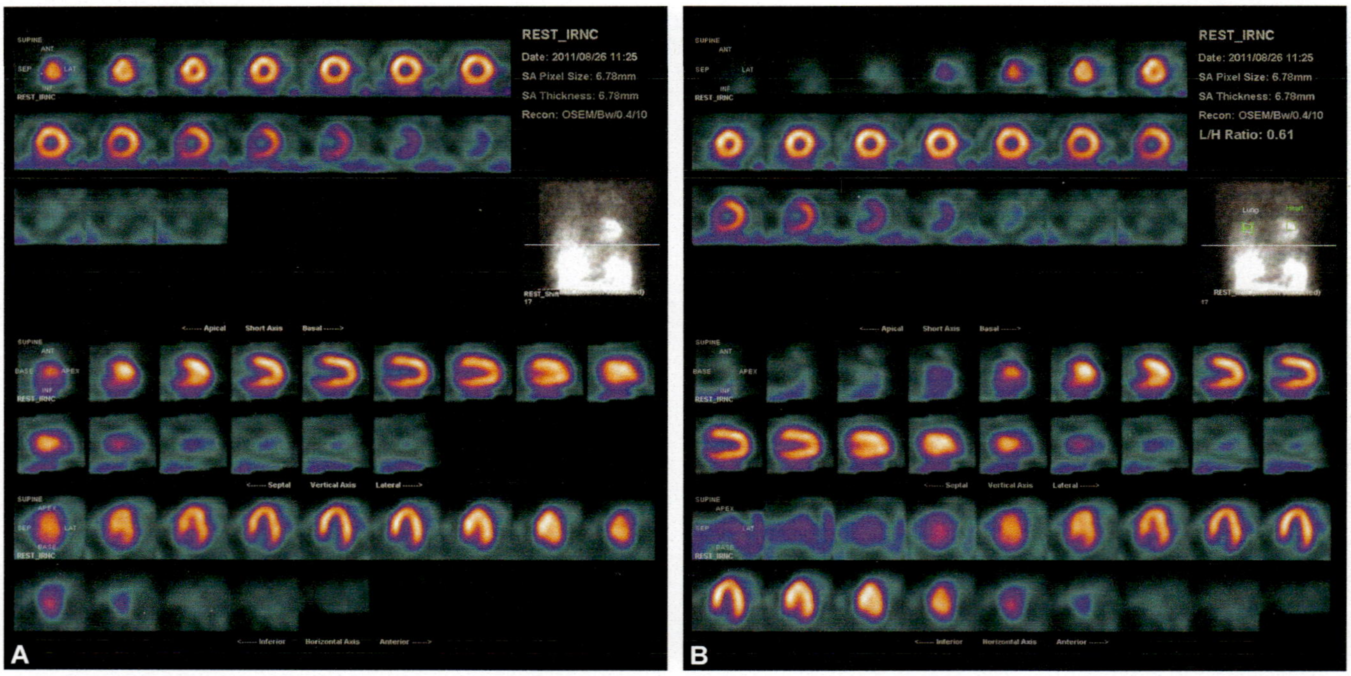

Figs. 1A and B: A 65-year-old female with coronary artery disease risk factors and exertional dyspnea.
Imaging protocol: Rest/stress technetium-99m sestamibi.
Stress modality: Regadenoson. The patient experienced no chest pain during pharmacologic stress, and there were no ST segment abnormalities.

CASE 20: HIATAL HERNIA; NORMAL MYOCARDIAL PERFUSION

Stress and rest perfusion tomograms (A) demonstrate normal myocardial perfusion. In the resting vertical long-axis tomograms, there is focal accumulation posterior to the base of the inferior wall of the left ventricle. In planar projection images, this activity is noted to be due to radiotracer concentration in the fundus of the stomach extending caudally posterior to the heart. These findings are therefore due to a hiatal hernia containing radiotracer excreted by the hepatobiliary system into the duodenum, having refluxed into the stomach. Functional images (B) demonstrate normal left ventricular volume and ejection fraction (60%) (Figs. 1A and B).

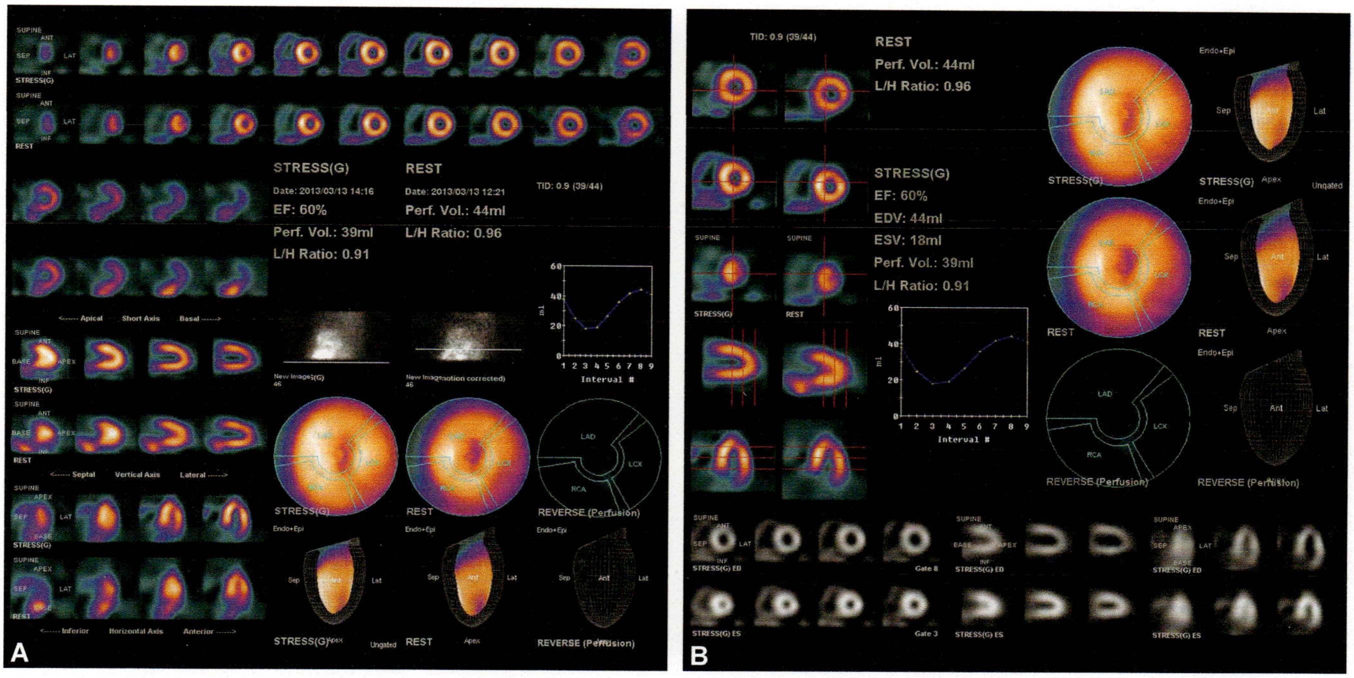

Figs. 1A and B: A 66-year-old female with coronary artery disease risk factors and nonanginal chest pain.

Imaging protocol: Rest/stress technetium-99m sestamibi.

Stress modality: Regadenoson. The patient experienced no chest pain during pharmacologic stress, and there were no ST segment abnormalities.

Advanced Cases

CASE 1: INFEROLATERAL BREAST ATTENUATION ARTIFACT; DIFFUSE NONISCHEMIC CARDIOMYOPATHY

Stress and rest perfusion images (A) demonstrate a moderately extensive, moderately severe fixed perfusion defect in the inferolateral wall of the left ventricle. The defect is somewhat more marked in the resting images, a finding particularly evident in the polar plots. In the stress and rest planar projection images, there is a dense "shadow" overlying the inferolateral wall of the left ventricle caused by attenuation by the patient's large, pendulous breasts, lying posterolaterally on the chest wall with the patient in the supine position. Functional images (B) demonstrate that the left ventricle is moderately dilated (end-diastolic volume = 168 cc, end-systolic volume = 99 cc) with a moderately decreased left ventricular ejection fraction (41%). However, there is no regional inferolateral wall motion abnormality. These combined findings are consistent with a nonischemic cardiomyopathy. The fixed inferolateral defect is attributable to photon attenuation by the patient's pendulous left breast as evidenced by its worsening in the resting images and relatively preserved wall motion and wall thickening. Although inferolateral myocardial scarring cannot be totally excluded, it is much less likely (Figs. 1A and B).

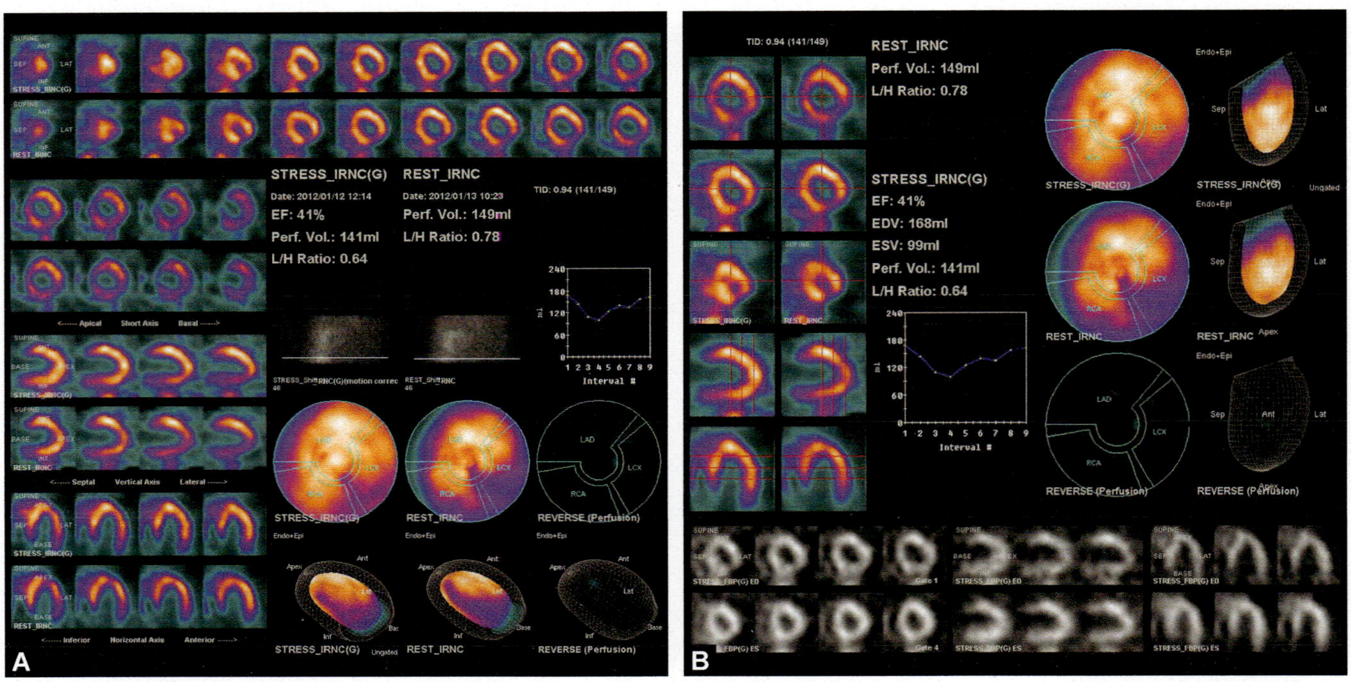

Figs. 1A and B: A 64-year-old female with coronary artery disease risk factors including long-standing hypertension and exertional dyspnea.
Imaging protocol: Rest/stress technetium-99m sestamibi.
Stress modality: Regadenoson. The patient experienced no chest pain or ST segment changes during pharmacologic stress.

CASE 2: D-SHAPED LEFT VENTRICLE; DILATED, HYPOKINETIC RIGHT VENTRICLE; PULMONARY HYPERTENSION DOCUMENTED BY ECHOCARDIOGRAPHY

Perfusion images (A) demonstrate normal stress and rest perfusion of the left ventricular myocardium. However, the right ventricle is dilated and there is moderate "flattening" of the septum (best noted in horizontal long-axis tomograms), giving the left ventricle a "D-shaped" configuration. These findings are better appreciated with the tomograms displayed in black and white (B). Functional images (C) demonstrate normal left ventricular volume and ejection fraction (60%). The right ventricle is dilated and moderately hypokinetic.

Increased right ventricular volume and/or pressure overload inhibits diastolic relaxation of the septum, resulting in "flattening" of the septum and a "D-shaped" configuration of the left ventricle. In this patient, these findings were confirmed by echocardiography (Figs. 1A to C).

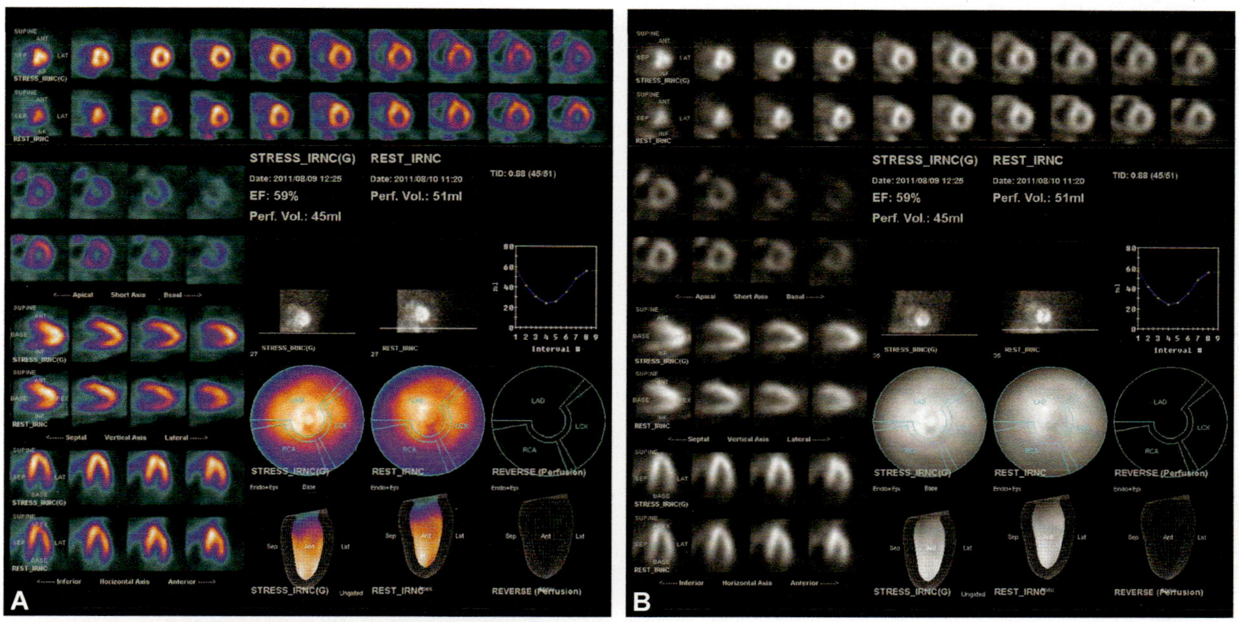

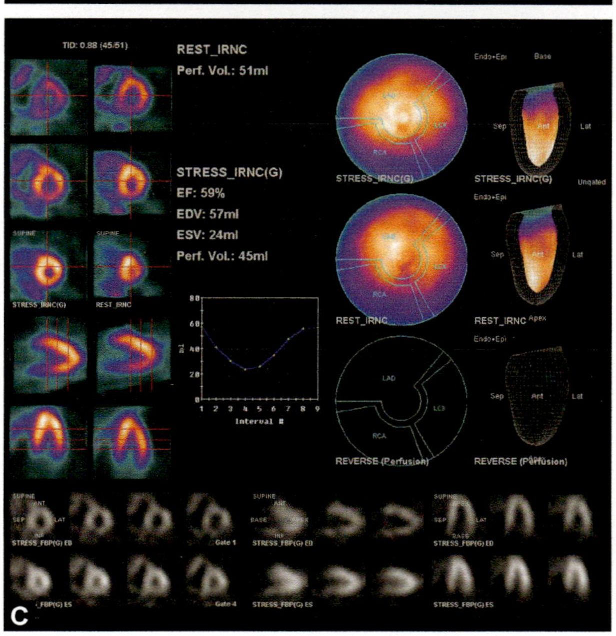

Figs. 1A to C: A 66-year-old female with pulmonary hypertension and atypical chest pain.
Imaging protocol: Rest/stress technetium-99m sestamibi.
Stress modality: Regadenoson. The patient experienced no chest pain or ST segment changes during pharmacologic stress.

CASE 3: MILD REVERSIBLE APICAL DEFECT WITH MODERATE TID (1.25); CATHETERIZATION DEMONSTRATED MULTIVESSEL DISEASE CONSISTENT WITH "BALANCED ISCHEMIA"

Perfusion images (A) demonstrate only a small, moderately severe reversible apical perfusion defect. Tracer distribution is otherwise normal throughout the left ventricular myocardium. However, there is mild/moderate TID (TID ratio = 1.21). Functional images (B) demonstrate normal left ventricular volume and a borderline-low left ventricular ejection fraction (51%).

Subsequent coronary angiography in this patient demonstrated significant multivessel coronary disease. The extent of coronary artery disease was significantly underestimated in the perfusion scan, which demonstrated only a small area of stress-induced apical ischemia. However, TID suggested more extensive stress-induced ischemia. Even occasionally in patients with entirely normal myocardial perfusion scans TID is present and may be indicative of underlying multivessel disease (Figs. 1A and B).

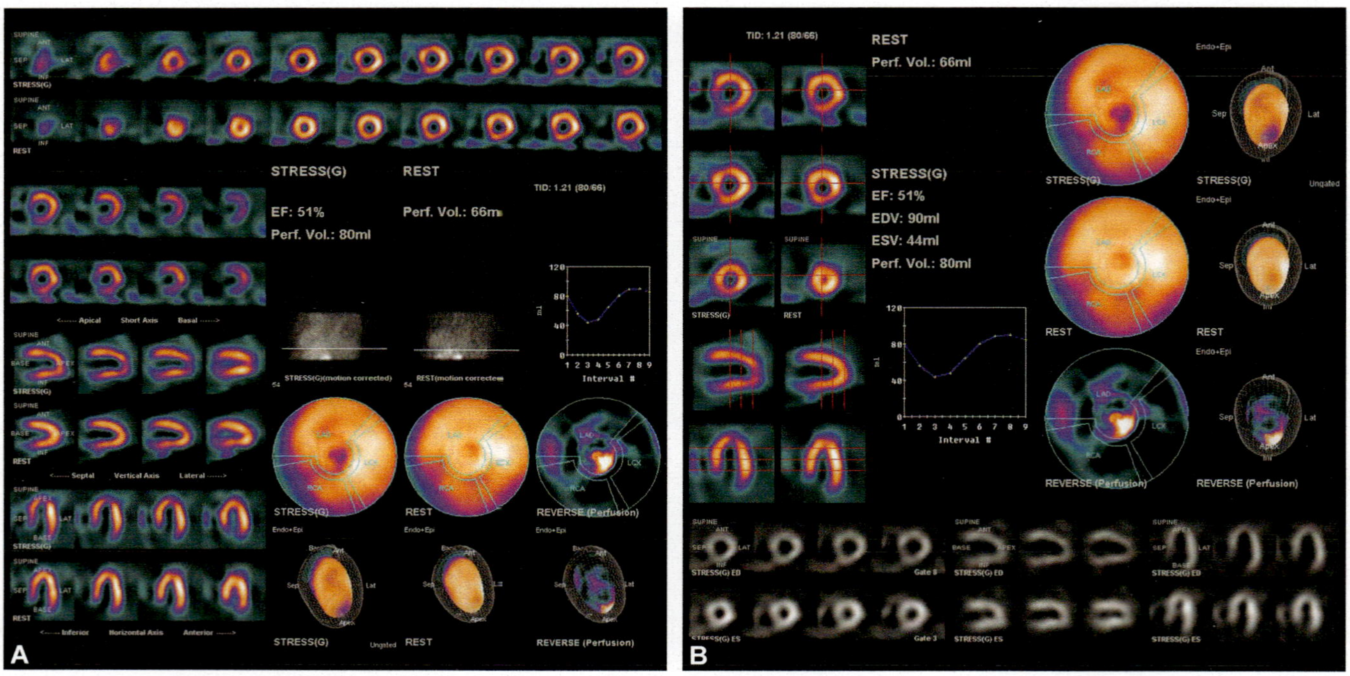

Figs. 1A and B: A 73-year-old male with coronary artery disease risk factors and atypical angina.
Imaging protocol: Rest/stress technetium-99m sestamibi.
Stress modality: Treadmill exercise. The patient developed dyspnea during exercise. There was 1 mm horizontal ST segment compression in leads II, III, aVF, and V1–V2.

CASE 4: MULTIPLE AXILLARY NODES FROM BREAST CANCER; NORMAL PERFUSION SCAN

Perfusion images (A) are normal. Anterior planar projection images (A) demonstrate several small focal areas of radiotracer concentration in the left axilla. These are appreciated better in LAO (B) and left lateral (C) planar projection images. These abnormalities correspond to known axillary lymph node metastases in this patient with breast cancer. Axillary lymph node uptake of Tc-99m sestamibi and tetrofosmin is much more commonly associated with infiltration of the injected radiopharmaceutical dose and migration to axillary lymph nodes via lymphatic channels (Figs. 1A to C).

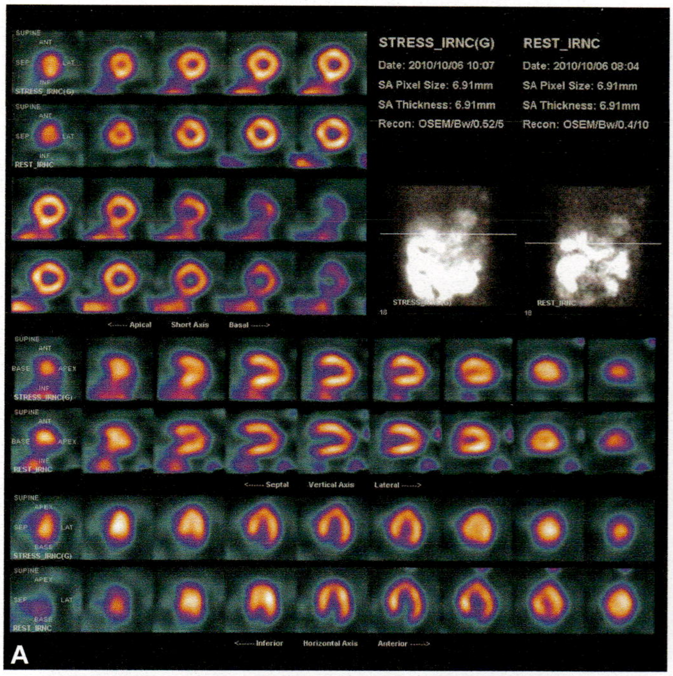

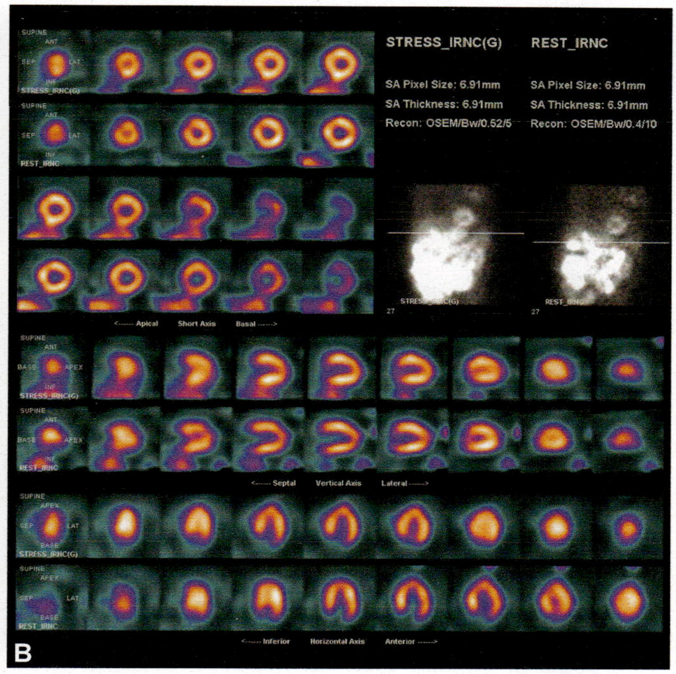

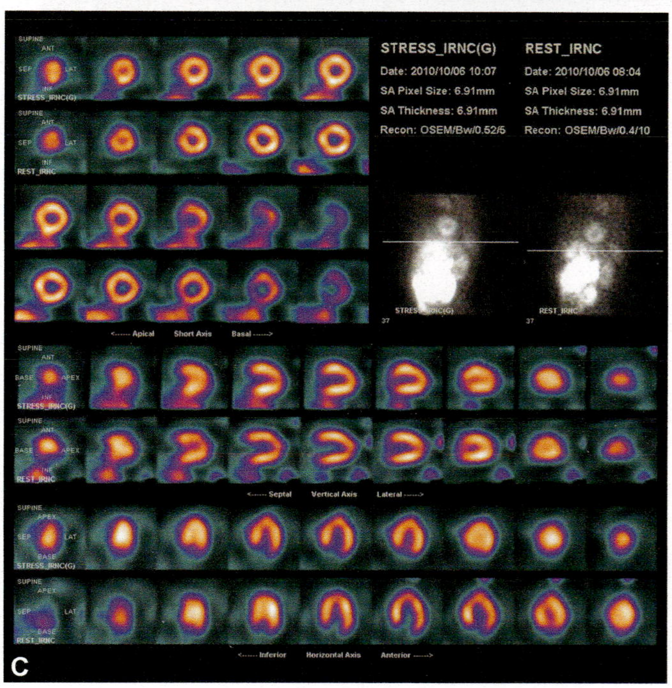

Figs. 1A to C: A 56-year-old female with coronary artery disease risk factors, breast cancer, and atypical chest pain.
Imaging protocol: Rest/stress technetium-99m sestamibi.
Stress modality: Regadenoson. The patient experienced no chest pain or ST segment changes during pharmacologic stress.

CASE 5: PERICARDIAL EFFUSION WITH SEPTAL AKINESIS; MULTIVESSEL ISCHEMIA

In the stress perfusion images (A) there is a moderately extensive, severe decrease in tracer concentration in the anteroseptal wall of the left ventricle and a severe, extensive abnormality in the inferolateral wall. In resting images, there is moderate-to-nearly complete reversibility of the anteroseptal defect and moderate, partial reversibility of the inferolateral defect. These findings are consistent with ischemia with mild underlying scarring in the anteroseptal wall in the LAD territory and scarring with moderate stress-induced peri-infarct ischemia in the inferolateral wall in the right coronary artery (RCA) distribution. Close inspection of the planar projection images displayed in black and white (B) demonstrates a faint "halo" of markedly diminished tracer concentration surrounding the heart. This was demonstrated by echocardiography to represent a pericardial effusion. Functional images (C) demonstrate localized distal anterior moderate hypokinesis and inferolateral marked hypokinesis, consistent with scarring in these regions. Left ventricular volume is normal, and left ventricular ejection fraction is low-normal (51%) (Figs. 1A to C).

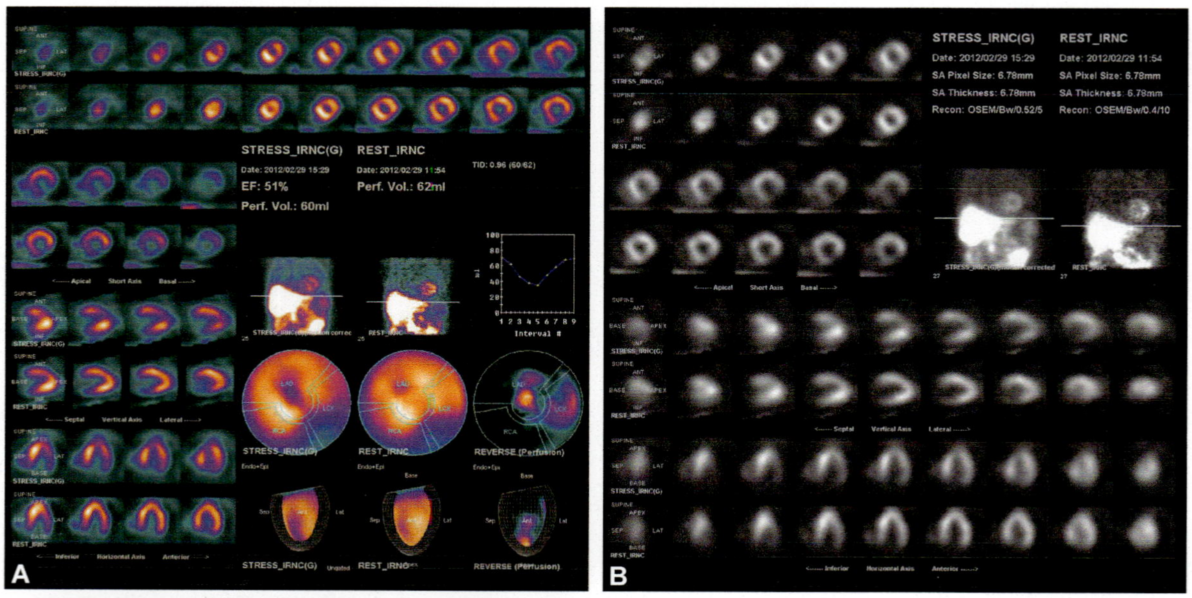

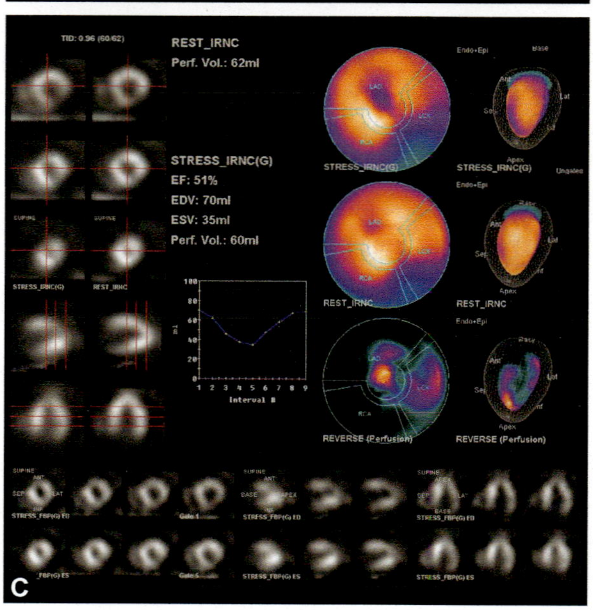

Figs. 1A to C: A 63-year-old male with prior myocardial infarction now presents with atypical chest pain and exertional dyspnea.
The resting electrocardiogram demonstrated Q waves in leads II and III. No additional ST segment abnormalities occurred during pharmacologic stress.

CASE 6: REVERSE TID DUE TO HIGH POST-STRESS HEART RATE

Stress and rest tomographic images (A) demonstrate normal perfusion. Of note, the left ventricular cavity is considerably smaller in the stress images than in the rest images. The TID ratio = 0.32 (normal = <1.12, and usually 0.95–1.05). Functional images (B) demonstrate a hypercontractile left ventricle with an ejection fraction of 91%. In this patient, "reverse TID" and hyperdynamic function resulted from persistent tachycardia following treadmill exercise stress, which persisted until and during the post-stress SPECT acquisition (Figs. 1A and B).

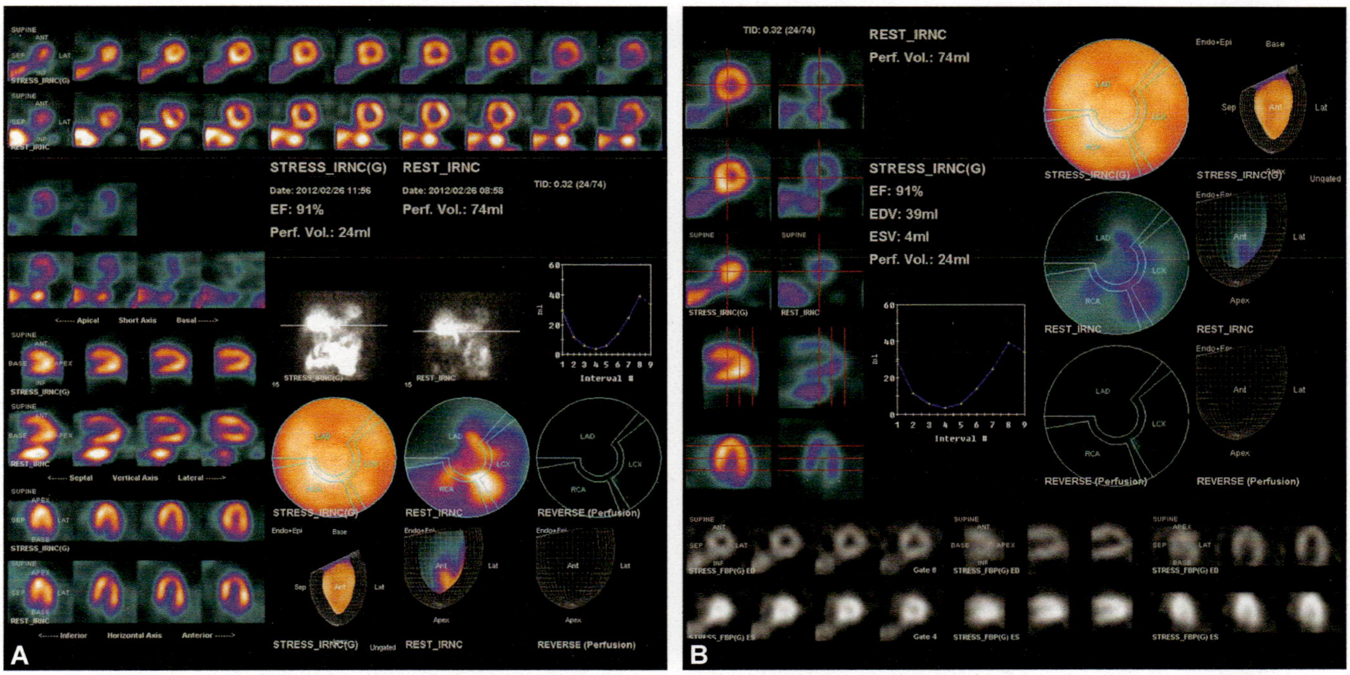

Figs. 1A and B: A 55-year-old male with coronary artery disease risk factors and nonanginal chest pain.
Imaging protocol: Rest/stress technetium-99m sestamibi.
Stress modality: Treadmill exercise. The patient developed no chest pain and no ST segment abnormalities during exercise.

CASE 7: NON-INJECTED STRESS DOSE

With a single-day 10 mCi rest/32 mCi stress Tc-99m sestamibi protocol, which was used in this patient, the count density of stress images should be at least three times greater than that of the resting images. However, in this case, the count density of the stress planar projection image is no greater than and in fact slightly less than that of the resting planar projection image. Also, the quality of the stress perfusion tomograms is poor then that of the resting tomograms. This resulted from total infiltration of the stress radiopharmaceutical dose. Therefore, the "stress" images were really only partially decayed resting images, and the study was nondiagnostic. The interpreting physician should always visually assess the count density of the stress and rest planar projection images to assure that stress count density is significantly higher than that at rest. Some myocardial perfusion SPECT processing software programs display maximal myocardial count densities for the stress and rest tomograms (Fig. 1)

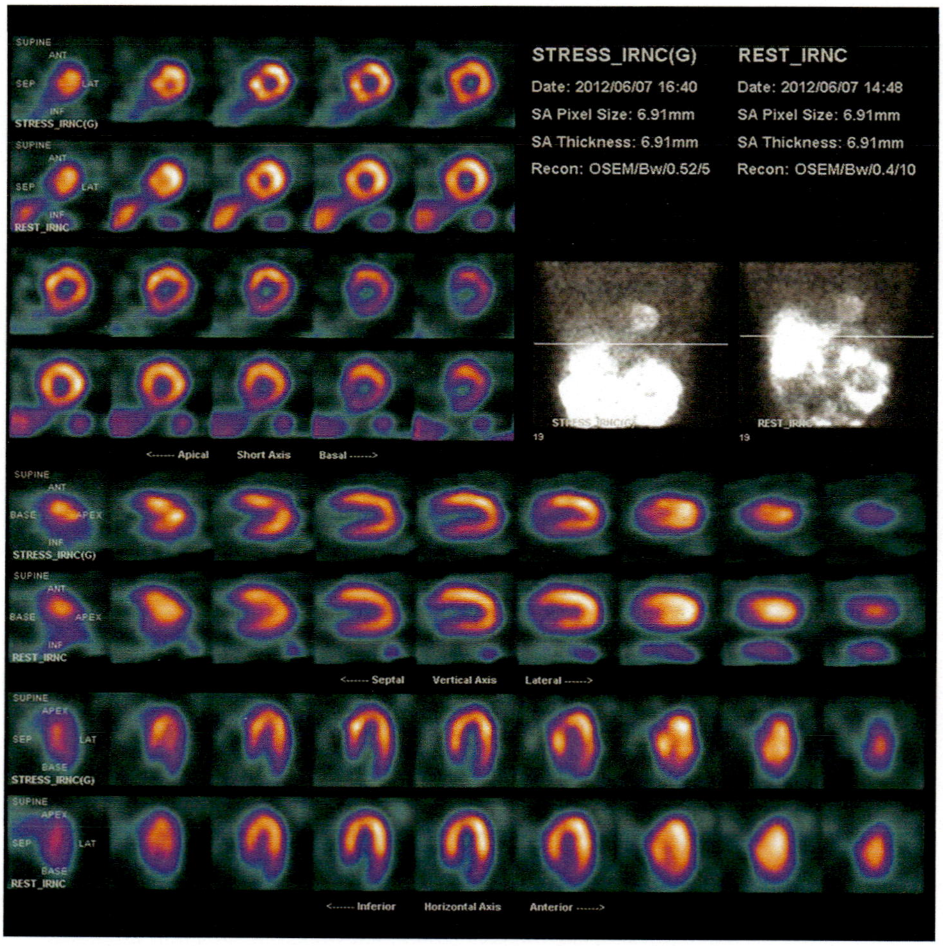

Fig. 1: A 61-year-old male with coronary artery disease risk factors and atypical angina. Imaging protocol: Rest technetium-99m tetrofosmin/ stress technetium-99m sestamibi.
Stress modality: Dipyridamole.
Imaging protocol: Rest/stress technetium-99m sestamibi.
Stress modality: Treadmill exercise. The patient developed no chest pain and no ST segment abnormalities during exercise.

CASE 8: NORMAL SCAN, GOITER

Perfusion tomograms demonstrate a small, moderately severe reversible anteroapical defect, consistent with localized stress-induced ischemia in the distal LAD territory. Incidentally noted in the stress and rest planar projection images is a large focus of increased tracer concentration in the neck. Of note, the neck is usually not included in the SPECT imaging field-of-view but was in this particular patient, who was unusually short. Tc-99m is physiologically taken up by the thyroid gland. This patient had a diffuse toxic goiter and a markedly elevated radioiodine uptake, accounting for the marked increase in sestamibi concentration in the thyroid gland. Therefore, Tc-99m sestamibi and tetrofosmin localization in the neck and upper mediastinum may be due to physiologic uptake in the thyroid or uptake in benign or malignant neoplasms (Fig. 1).

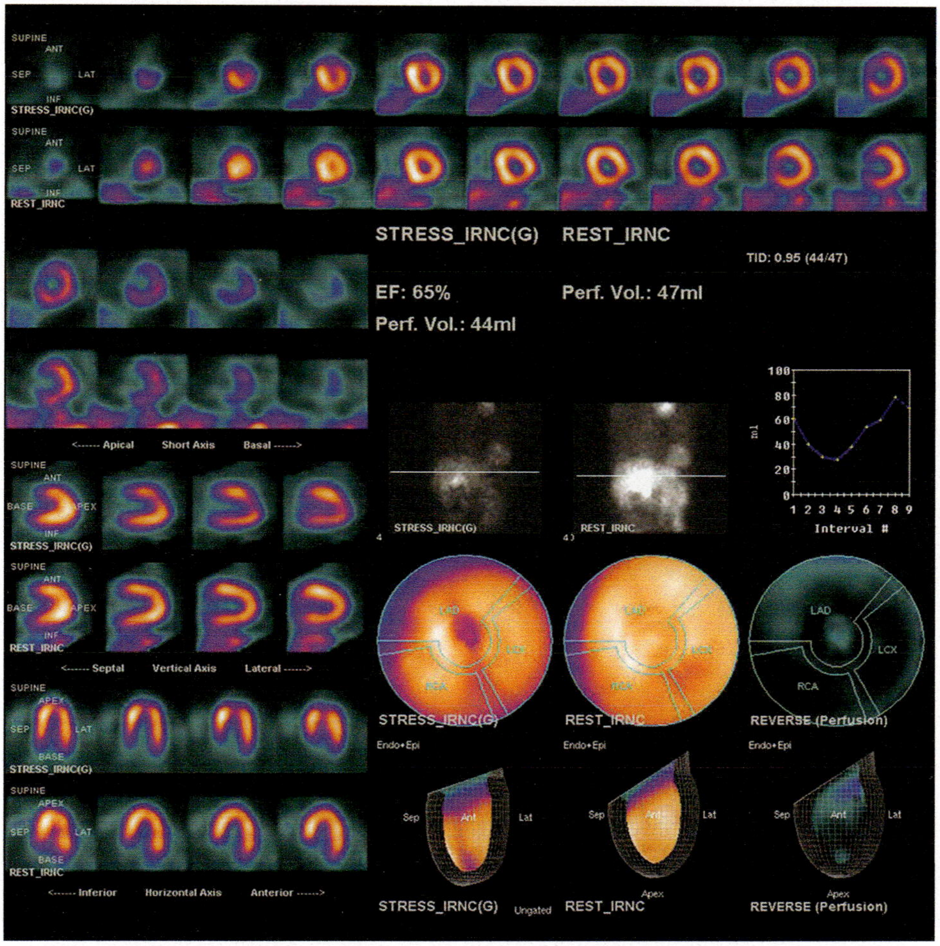

Fig. 1: A 51-year-old male with coronary artery disease risk factors, hyperthyroidism, and arrhythmia.
Imaging protocol: Rest/stress technetium-99m sestamibi.
Stress modality: Treadmill exercise. The patient developed no chest pain and no ST segment abnormalities during exercise.

CASE 9: THREE-VESSEL ISCHEMIA

Stress perfusion images (A) demonstrate an extensive, severe decrease in tracer concentration throughout the lateral wall; an extensive, moderately severe decrease in tracer concentration in the anterior wall; and an extensive, moderately severe decrease in the inferior wall. These abnormalities are completely reversible in resting images, consistent with stress-induced ischemia in a multivessel distribution involving the left anterior descending, circumflex, and right coronary arteries. Of note, despite multivessel stress-induced ischemia there is no significant TID (TID ratio = 1.05). Functional images (B) demonstrate borderline left ventricular dilatation (end-diastolic volume = 114 cc, end-systolic volume = 49 cc) and a normal post-stress left ventricular ejection fraction (57%) (Figs. 1A and B).

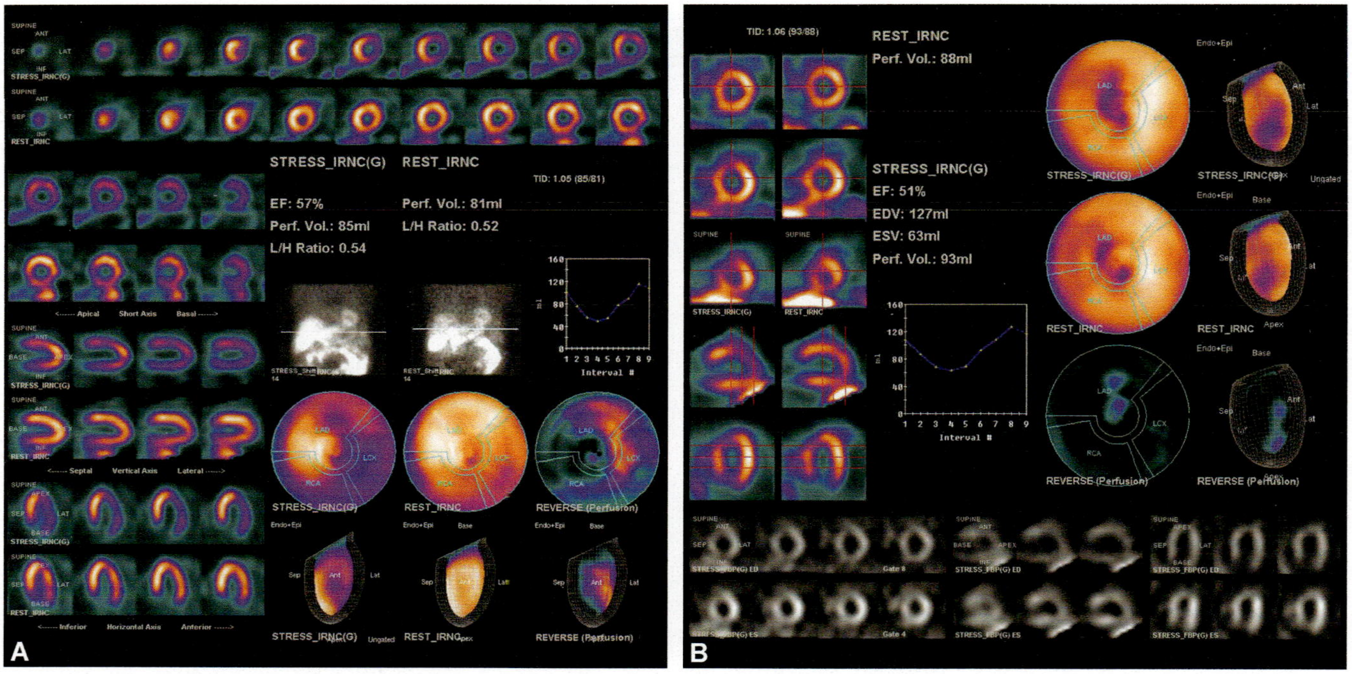

Figs. 1A and B: A 71-year-old male with coronary artery disease risk factors and typical angina.
Imaging protocol: Rest/stress technetium-99m sestamibi.
Stress modality: Regadenoson. During exercise the patient developed typical angina, and there were 1–2 mm of ST segment depression in the inferior and lateral precordial leads.

CASE 10: SEVERE ANTERIOR AND SEPTAL SCAR, INCREASED L/H RATIO, LEFT PLEURAL EFFUSION

Perfusion tomograms (A) demonstrate a very extensive, very severe fixed defect involving the anterior wall, apex, and septum. There is no evidence of defect reversibility in resting images. Planar projection images displayed in the left lateral view demonstrate a curvilinear photopenic defect in the base of the left lung, consistent with a left pleural effusion demonstrated radiographically. Functional images (B) demonstrate a markedly dilated left ventricle (end-diastolic volume = 201 cc, end-systolic volume = 173 cc) and a markedly decreased left ventricular ejection fraction (14%). The L/H ratio (C) is 0.85 in the stress anterior planar projection image, and 0.61 in the resting planar projection image (normal = <0.42 for Tc-99m sestamibi) (Figs. 1A to C).

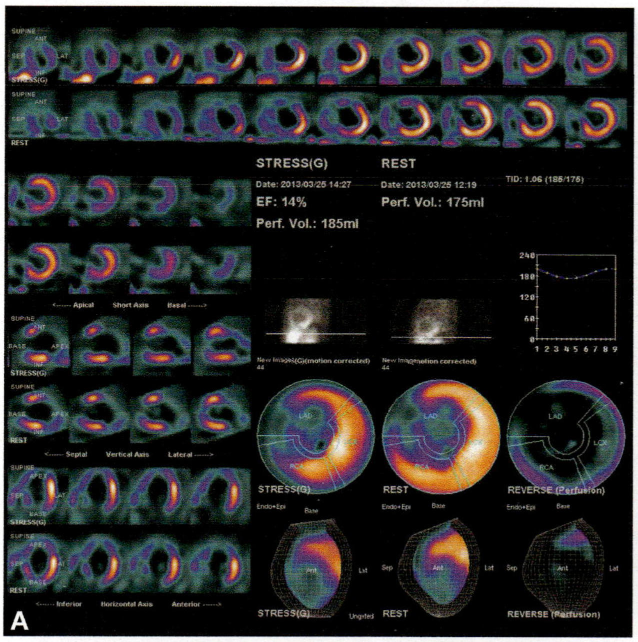

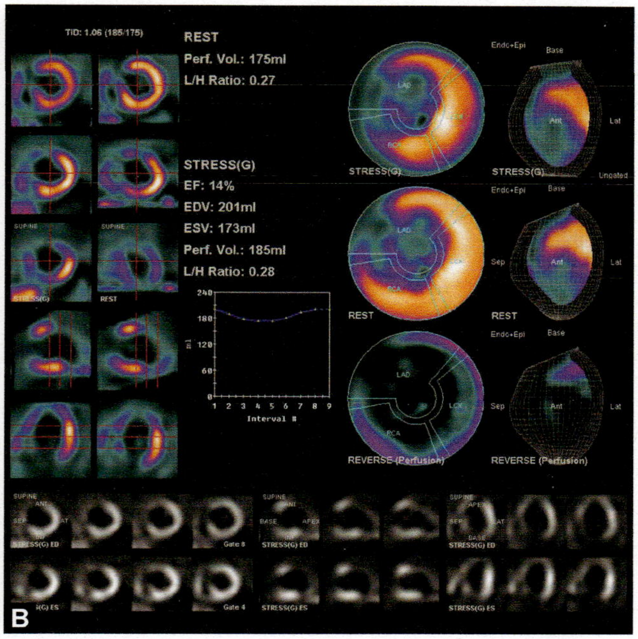

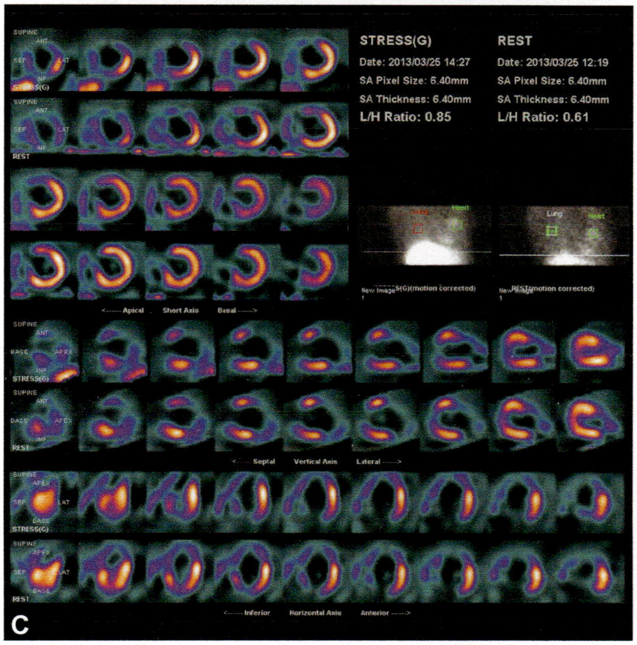

Figs. 1A to C: A 69-year-old female with prior myocardial infarction and congestive heart failure, now presents with worsening dyspnea.
Imaging protocol: Rest technetium-99m tetrofosmin/stress technetium-99m sestamibi.
Stress modality: Dipyridamole. The patient experienced no chest pain, and there were no ST segment changes during pharmacologic stress.

CASE 11: HERNIATED BOWEL; NORMAL MYOCARDIAL PERFUSION

Perfusion images (A) are normal. Anterior planar projection images suggest the presence of radiotracer concentration in the left hemithorax exterior to the heart. Projection images in the LAO (B) and left lateral (C) views clearly demonstrates the location of this extra-cardiac activity posterior to the heart, which is nearly as intense as the left ventricular myocardium. Further radiographic evaluation demonstrated herniation of bowel into the posterior left hemithorax. Tc-99m sestamibi is physiologically excreted into the bowel via the hepatobiliary system (Figs. 1A to C).

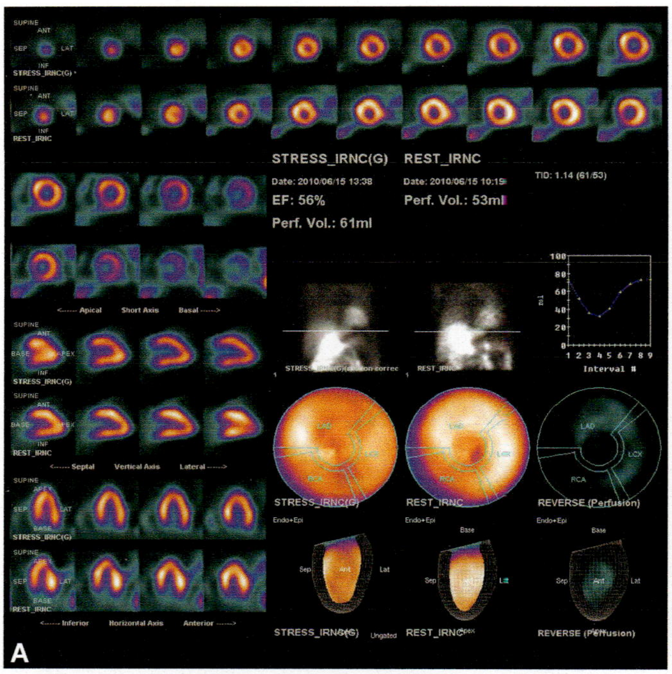

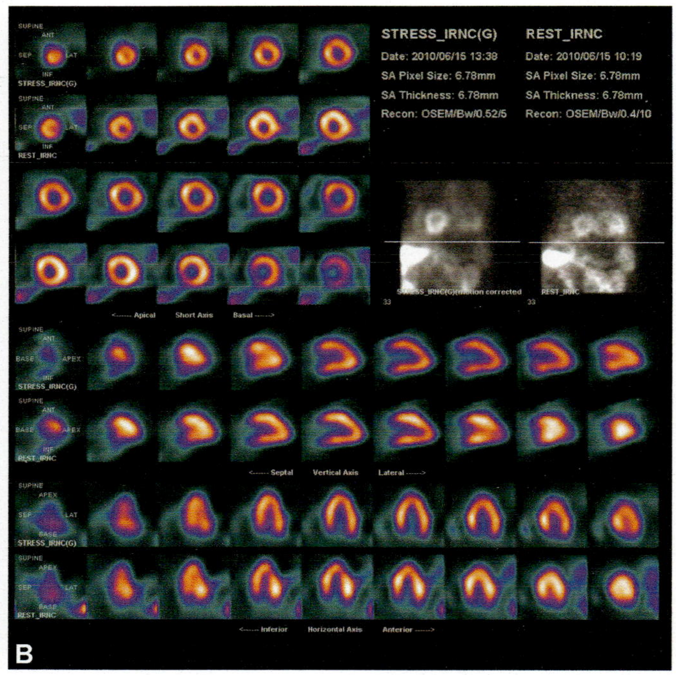

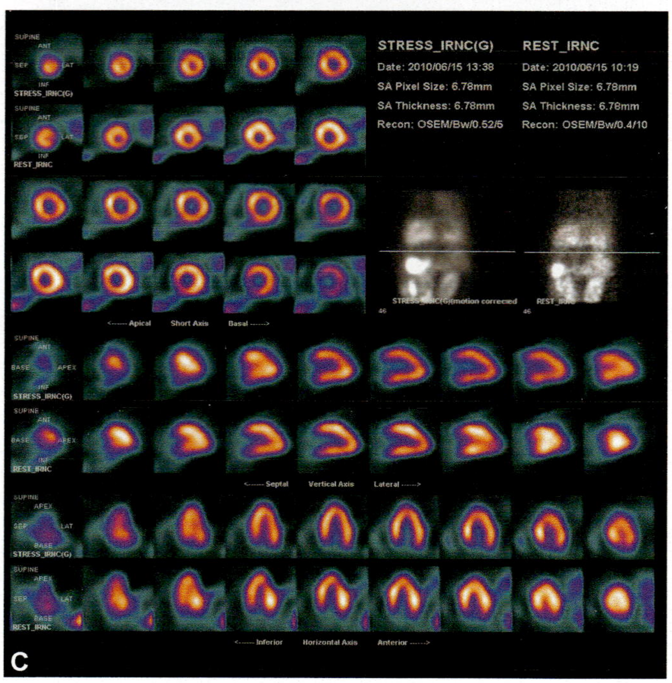

Figs. 1A to C: An 89-year-old male with coronary artery disease risk factors and nonanginal chest pain.
Imaging protocol: Rest technetium-99m tetrofosmin/stress technetium-99m sestamibi.
Stress modality: Dipyridamole. The patient experienced no chest pain, and there were no ST segment changes during pharmacologic stress.

Section 3

PET/CT

Amir Kashefi, Munir Ghesani

Chest Cases

CASE 1: DETECTION OF DISTANT METASTASES IN ESOPHAGEAL CANCER WITH RADIOGRAPHICALLY OPERABLE DISEASE

Brief History

A 51-year-old male with adenocarcinoma of the gastroesophageal junction underwent neoadjuvant chemoradiation therapy prior to surgical resection. Positron emission tomography/computed tomography (PET/CT) imaging was then pursued for surveillance of response to therapy and preoperative restaging.

Findings

Findings are shown in Figures 1 to 3.

Due to evolution of distant metastatic disease, the patient was no longer a surgical candidate and continued on to pursue a more aggressive chemotherapy regimen.

Main Teaching Point

- Positron emission tomography imaging is a powerful adjunct to anatomical modalities in identifying metastatic disease, especially when little anatomic correlation is seen.

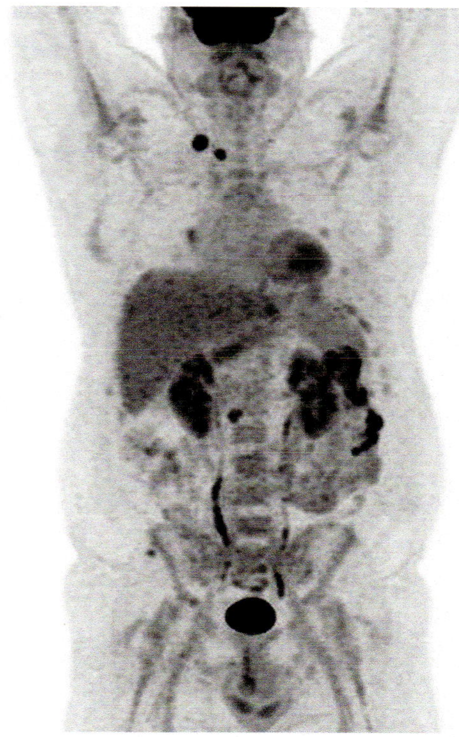

Fig. 1: Maximum intensity projection whole body image demonstrates two intense foci of radiotracer accumulation projecting over the right upper chest.

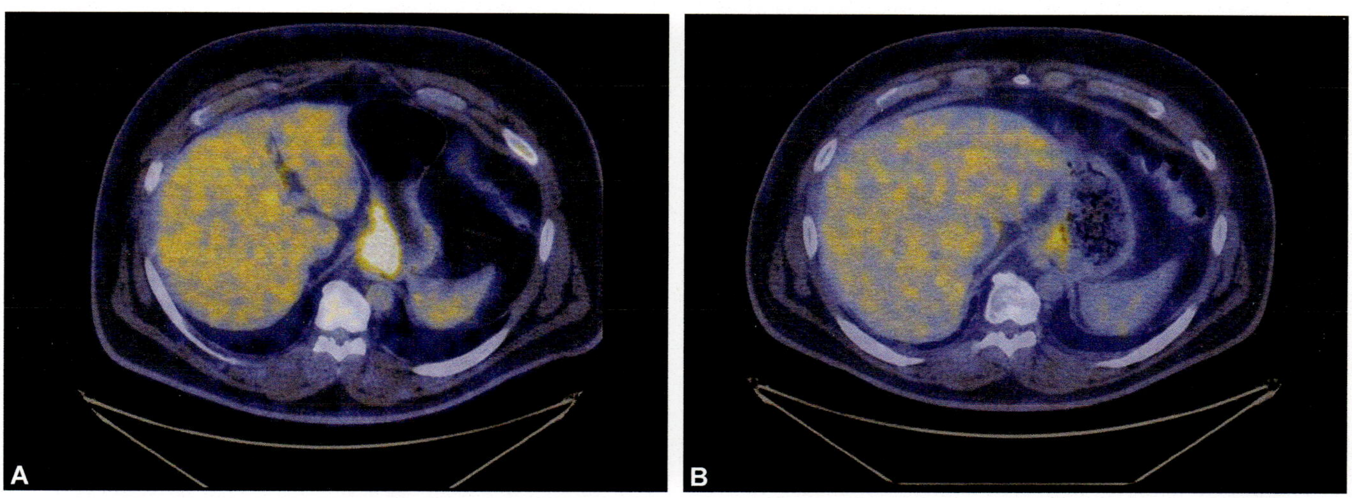

Figs. 2A and B: PET/CT images demonstrate significant interval improvement in both size and metabolic activity of the primary tumor as well as associated gastric thickening, indicating a favorable response to chemoradiation therapy. (A) Baseline study prior to radiation therapy; (B) Postradiation therapy.

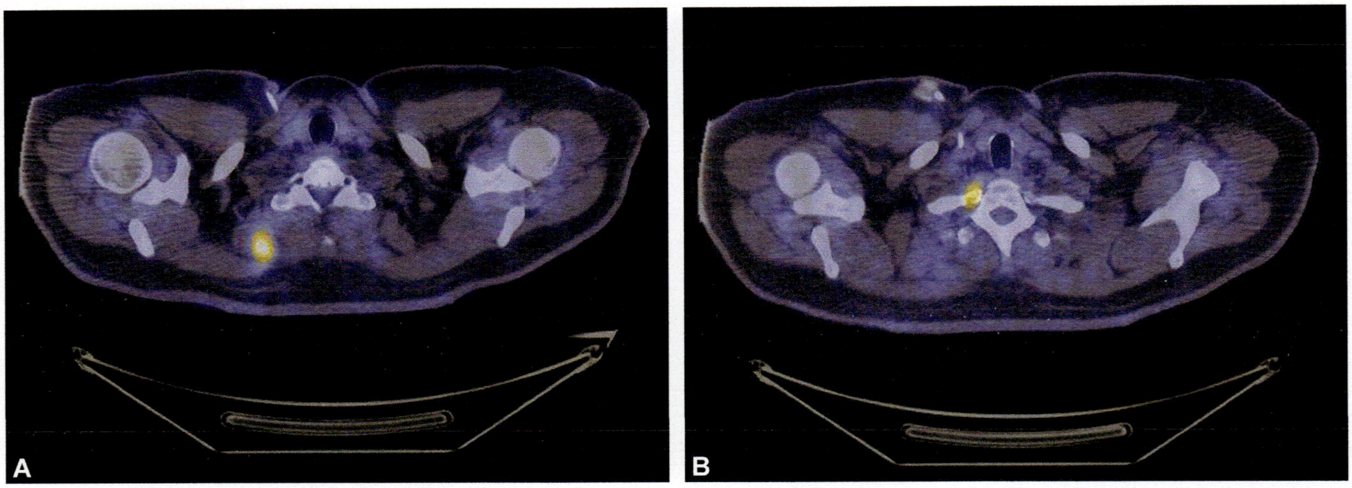

Figs. 3A and B: A new focus of ^{18}F fluorodeoxyglucose (FDG) accumulation is identified within the right posterior paraspinal musculature, which is highly concerning for metastasis. Additionally, a new hypermetabolic lytic rib lesion is observed that represents osseous metastasis with high certainty. (A) Paraspinal muscular metastasis; (B) Rib metastasis.

CASE 2: ASSESSMENT OF RECURRENCE OF PULMONARY MALIGNANCY

Brief History

A 69-year-old female with stage IA squamous cell carcinoma of the right lower lung lobe, status post video-assisted thoracoscopic resection, was found to have two new right upper lobe pulmonary nodules by surveillance computed tomography (CT). She subsequently underwent positron emission tomography (PET/CT) imaging as scintigraphic assessment of these lesions and for restaging of her primary disease.

Findings

Findings are shown in Figures 1 to 3.

Two pulmonary nodules are identified within the right upper lobe. The larger nodule measures 0.8 cm and has SUV maximum of 3.5 g/mL, which is highly suspicious for recurrent metastatic disease. The smaller 0.4 cm nodule demonstrates no visibly elevated radiotracer accumulation, but is below threshold for reliable characterization by PET imaging.

Main Teaching Points

- Approximately 25% of patients treated for stage IA non-small cell lung cancer can develop recurrence of disease.
- Lesions less than 0.8 cm are too small to fully characterize by PET imaging and cannot be excluded as malignancy even when demonstrating background metabolic activity.

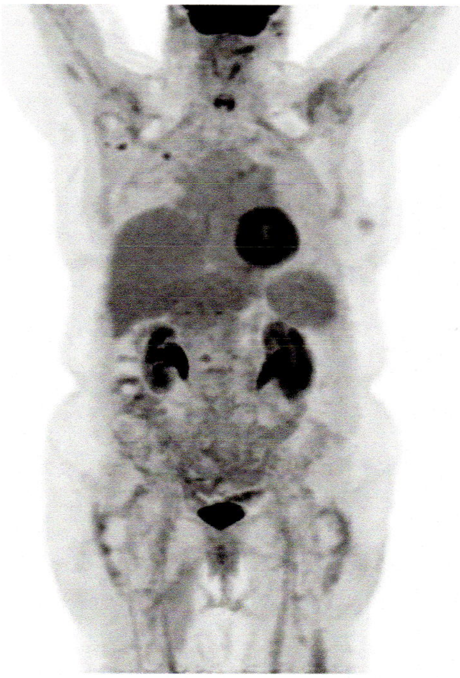

Fig. 1: Maximum intensity projection whole body image demonstrates abnormal foci of radiotracer activity projecting over the right chest and axilla.

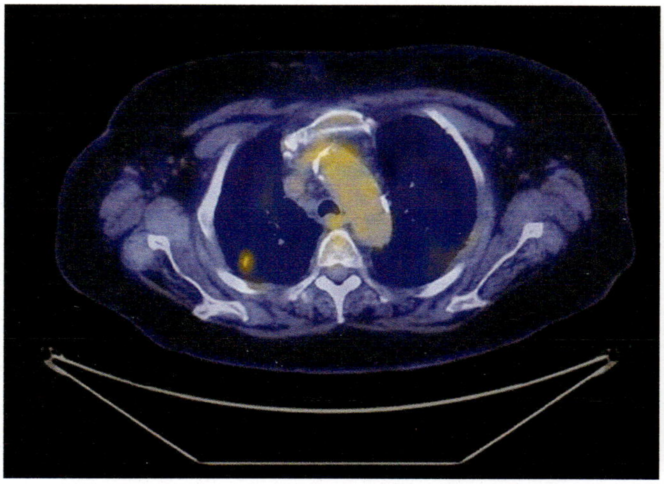

Fig. 2: The largest 0.8 cm nodule is identified in the posterior right upper lobe.

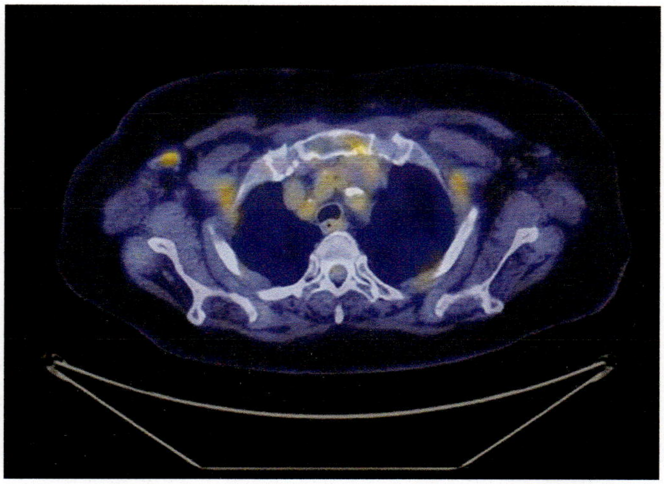

Fig. 3: Low-grade hypermetabolic lymphadenopathy is observed within the mediastinum and right axilla.

CASE 3: INCIDENTAL CANCER WHILE STAGING NEW PULMONARY MALIGNANCY

Brief History

A 74-year-old female with a history of pulmonary large cell neuroendocrine tumor, status post left upper lobectomy, was recently diagnosed with a new right upper lobe pulmonary squamous cell carcinoma. She underwent ^{18}F fluorodeoxyglucose (FDG) positron emission tomography/computed tomography (PET/CT) for initial staging of her disease.

Findings

Findings are shown in Figures 1 to 4.

Main Teaching Point

- Adrenal glucose metabolism greater than that of liver is worrisome for malignant involvement of either primary or metastatic nature.

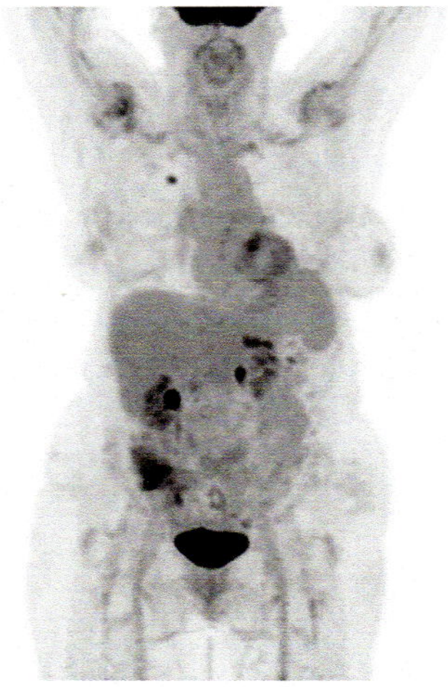

Fig. 1: Maximum intensity projection whole body image demonstrates the known right upper lobe squamous cell carcinoma. Additionally, focally increased radiotracer activity is noted within the right pelvis.

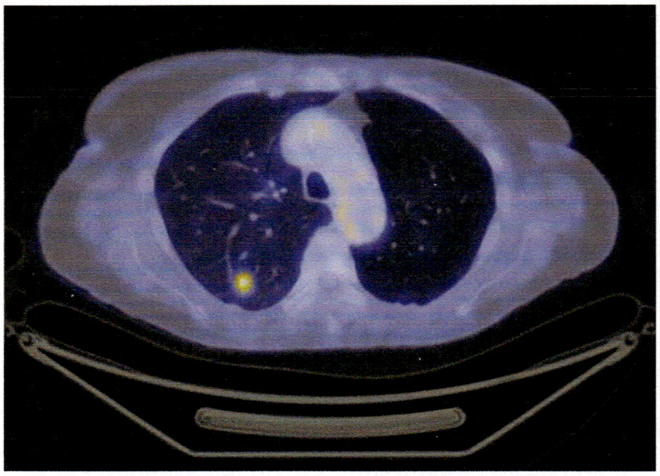

Fig. 2: A hypermetabolic right upper lobe nodule correlates to the biopsy-proven squamous cell carcinoma.

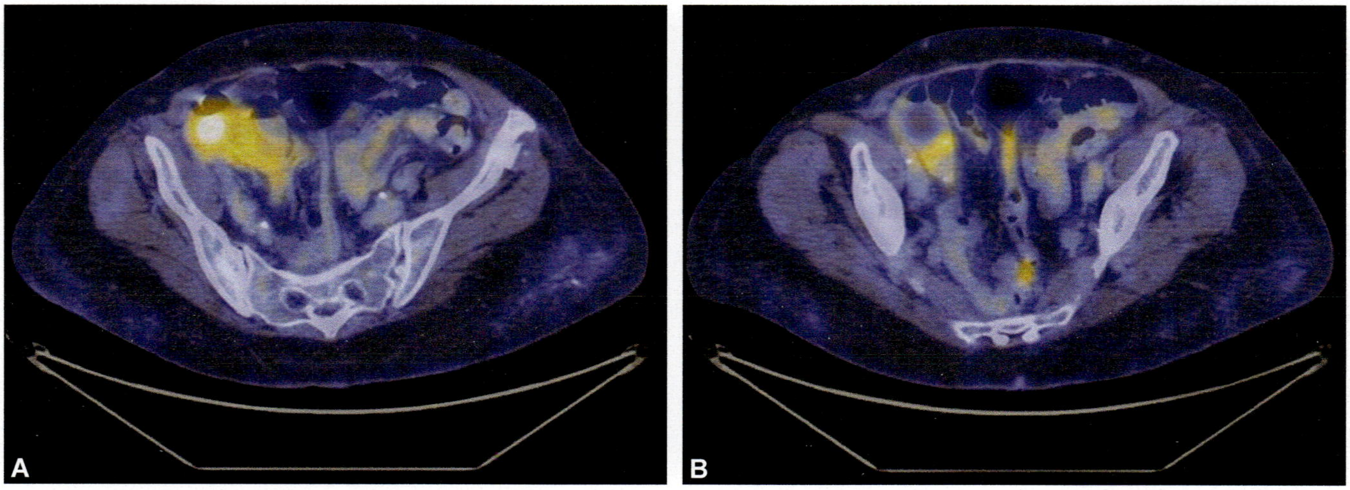

Figs. 3A and B: A large, variably hypermetabolic, mixed solid-cystic ovoid mass is identified in the right pelvis. The right ovary is not visualized and the mass directly abuts the cecum. Histologic origin could either be gastrointestinal or ovarian. (A) The inferior and solid portion of the mass is adjacent to the cecum. (B) Superiorly, a cystic component is seen with decreased radiotracer activity centrally and a hypermetabolic rim.

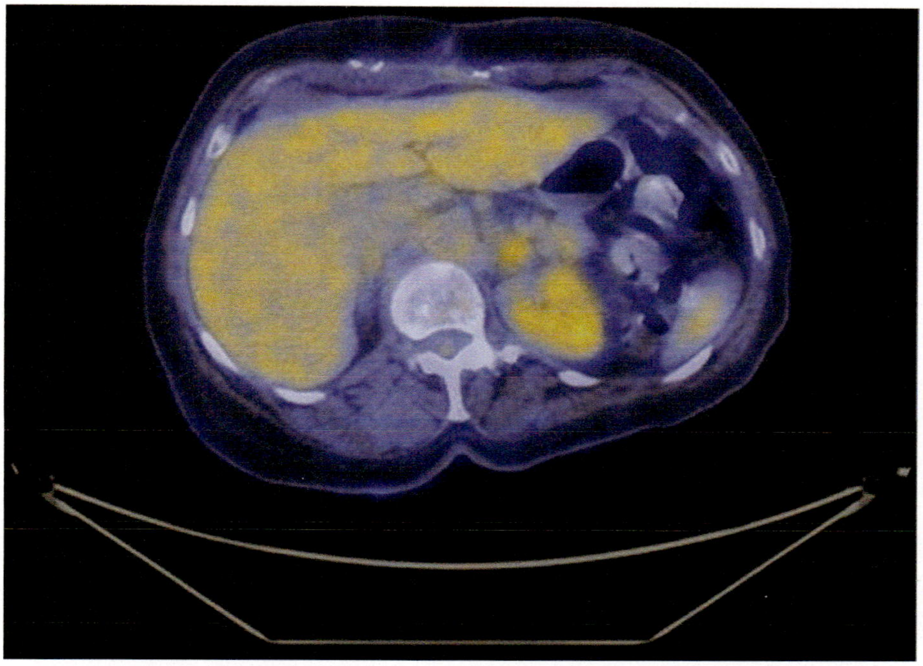

Fig. 4: Hypermetabolic fullness of the left adrenal gland demonstrates FDG avidity greater than normal adjacent liver parenchyma, which raises concern for malignant involvement.

CASE 4: MONITORING RESPONSE TO LUNG CANCER THERAPY

Brief History

A 67-year-old male with a history of laryngeal cancer was incidentally found to have lung cancer by baseline positron emission tomography/computed tomography (PET/CT) evaluation. He subsequently underwent definitive stereotactic body radiation therapy and required reimaging for evaluation of response.

Findings

Findings are shown in Figures 1A and B.

Main Teaching Points

- Radiotherapy-treated pulmonary masses can persist as scarred parenchymal lesions.
- Comparison of ^{18}F fluorodeoxyglucose (FDG) uptake of a treated pulmonary mass to adjacent or contralateral background lung activity can help to determine if it has been adequately treated.

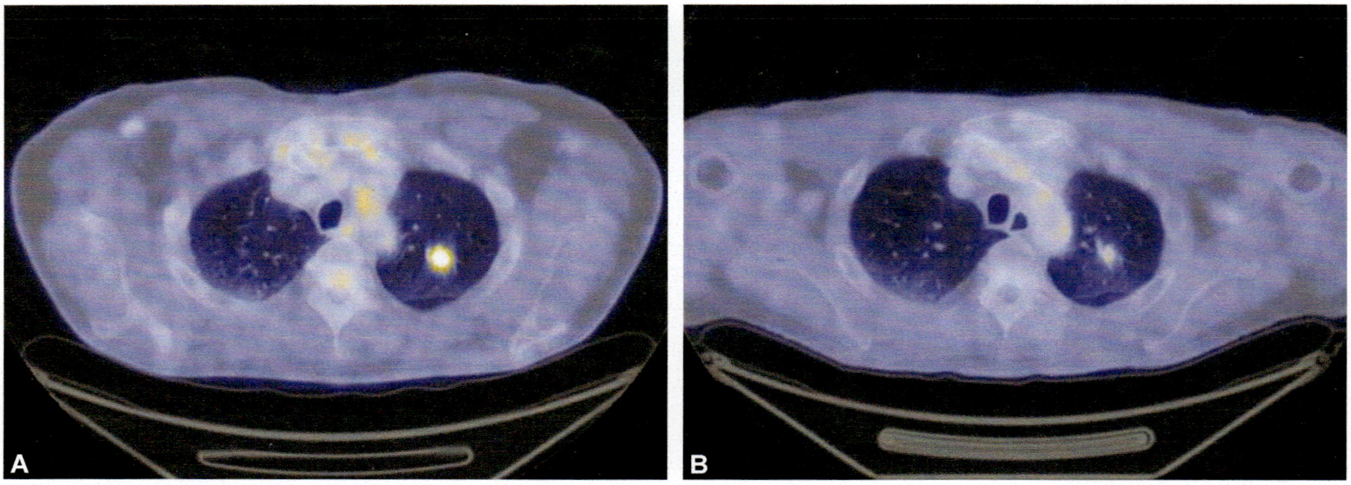

Figs. 1A and B: Interval decrease in metabolic activity in the left upper lobe pulmonary mass is appreciated. The lesion was originally a spiculated soft tissue density, but developed a more scarred, fibrotic appearance following radiation therapy. Visually, the metabolic activity has noticeably decreased, and the standard uptake value (SUV) maximum measurement has fallen from 5.6 g/mL to 1.8 g/mL. Adjacent background lung activity has a SUV maximum of 1.6 g/mL. (A) Baseline appearance prior to treatment; (B) Post-radiotherapy.

CASE 5: CHARACTERIZATION OF A SUSPICIOUS PULMONARY NODULE

Brief History

A 65-year-old female presented with computed tomography (CT) evidence of multiple pulmonary nodules, one of which had increased in size with a mildly spiculated appearance. She required ^{18}F fluorodeoxyglucose (FDG) positron emission tomography (PET)/CT imaging to evaluate the functional status of this lesion.

Findings

Findings are shown in Figures 1 and 2.

Main Teaching Points

- Positron emission tomography is a useful tool to assess the metabolic activity of a newly discovered lesion, especially when limited prior imaging is available.
- Pulmonary nodules on the border of PET resolution (0.8–1.0 cm) that demonstrate background activity favor benign etiology, but should still be followed with repeat imaging in 2–3 months.

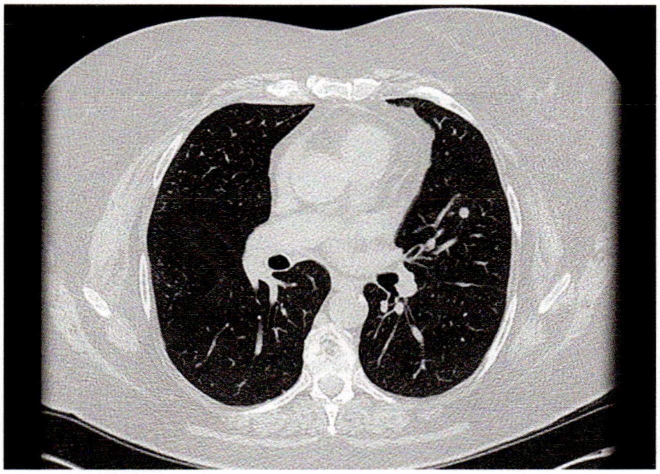

Fig. 1: Initial chest CT demonstrates an 8 mm pulmonary nodule within the lingual.

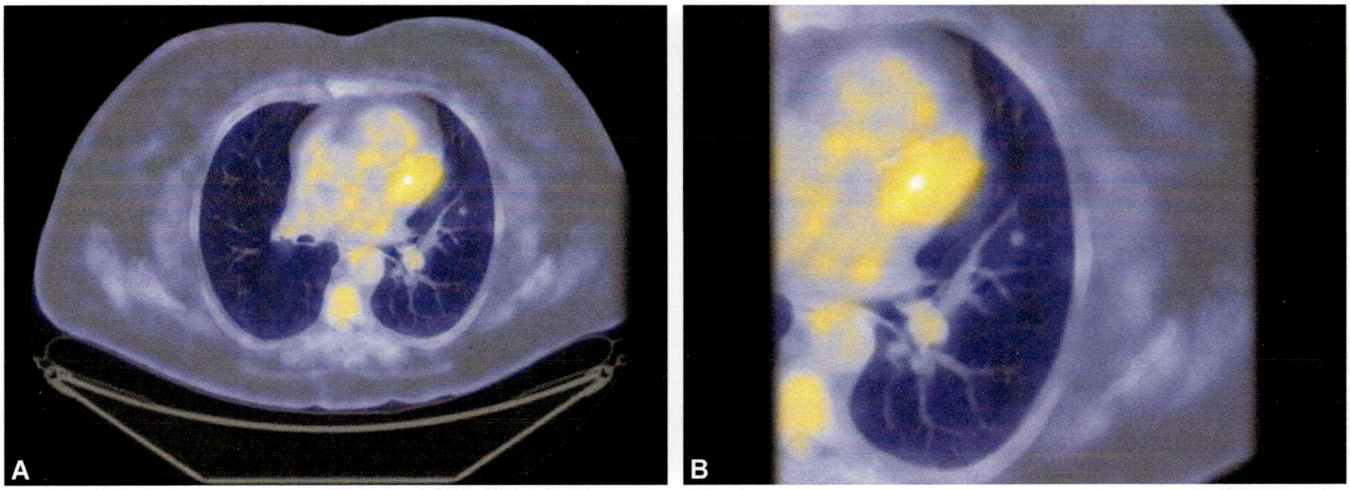

Figs. 2A and B: By PET/CT, the lesion of question demonstrates no abnormal FDG accumulation; however, the size of this lesion is on the border of reliable detection by PET resolution and should be followed with future imaging.

CASE 6: INITIAL STAGING OF PATHOLOGICALLY PROVEN PULMONARY MALIGNANCY

Brief History

A 65-year-old female presented with recently diagnosed pulmonary adenocarcinoma and required ^{18}F fluorodeoxyglucose (FDG) positron emission tomography/computed tomography (PET/CT) imaging for initial staging of her disease.

Findings

Findings are shown in Figures 1 to 6.

Main Teaching Points

- Tumoral encroachment on the spinal canal is an urgent finding, and the patient should be assessed clinically for neurologic impingement.
- Positron emission tomography/computed tomography can be used to identify hypermetabolic biopsy targets to help establish metastatic pathology.

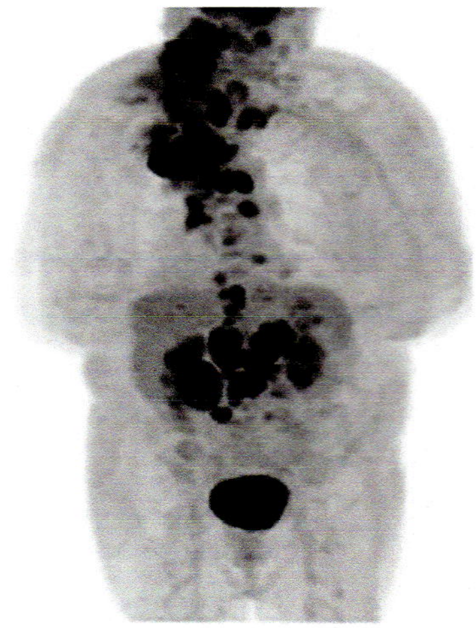

Fig. 1: Maximum intensity projection whole body image demonstrates extensive hypermetabolic metastases projecting of the right chest, right neck, and central abdomen.

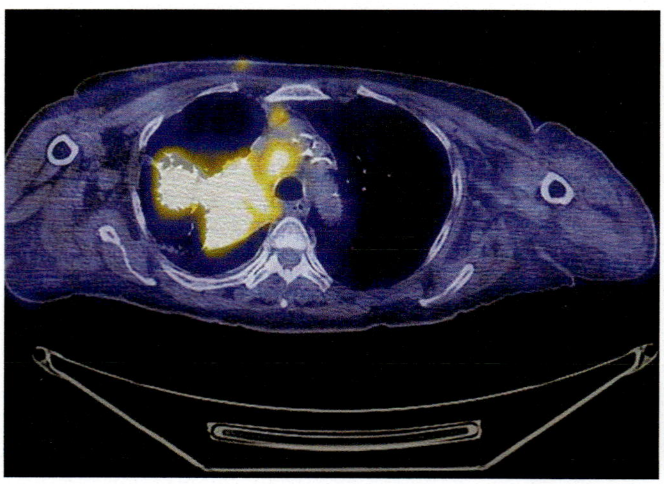

Fig. 2: A large hypermetabolic right upper lobe pulmonary mass is identified.

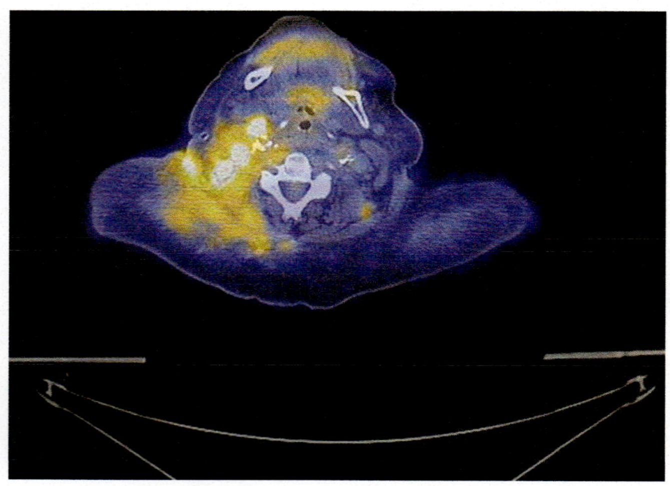

Fig. 3: Extensive conglomerate lymphadenopathy is seen throughout nearly all nodal stations of the mediastinum and neck.

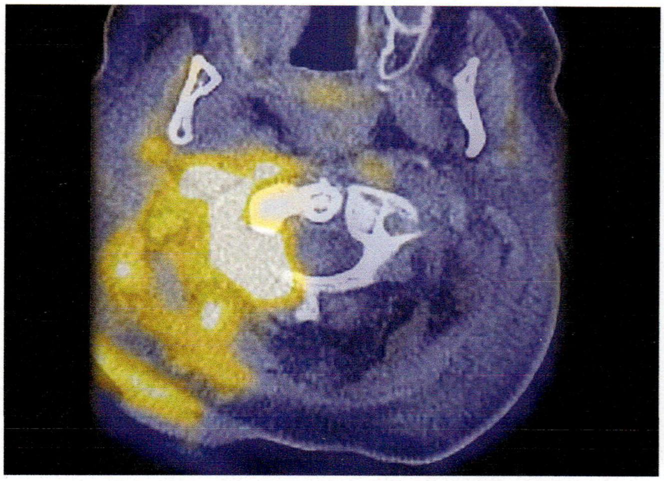

Fig. 4: Thickening of hypermetabolic right lateral paraspinal musculature is seen with direct extension between the C1/C2 interface with effacement of the thecal sac. No osseous destruction was appreciated at this location.

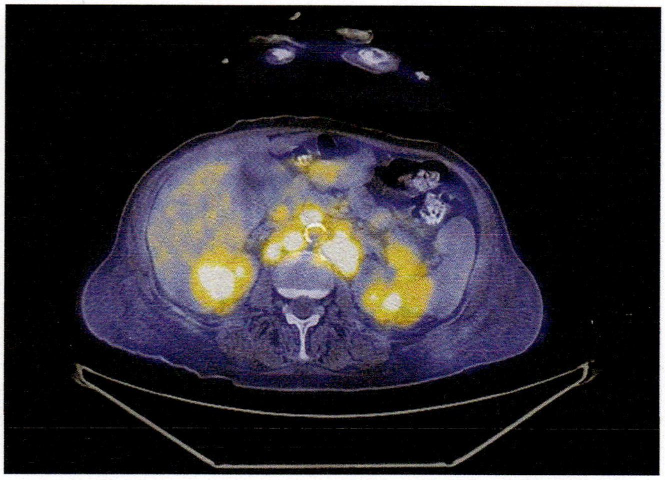

Fig. 5: Bulky retroperitoneal hypermetabolic lymphadenopathy represents significant metastatic spread inferior to the diaphragm.

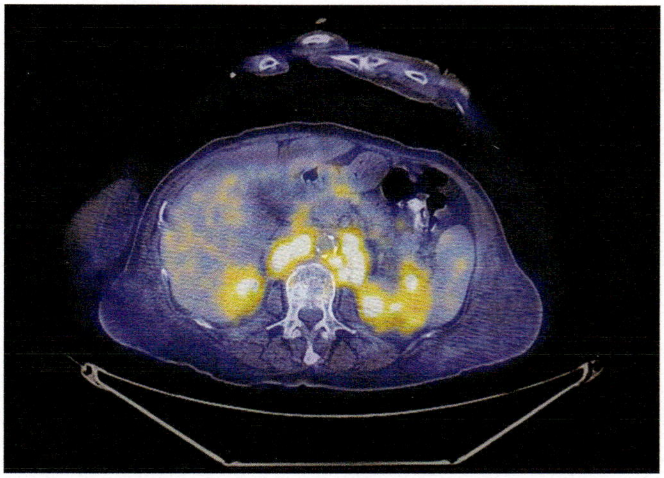

Fig. 6: A hypermetabolic left-sided retroperitoneal lymph node is identified that would be particularly amenable to image-guided biopsy, if clinically indicated.

CASE 7: BREAST CANCER EVALUATION AND RESPONSE TO THERAPY

Brief History

A 64-year-old female with stage IIIA breast cancer was treated with modified radical mastectomy, reconstruction, and adjuvant chemotherapy with good clinical response. She was without evidence of recurrent disease for over 10 years until she presented with cardiac chest pain and computed tomography (CT) imaging revealed incidental mediastinal lymphadenopathy. Subsequent ^{18}F fluorodeoxyglucose (FDG) positron emission tomography (PET/CT) confirmed abnormal hypermetabolism, and lymph node biopsy was consistent with recurrence of breast primary malignancy. She was initiated on chemotherapy and underwent repeat PET/CT imaging to evaluate response to treatment.

Findings

Findings are shown in Figures 1 to 4.

Main Teaching Points

- Direct comparison of Standard Uptake Value (SUV) maximum measurements for select index lesions can be used to assess interval response to therapy.
- Stable or improving metabolic activity with no newly identified lesions indicates favorable response to therapy.

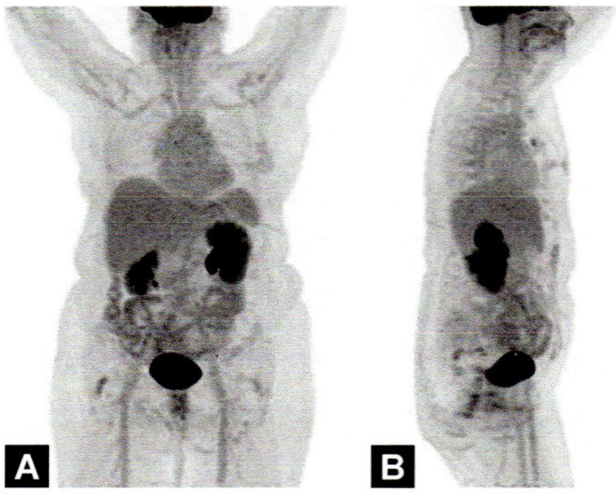

Figs. 1A and B: Maximum intensity projection whole body images demonstrate small subtle radiotracer-avid mediastinal lymph nodes. (A) The anterior view shows lymph nodes projecting over the central mediastinum. (B) The lateral view shows the most intense lesion is within the substernal anterior mediastinum.

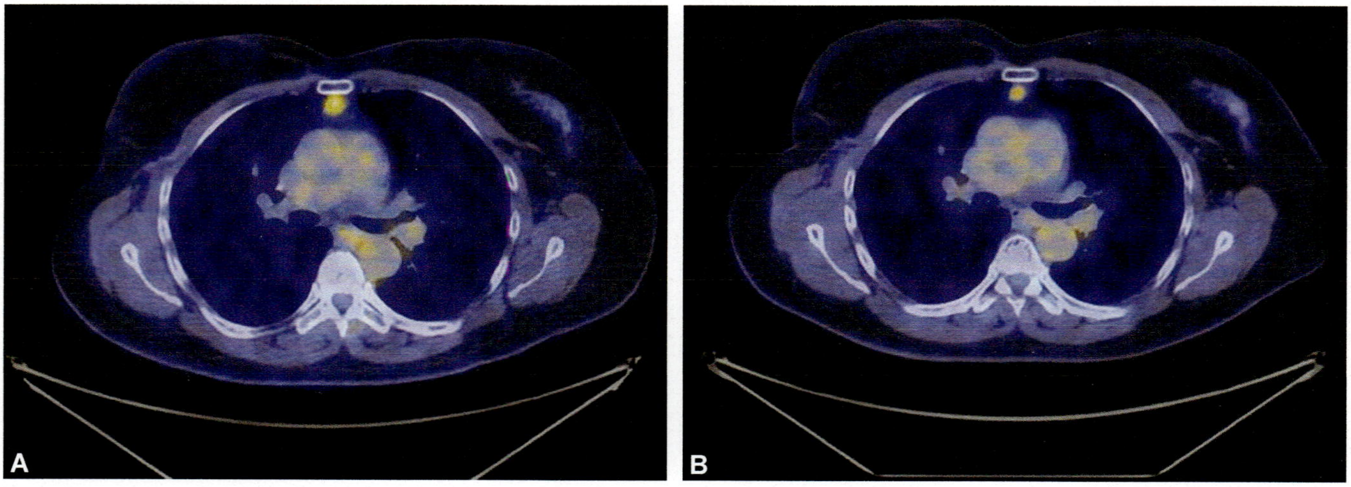

Figs. 2A and B: A hypermetabolic retrosternal anterior mediastinal lymph node has decreased in size from 1.1 x 1.5 cm to 0.8 x 1.1 cm. The SUV maximum measurement has also decreased from 4.7 g/mL to 2.4 g/mL. (A) Baseline study prior to chemotherapy. (B) Post-chemotherapy.

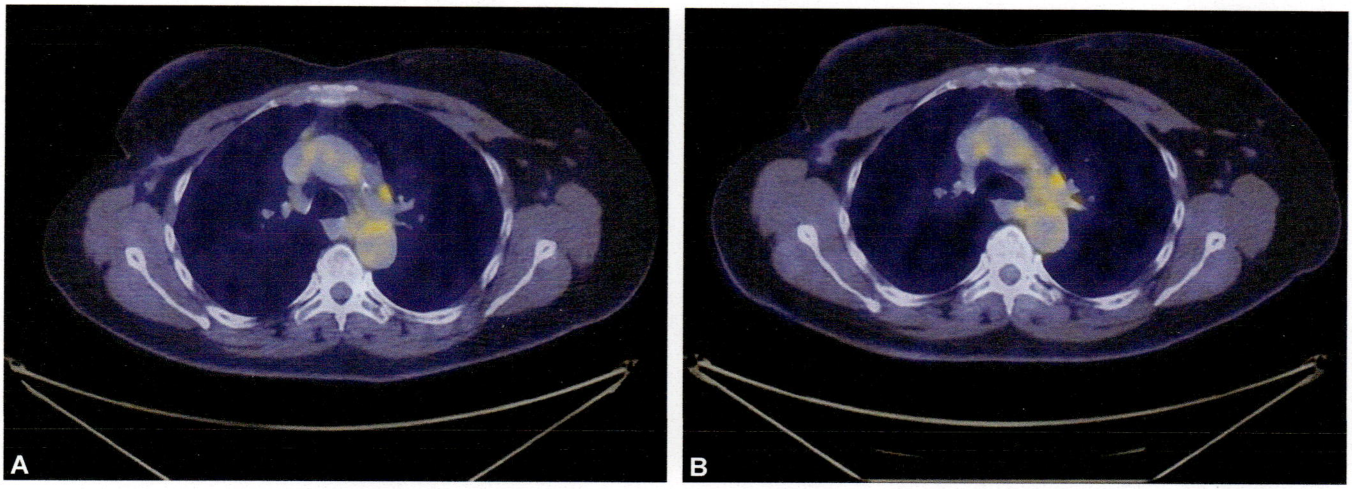

Figs. 3A and B: A persistent hypermetabolic lymph node in the left perihilar region is stable in both size and metabolic activity. (A) Baseline study prior to chemotherapy. (B) Post-chemotherapy.

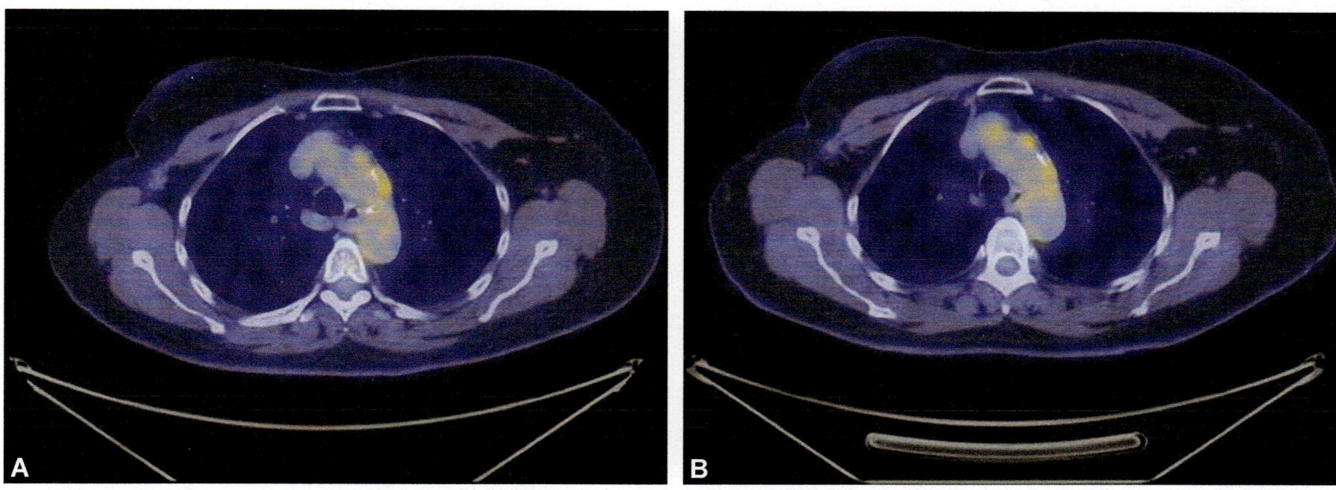

Figs. 4A and B: An aortopulmonary window hypermetabolic lymph nodes has decreased in standard uptake value (SUV) maximum measurement from 3.5 g/mL to 2.5 g/mL and visually appears slightly less intense. Anterior to this lesion is a hypermetabolic prevascular lymph node that has remained stable. (A) Baseline study prior to chemotherapy. (B) Post-chemotherapy.

CASE 8: INCIDENTAL LUNG CANCER WHILE STAGING ANOTHER MALIGNANCY

Brief History

A 57-year-old female with a history of breast carcinoma that was treated with mastectomy, reconstruction, and adjuvant chemotherapy 7 years ago, underwent positron emission tomography/computed tomography (PET/CT) imaging for surveillance of her disease.

Findings

Findings are shown in Figures 1 to 3.

No abnormal ^{18}F fluorodeoxyglucose (FDG) accumulation is identified in the breasts to suggest active or recurrent disease at that location. This finding further reinforces the likelihood of a metachronous primary cancer.

Main Teaching Points

- Subcarinal lung cancer metastasis qualifies for N2 and stage III disease, which has a 5-year survival rate of 80%.
- The risk of stage III breast cancer recurrence 5 years after resection and adjuvant chemotherapy is approximately 13%.
- A large solitary pulmonary mass favors new primary malignancy over breast cancer recurrence in the absence of active or recurrent breast lesions.

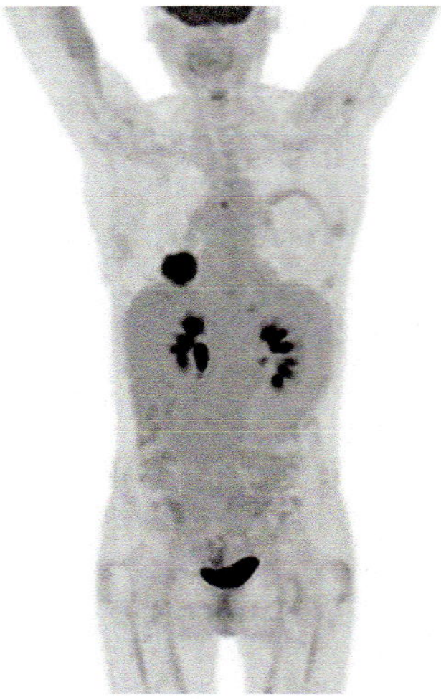

Fig. 1: Maximum intensity projection whole body image demonstrates a large intensely-hypermetabolic mass projecting over the right inferior lung, as well as a small central mediastinal hypermetabolic lymph node.

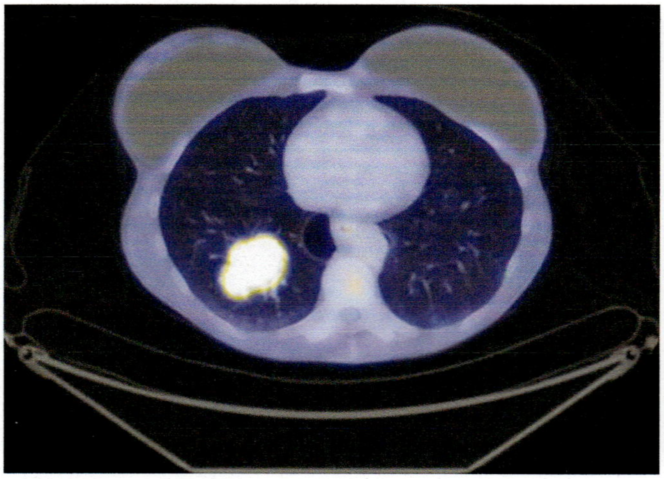

Fig. 2: A new large hypermetabolic mass is discovered in the right upper lung lobe. This lesion is mildly spiculated in appearance and is worrisome for a new primary pulmonary malignancy.

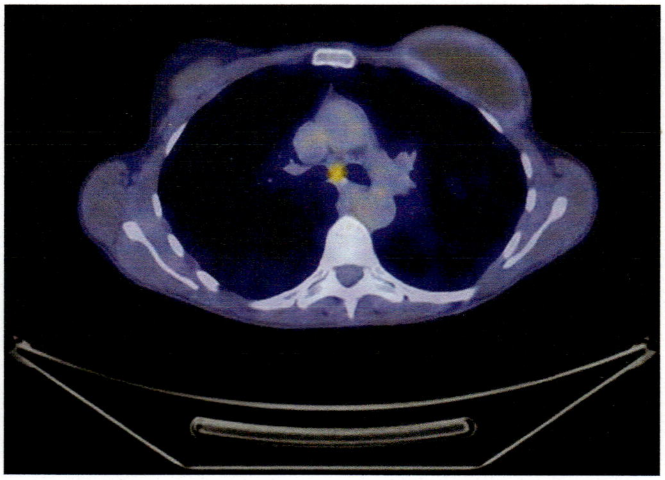

Fig. 3: A solitary hypermetabolic subcarinal lymph node is seen that likely represents regional spread of malignancy.

CASE 9: INITIAL STAGING OF BREAST CANCER

Brief History

A 44-year-old female with newly diagnosed invasive ductal carcinoma of the left breast and left chest wall pain required ^{18}F fluorodeoxyglucose (FDG) positron emission tomography/computed tomography (PET/CT) imaging for initial radiographic staging of her disease.

Findings

Findings are shown in Figures 1 to 3.

Main Teaching Points

- Patients with breast cancer metastases to bone have M1 or stage IV disease.
- Approximately 9% of patients with new diagnosis breast cancer present with distant metastases.

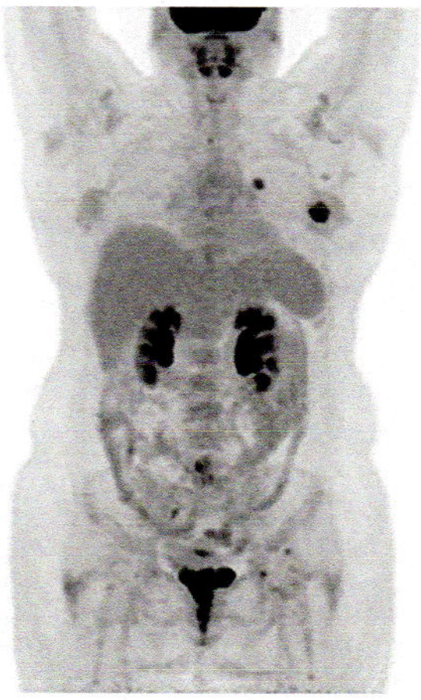

Fig. 1: Maximum intensity projection whole body image demonstrates multiple foci radiotracer activity projecting over the left breast and medial left chest.

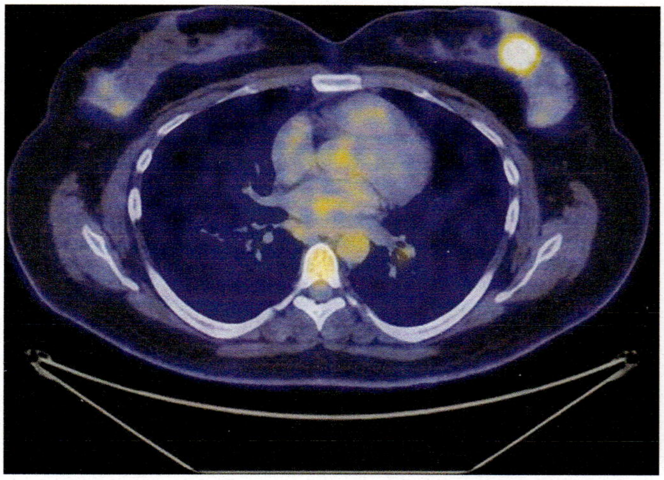

Fig. 2: A 12 o'clock hypermetabolic left breast mass is demonstrated consistent with the known primary malignancy.

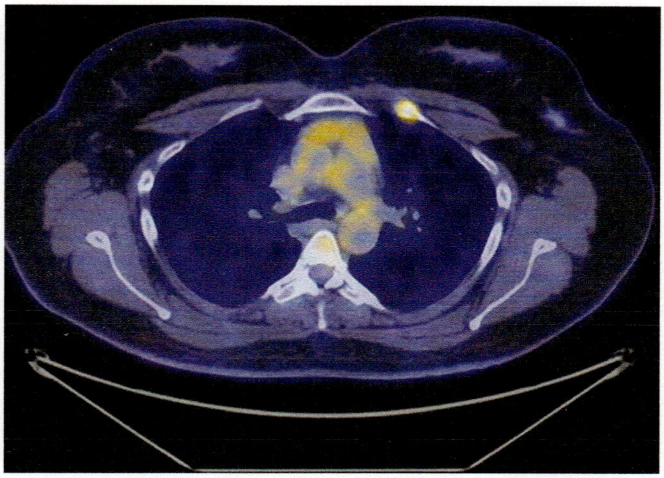

Fig. 3: A hypermetabolic lesion is observed in the left anterior second rib that corresponds to an expansile lytic osseous lesion and represents a solitary bone metastasis. No other metastatic foci are identified.

CASE 10: RESTAGING OF ESOPHAGEAL CANCER AFTER CHEMORADIATION THERAPY

Brief History

A 57-year-old male with metastatic esophageal cancer was treated with esophagectomy, gastric pull-up, and adjuvant chemoradiation therapy. On surveillance imaging, he was discovered to have distant metastases to the retroperitoneum, lungs and bone. He was subsequently initiated on a new chemotherapy regimen, and now requires ^{18}F fluorodeoxyglucose (FDG) positron emission tomography/computed tomography (PET/CT) for evaluation of response.

Findings

Findings are shown in Figures 1 to 4.

Incidental note is made of increased cardiac glucose metabolism between the examinations explained by difference in patient's fasting preparation. (A) Prior chemotherapy. (B) Postchemotherapy).

Significantly decreased activity is seen in a persistent para-aortic lymph node.

Main Teaching Points

- The 5-year survival rate of metastatic esophageal cancer is approximately 48%.
- There is no difference in survival rate between esophageal cancer patients with regional versus distant metastatic disease.

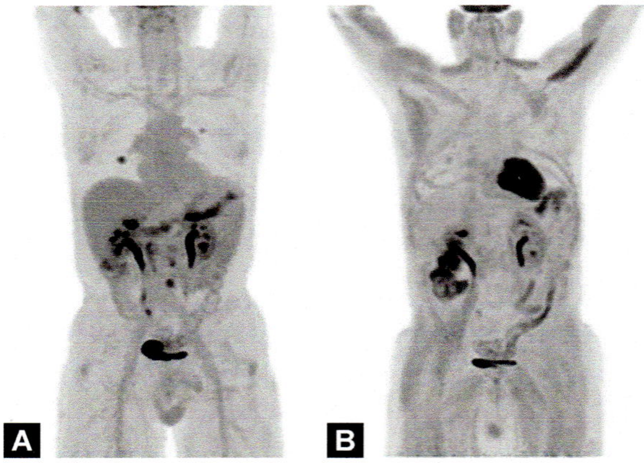

Figs. 1A and B: (A) Baseline maximum intensity projection whole body image prior to chemotherapy administration demonstrates multiple radio-tracer avid metastases projecting over the chest and central abdomen. (B) Followup imaging after chemotherapy shows resolution of abnormal activity within the prior metastases. Incidental note of skeletal and cardiac muscular uptake is attributable to differences in the patient's fasting preparation.

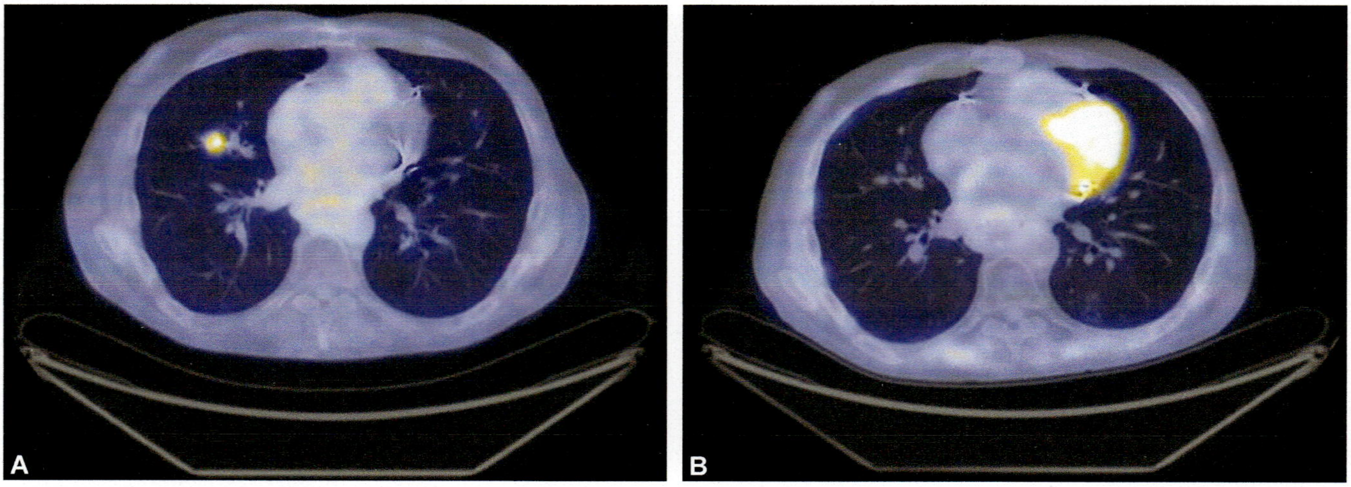

Figs. 2A and B: Interval resolution of FDG accumulation is seen in a right middle lobe nodule. The CT correlate to this lesion has shrunken in size and has a scarred appearance. (A) Baseline examination prior to chemotherapy; (B) Post chemotherapy.

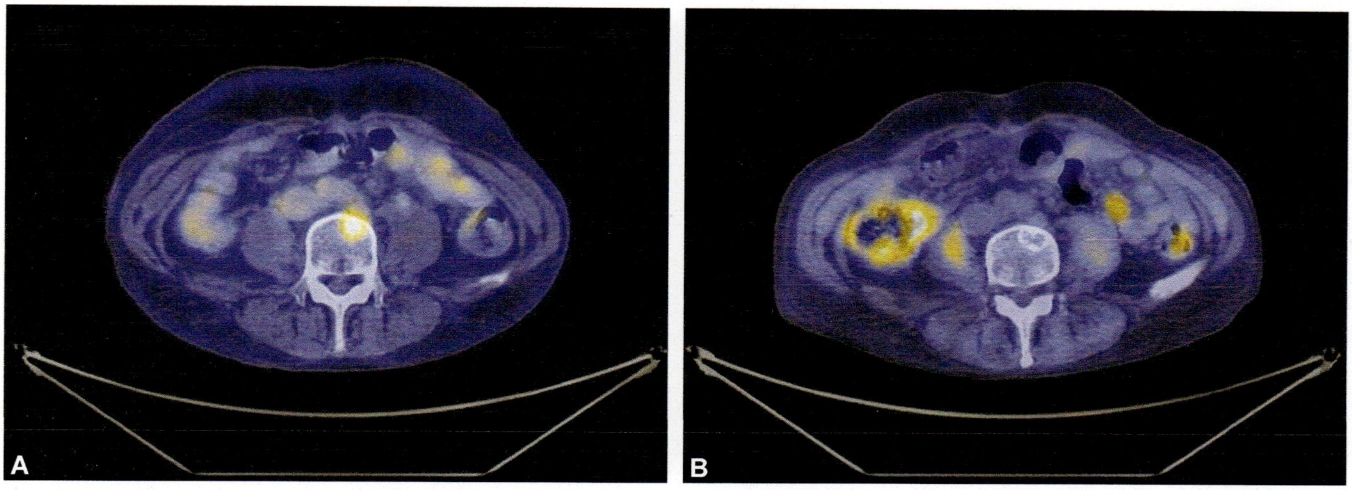

Figs. 3A and B: Interval resolution of FDG accumulation is seen in an L4 vertebral body metastasis. Previously, this finding had no CT correlate but now appears as a mixed lytic-sclerotic lesion. (A) Baseline examination prior to chemotherapy; (B) Post-chemotherapy.

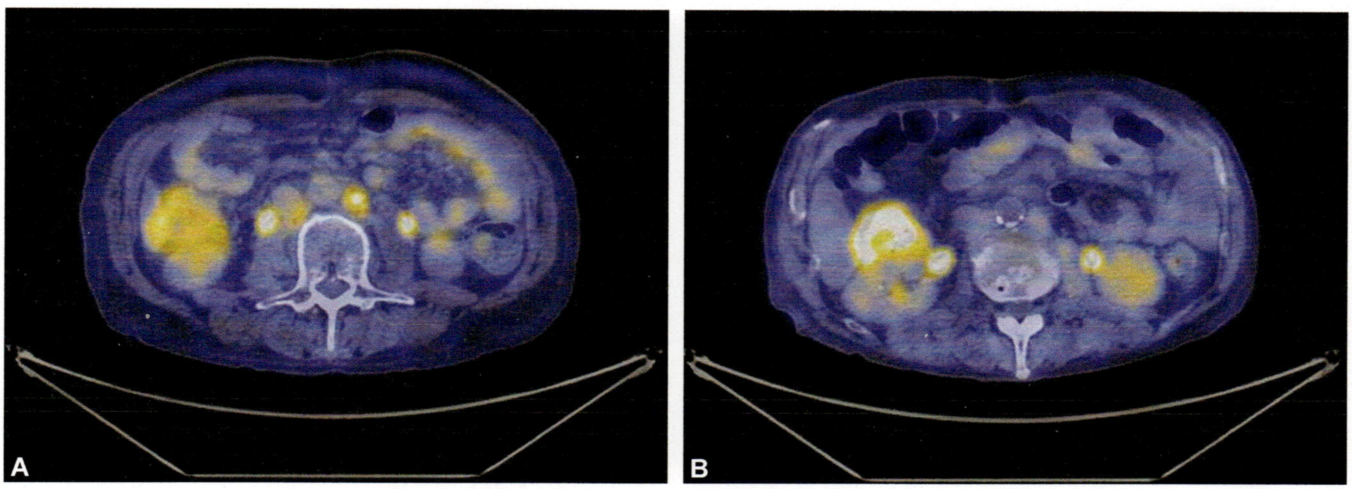

Figs. 4A and B: Significantly decreased activity is seen in a persistent para-aortic lymph node. Incidental interval development of ascending colitis was also noted. (A) Baseline examination prior to chemotherapy; (B) Post-chemotherapy.

CASE 11: POTENTIALLY RESECTABLE ESOPHAGEAL CANCER WITH NO DISTANT METASTASES

Brief History

A 51-year-old male presented with dysphagia and stricture on esophagram who was subsequently diagnosed with poorly differentiated esophageal adenocarcinoma. He required baseline ^{18}F fluorodeoxyglucose (FDG) positron emission tomography/computed tomography (PET/CT) for initial staging of his disease and evaluation for surgical candidacy.

Findings

Findings are shown in Figures 1 and 2.

Main Teaching Points

- Symptomatic esophageal cancer often presents with submucosal invasion, which carries a 50% chance of metastasis at the time of diagnosis.
- Malignancies detected early that only have mucosal-depth invasion have metastasized in up to 10% of cases.
- The chance of early metastasis is increased in squamous cell over adenocarcinoma subtypes.
- Overt metastatic disease precludes candidacy from surgical resection, and medical management must be pursued.

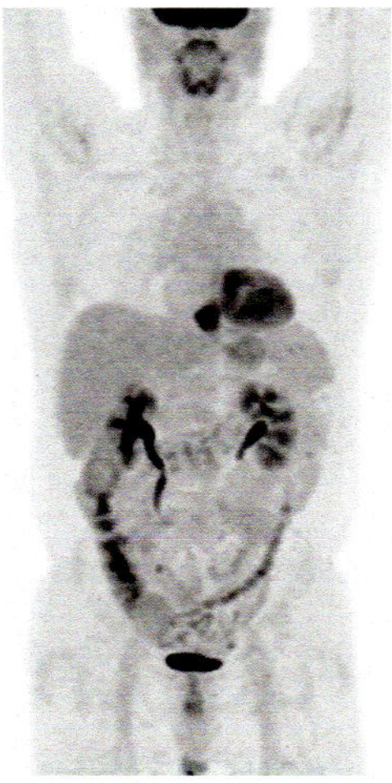

Fig. 1: Maximum intensity projection whole body image demonstrates a large hypermetabolic mass projecting over the distal esophagus. No other abnormality is identified to suggest locoregional spread or distant metastasis.

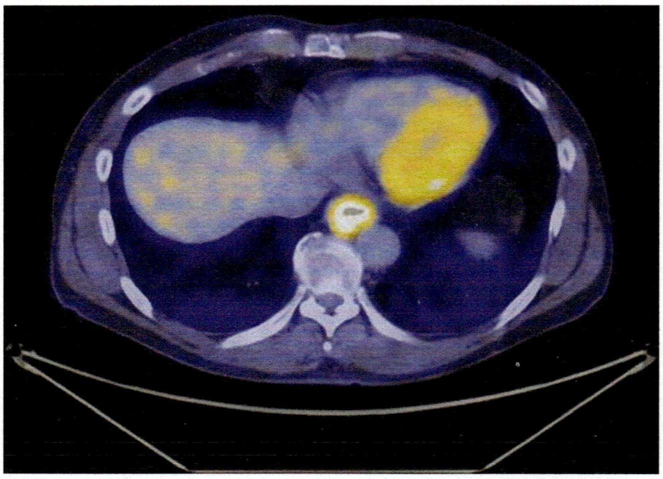

Fig. 2: Intensely hypermetabolic distal esophageal wall thickening correlates to biopsy-proven adenocarcinoma.

CASE 12: RESOLVING EQUIVOCAL BREAST FINDINGS ON ANATOMICAL IMAGING

Brief History

A 64-year-old female being evaluated for potential kidney transplant donation was found to have left axillary lymphadenopathy and underwent positron emission tomography/computed tomography (PET/CT) imaging to evaluate for indolent malignancy.

Findings

Findings are shown in Figures 1A to E.

No hypermetabolic focus is identified to suggest underlying malignancy.

Main Teaching Points

- Positron emission tomography/computed tomography is a useful tool to distinguish borderline or equivocal findings on anatomical imaging.
- Lymphadenopathy demonstrating low-grade metabolic activity favors reactive or inflammatory etiology.

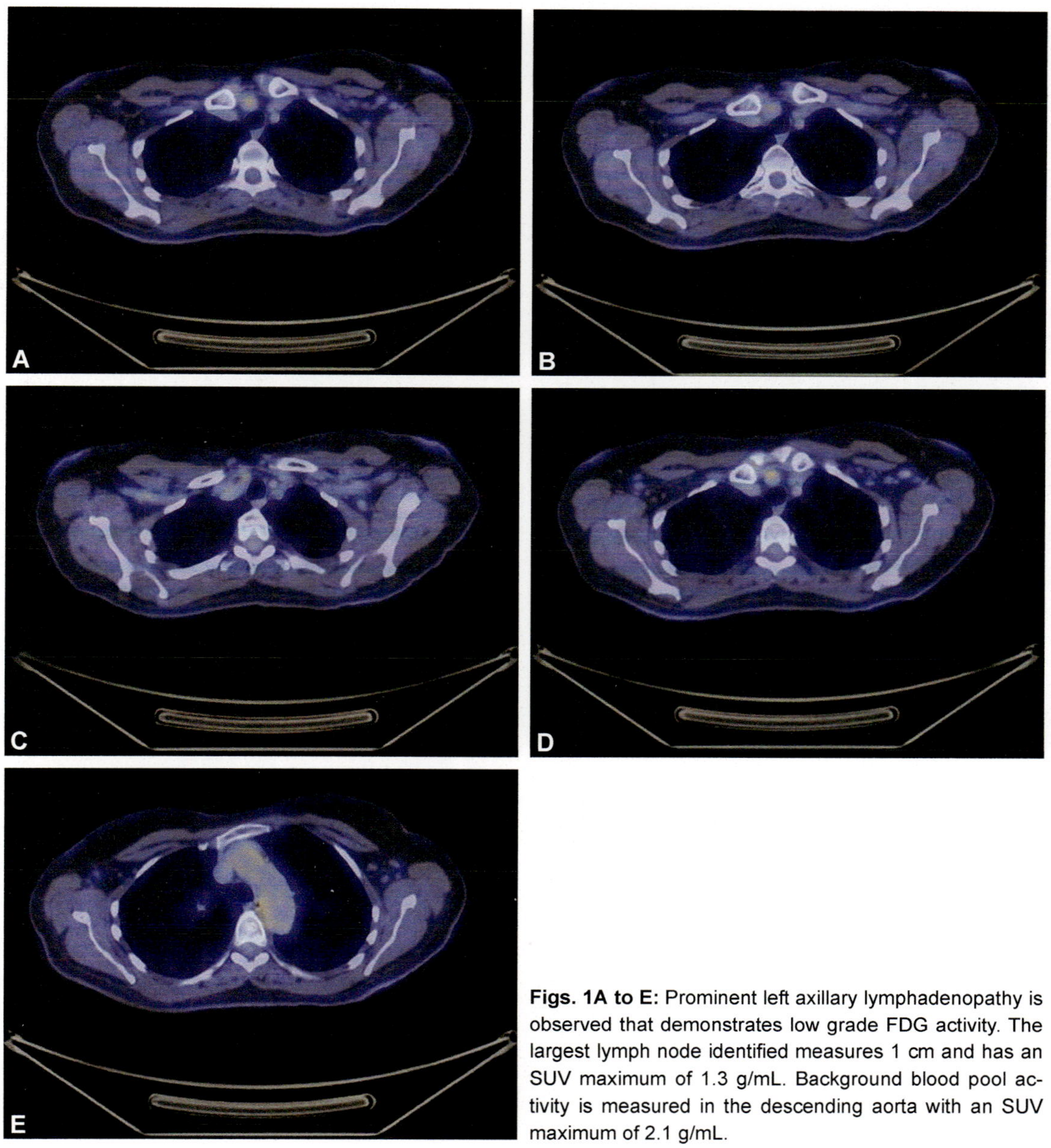

Figs. 1A to E: Prominent left axillary lymphadenopathy is observed that demonstrates low grade FDG activity. The largest lymph node identified measures 1 cm and has an SUV maximum of 1.3 g/mL. Background blood pool activity is measured in the descending aorta with an SUV maximum of 2.1 g/mL.

CASE 13: BENIGN ETIOLOGY WITH SIMILAR APPEARANCE TO CANCER

Brief History

A 46-year-old man with AIDS and Hodgkin's lymphoma, status post chemotherapy, received a follow-up ^{18}F fluorodeoxyglucose (FDG) positron emission tomography/ computed tomography (PET/CT) examination for surveillance of his disease.

Findings

Findings are shown in Figures 1A and B.

The patient subsequently underwent endoscopic biopsy that revealed mild chronic inflammation of the esophageal mucosa.

Main Teaching Points

- Over 30% of patients with AIDS experience esophageal symptoms at some point during their infection.
- Etiology of esophagitis in AIDS:
  - *Common*: Candida, cytomegalovirus (CMV), herpes simplex virus type II, and Idiopathic esophageal ulcer.
  - *Uncommon*: Antiretroviral therapy-induced or gastroesophageal reflux disease.
  - *Rare*: Epstein-Barr virus, Papovavirus, Human herpesvirus 6, *Histoplasma capsulatum, Penicillium chrysogenum, Exophiala jeanselmei, Cryptococcus neoformans, mucormycosis, Aspergillus fumigatus, Cryptosporidium parvum, Leishmania donovani, Pneumocystis carinii, Mycobacterium avium complex, Mycobacterium tuberculosis, Rochalimae henselae, Nocardia asteroides, Actinomyces israelii,* Non-Hodgkin lymphoma, Kaposi sarcoma, squamous cell carcinoma, adenocarcinoma, and lymphomatoid granulomatosis.

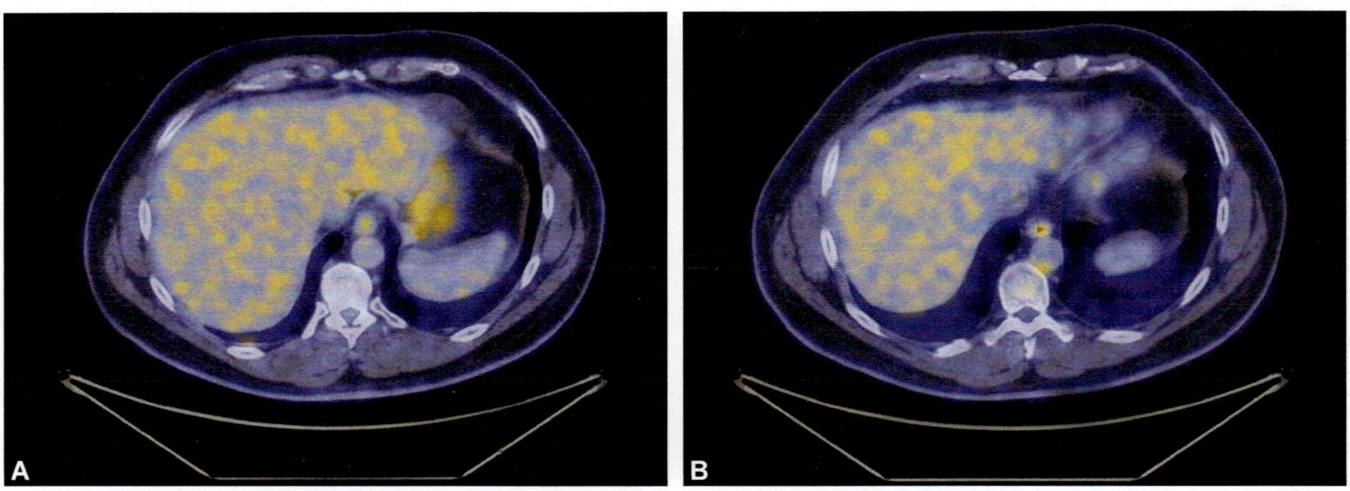

Figs. 1A and B: Incidental diffuse increased activity is observed within the esophageal mucosa, ascending proximally from the gastroesophageal junction. No focal mass or hiatal hernia is identified. (A) Inferior distal esophagus; (B) Superior distal esophagus.

CASE 14: INCIDENTAL BREAST CANCER DURING SURVEILLANCE OF OTHER MALIGNANCIES

Brief History

A 92-year-old female with a history of endometrial cancer underwent ^{18}F fluorodeoxyglucose (FDG) positron emission tomography/computed tomography (PET/CT) imaging for surveillance of her disease.

Findings

Findings are shown in Figures 1 and 2.

Main Teaching Points

- Positron emission tomography/computed tomography carries high sensitivity for the detection of breast malignancy, which can be discovered during routine surveillance for other malignancies.
- When reporting a finding suspicious for new diagnosis breast cancer, clinical correlation should be recommended with physical examination, mammography and biopsy.

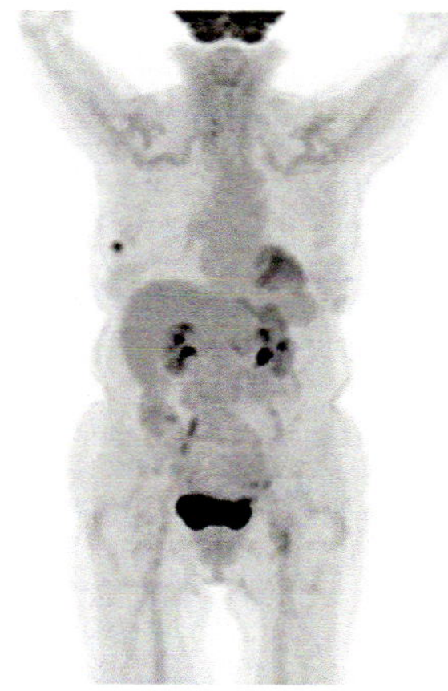

Fig. 1: Maximum intensity projection whole body image demonstrates hazy radiotracer uptake within the pelvis, as well as an intense focus of activity projecting over the right breast.

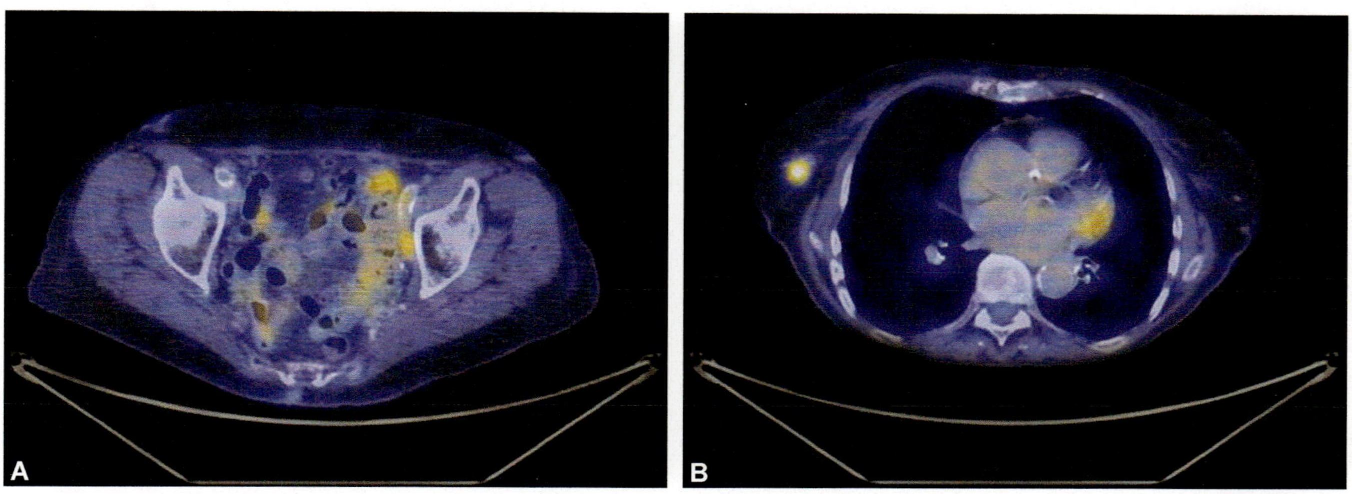

Figs. 2A and B: (A) Diffuse FDG activity is observed throughout the low pelvis with multiple hypermetabolic peritoneal implants, consistent with recurrence of endometrial carcinoma. (B) Within the upper outer quadrant of the right breast, a new hypermetabolic nodule is discovered. The lesion is very superficial and is likely palpable on physical examination.

CASE 15: DISCRIMINATION OF POST-RADIOTHERAPY ESOPHAGEAL TUMOR MASS

Brief History

A 75-year-old female with adenocarcinoma of the distal esophagus underwent preoperative chemoradiation therapy and required ^{18}F fluorodeoxyglucose (FDG) positron emission tomography/computed tomography (PET/CT) for restaging of her disease.

Findings

Findings are shown in Figures 1A to D.

Main Teaching Points

- Computed tomography evaluation of the distal esophagus can be limited due to compression by adjacent structures and lack of intraluminal contrast.
- Malignancy that presents as subtle esophageal wall thickening by CT can have striking metabolic activity on PET imaging.

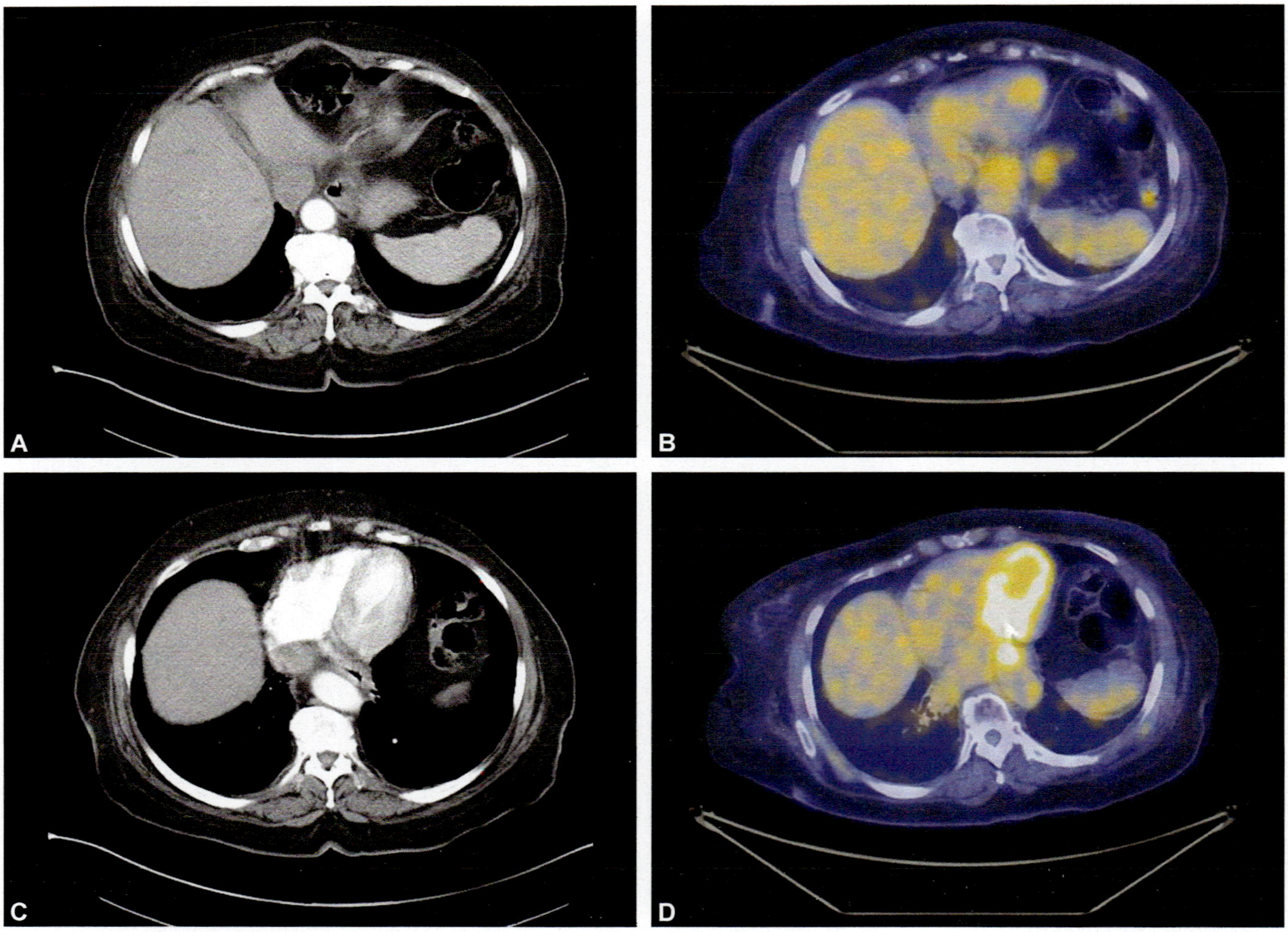

Figs. 1A to D: Borderline thickening of the esophageal wall is noted by contrast computed tomography (CT) with no discrete mass or abnormality identified. The separate noncontrast positron emission tomography (PET/CT) study shows significant FDG accumulation in the distal esophagus and gastroesophageal junction, consistent with the biopsy-proven malignancy. (A) Contrast CT of gastroesophageal junction; (B) PET/CT of gastroesophageal junction; (C) Contrast CT of distal esophagus; (D) PET/CT of distal esophagus.

CASE 16: COMPLEMENTARY ROLE OF BONE SCAN AND POSITRON EMISSION TOMOGRAPHY/ COMPUTED TOMOGRAPHY (PET/CT) FINDINGS IN BREAST CANCER

Brief History

A 73-year-old female with breast cancer, status post-mastectomy and adjuvant chemotherapy, developed increasing back pain after several years of being clinically disease free. Bone scan revealed two foci of uptake within the T8 and T11 vertebral bodies suspicious for osseous recurrence of malignancy. She subsequently underwent ^{18}F fluorodeoxyglucose (FDG) PET/CT imaging for restaging of her disease.

Findings

Findings are shown in Figures 1 to 4.

Main Teaching Points

- Bone scan imaging is highly sensitive for detecting increased osseous turnover and is a useful screening tool in patients with bone pain and an oncologic history.
- High resolution PET/CT can be used to further characterize positive findings on bone scan and can uncover additional metastatic foci in recurrent malignancies that present only with new bone pain.

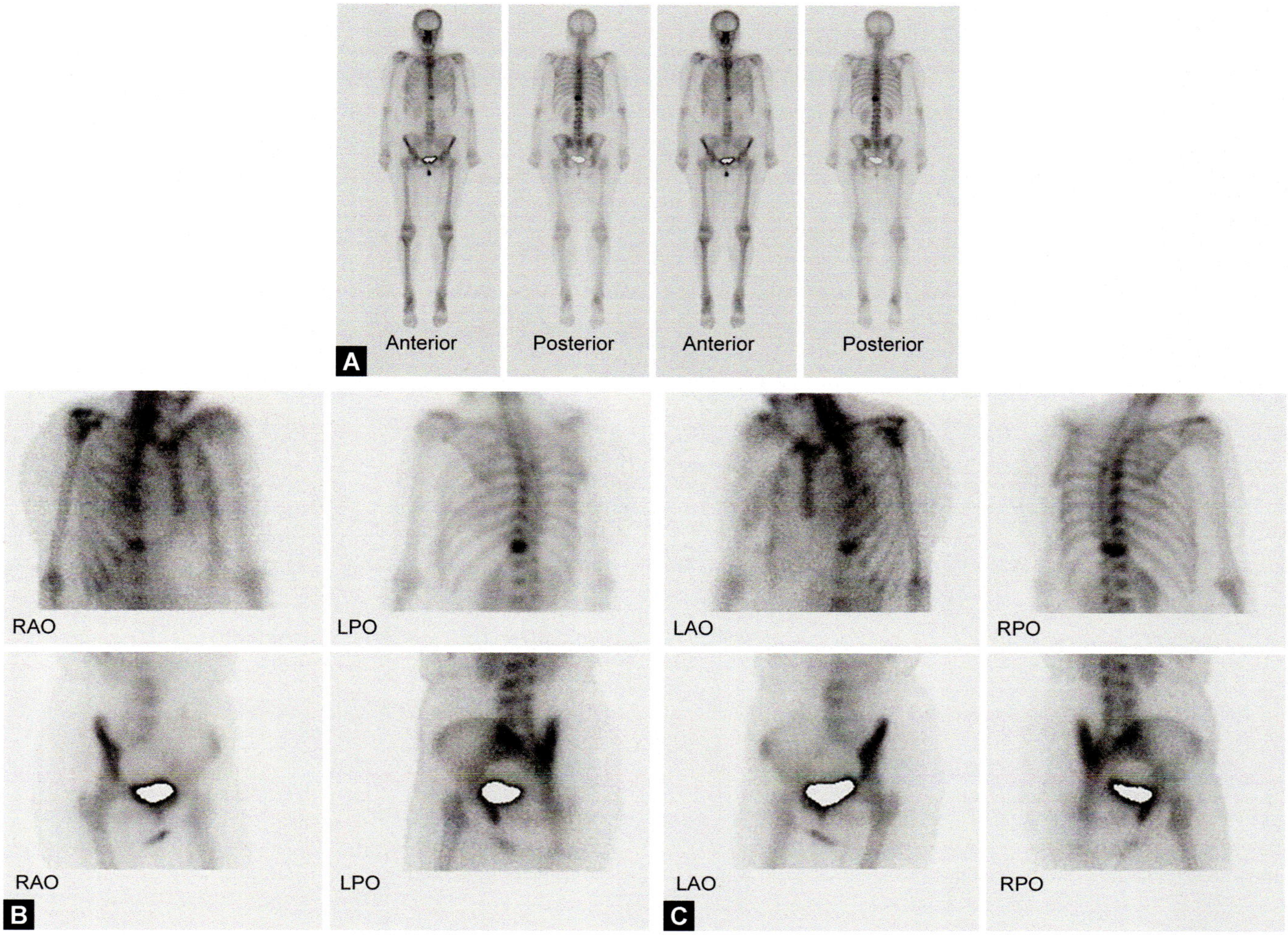

Figs. 1A to C: Prior bone scan demonstrating significant osseous turnover in the T11 vertebral body with a subtle focus of uptake within the T8 vertebral body.

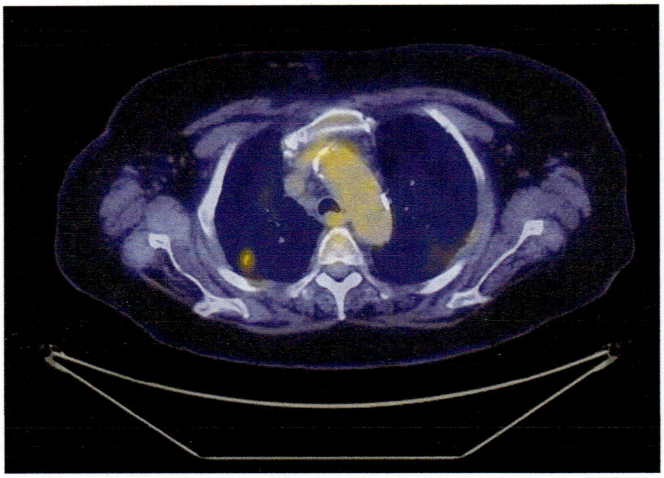

Fig. 2: By positron emission tomography/computed tomography, a large hypermetabolic sclerotic lesion is identified encompassing the entire T11 vertebral body, which is highly concerning for recurrent breast carcinoma.

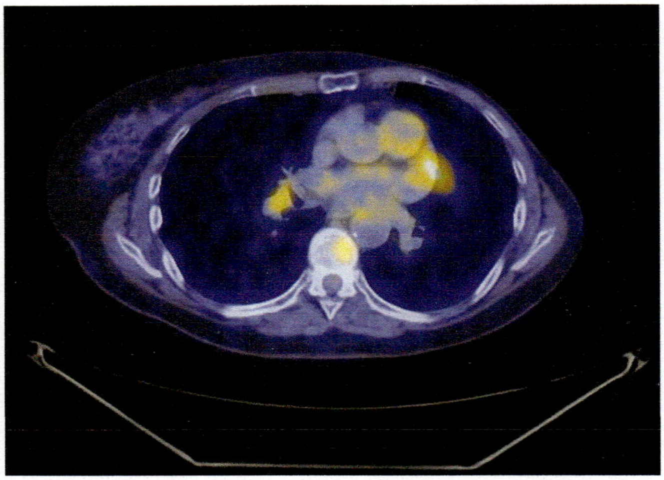

Fig. 3: The T8 vertebral body contains a smaller hypermetabolic focus representing a second bone metastasis.

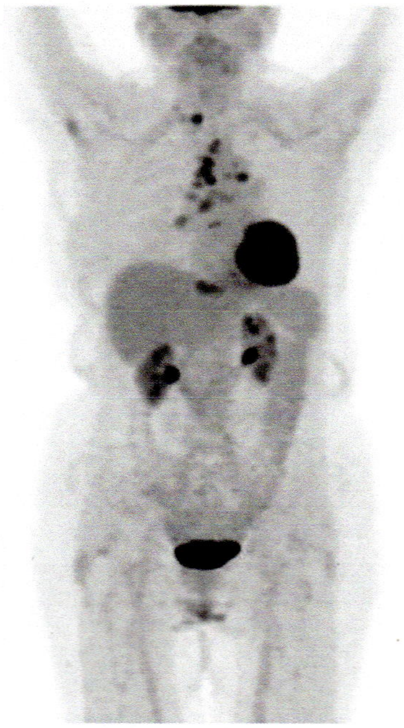

Fig. 4: Significant hypermetabolic mediastinal lymphadenopathy was also discovered.

CASE 17: PHYSIOLOGIC OVARIAN ACTIVITY

Brief History

A 49-year-old female with breast cancer status postsurgical resection and chemotherapy presented for surveillance imaging of her disease.

Findings

Findings are shown in Figures 1 to 4.

Main Teaching Points

- Physiologic ovarian activity can be appreciated in premenopausal women as diffuse homogenous bilateral ^{18}F fluorodeoxyglucose (FDG) accumulation. Occasionally, an active follicle can be seen. Recommending clinical correlation with menstrual cycle is useful, and if any suspicion remains, pelvic ultrasound can be pursued for further characterization.
- If follow-up positron emission tomography/computed tomography (PET/CT) imaging is scheduled on an off-cycle date, often resolution of ovarian activity is observed.

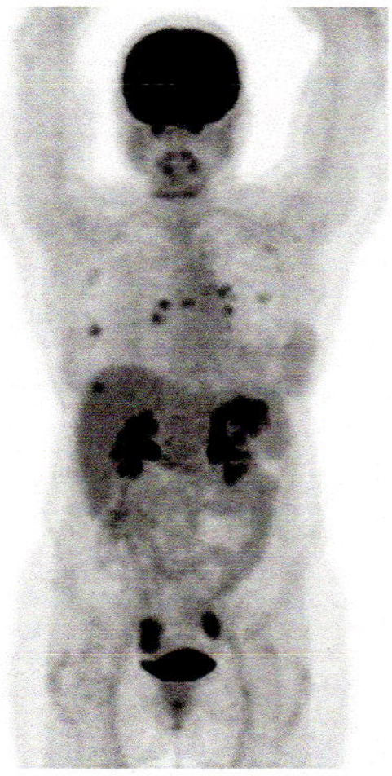

Fig. 1: Maximum intensity projection whole body image demonstrates multiple small foci of radiotracer uptake projecting over the chest. Two larger foci are seen within the pelvis.

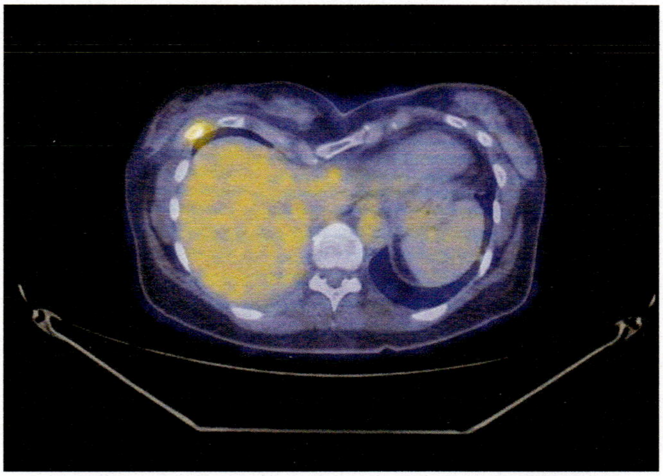

Fig. 2: Multiple worrisome FDG-avid foci are identified in the ribs and mediastinal lymph nodes. No abnormal FDG uptake is seen inferior to this rib at the level of the diaphragm.

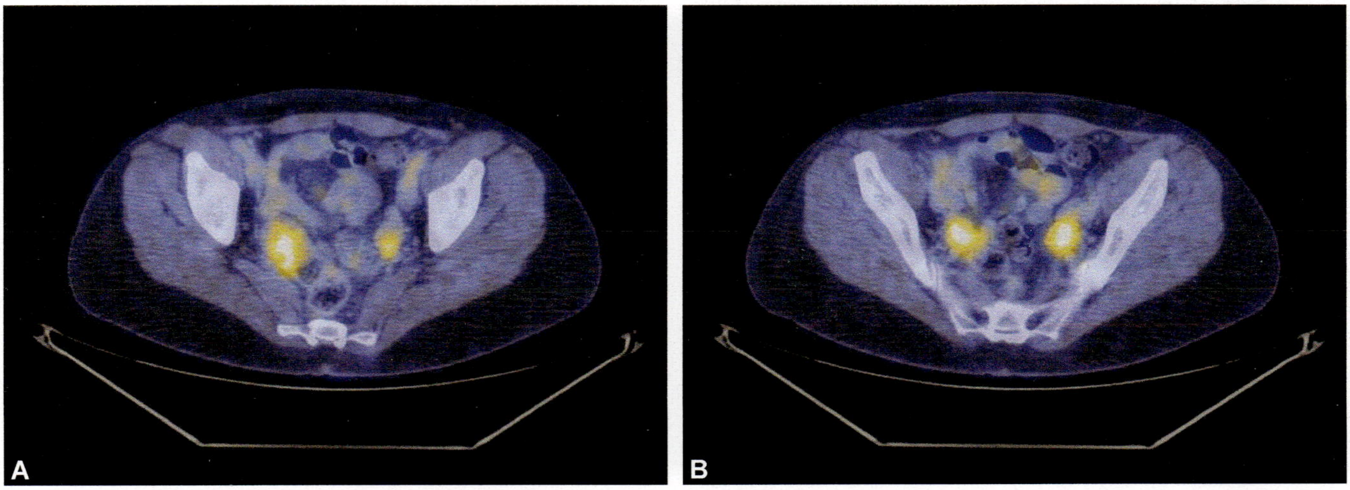

Figs. 3A and B: Significant physiologic FDG accumulation is noted in the bilateral ovaries.

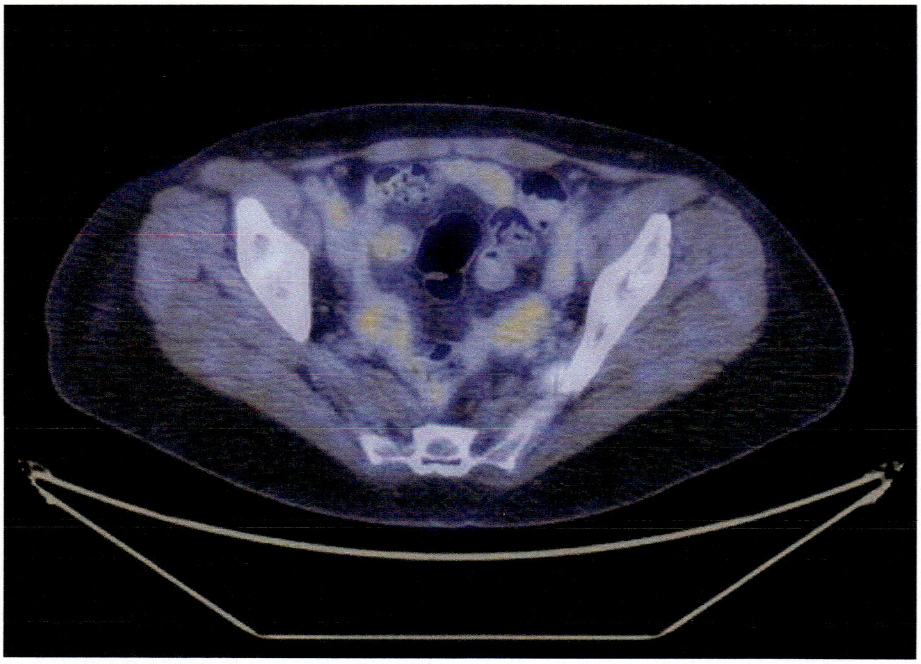

Fig. 4: Follow-up positron emission tomography/computed tomography 10 weeks later reveals resolution of ovarian activity.

CASE 18: INITIAL STAGING OF LYMPHOMA

Brief History

A 14-year-old male with new diagnosis of nodular sclerosing Hodgkin's disease underwent ^{18}F fluorodeoxyglucose (FDG) positron emission tomography/computed tomography (PET/CT) imaging for initial staging of his disease.

Findings

Findings are shown in Figures 1 to 4.

Main Teaching Points

- ^{18}F fluorodeoxyglucose (FDG) PET/CT is an effective diagnostic tool for initial staging of many malignancies, and can help in assessment of candidacy for external beam radiation therapy.
- Demonstration of distant metastasis below th diaphragm is important both prognostically and for management decisions.

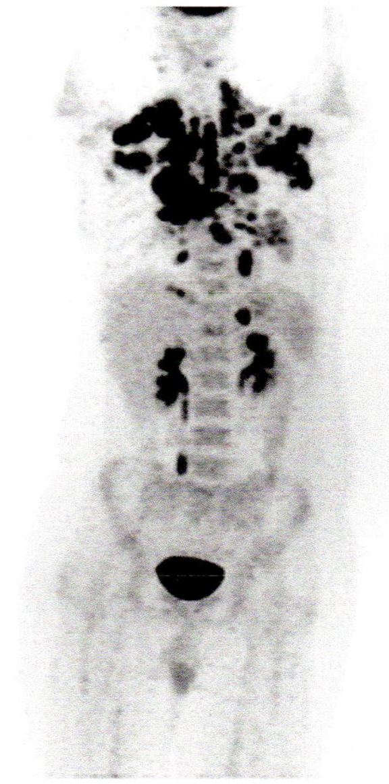

Fig. 1: Maximum intensity projection whole body image demonstrates extensive hypermetabolic adenopathy projecting over the lower neck and upper chest. Focal radiotracer activity is also noted in the region of the left adrenal gland.

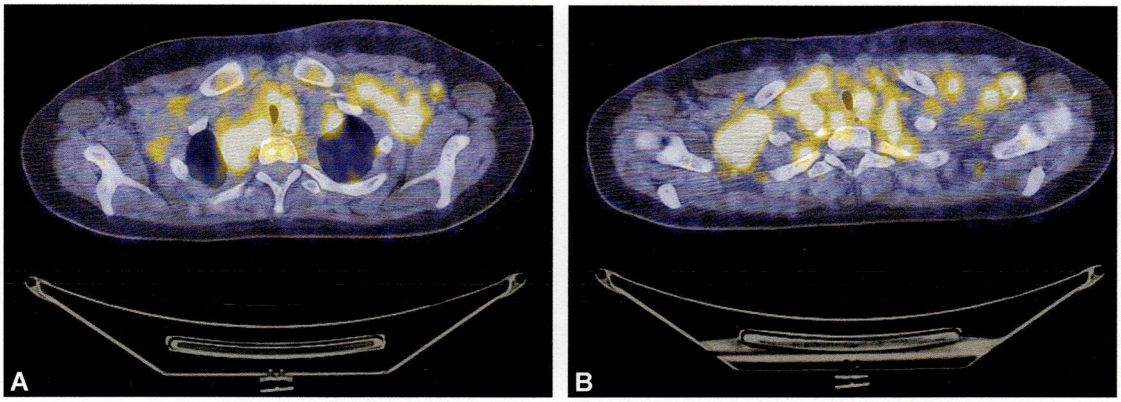

Figs. 2A and B: Significant hypermetabolic lymphadenopathy is identified throughout the lower neck and upper mediastinum.

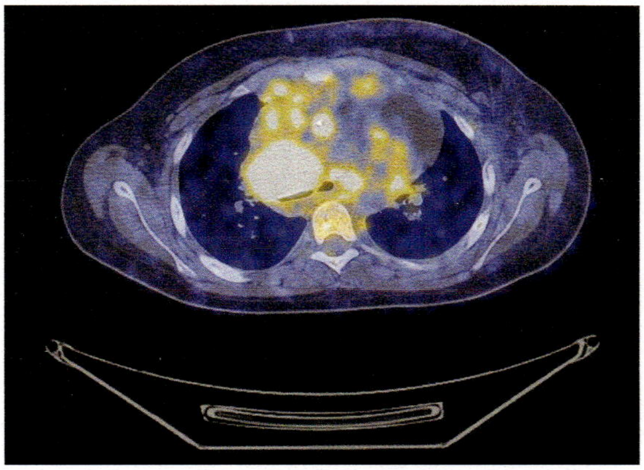

Fig. 3: A massive conglomeration of malignant soft tissue is abutting the right heart in the mediastinum and is causing compression by mass effect on the right mainstem bronchus.

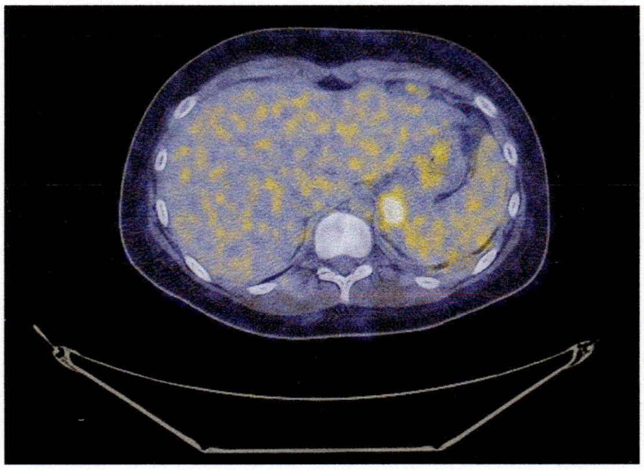

Fig. 4: A large periadrenal lymph node offers evidence of metastatic disease below the diaphragm.

CASE 19: EVALUATION OF RESPONSE TO LYMPHOMA THERAPY

Brief History

A 12-year-old female with Hodgkin's lymphoma of the right neck underwent systemic chemotherapy and required ^{18}F fluorodeoxyglucose (FDG) positron emission tomography/computed tomography (PET/CT) imaging to evaluate her response.

Findings

Findings are shown in Figures 1 to 4.

Main Teaching Points

- ^{18}F fluorodeoxyglucose (FDG) PET/CT is a useful tool to follow the pathological response to chemotherapy.
- Brown fat activation is a physiologic mechanism to generate body heat and can present as a characteristic scattered pattern of intense FDG accumulation through the neck and upper chest. Radiotracer activity is localized to adipose tissue by CT. This phenomenon can decrease the sensitivity for detecting small adjacent malignancy and can be avoided by keeping the patient warm during the uptake portion of the examination.

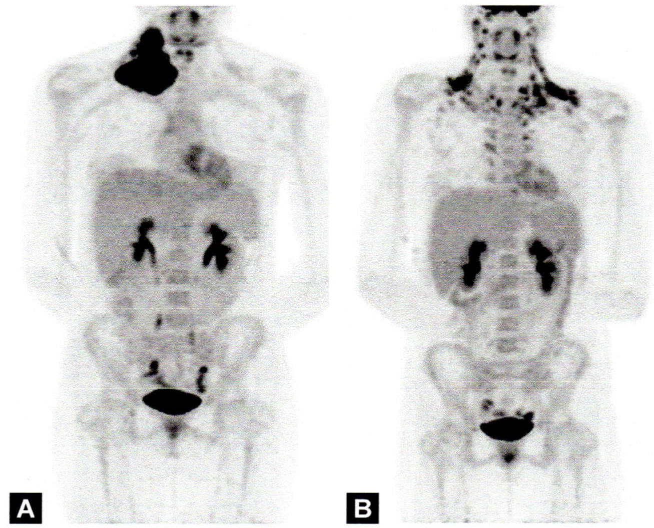

Figs. 1A and B: Baseline maximum intensity projection whole body image obtained prior to chemotherapy demonstrates bulky hypermetabolic adenopathy in the right neck. (1B) Post chemotherapy image shows significant reduction in size of the baseline disease, but new symmetrical bilateral cervical uptake has appeared.

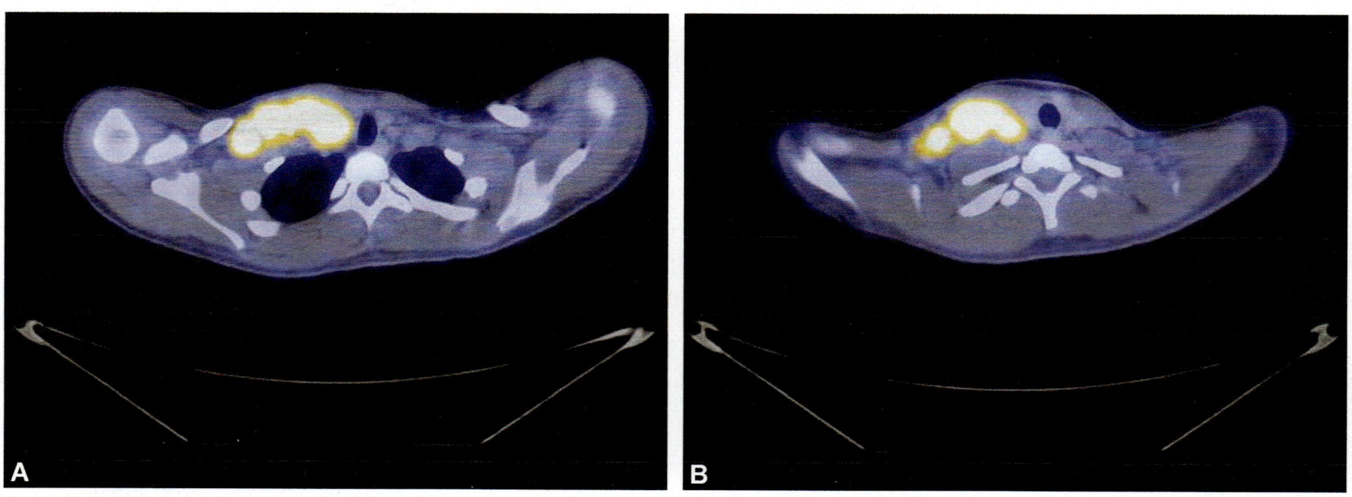

Figs. 2A and B

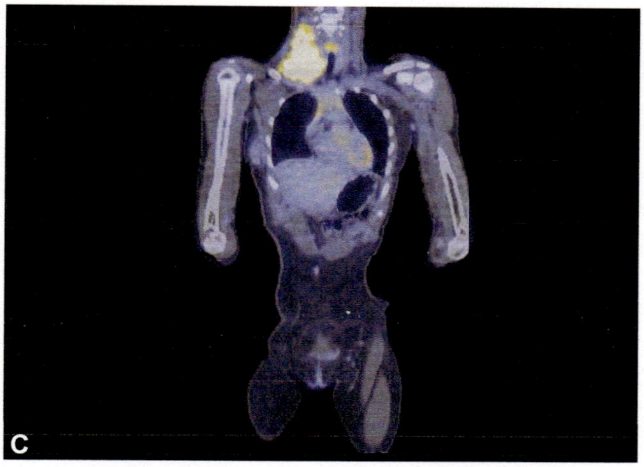

Figs. 2A to C: Baseline FDG positron emission tomography/computed tomography (PET/CT) imaging demonstrates hypermetabolic bulky lymphadenopathy within the right neck extending inferiorly to the supraclavicular region.

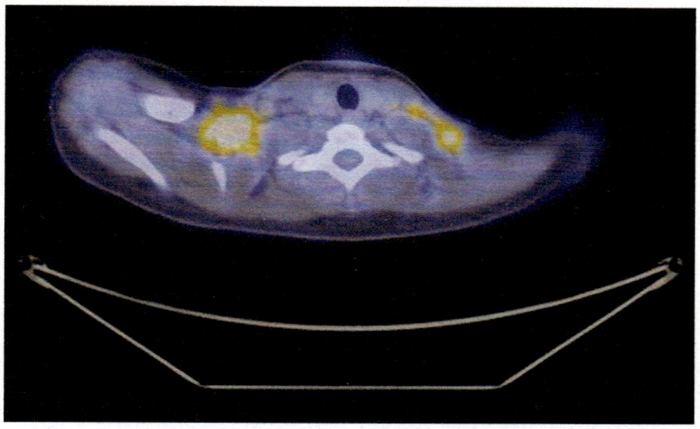

Fig. 3: Following two cycles of chemotherapy, dramatic improvement in size and FDG activity of the persistent primary mass is demonstrated on follow-up positron emission tomography/computed tomography (PET/CT) imaging.

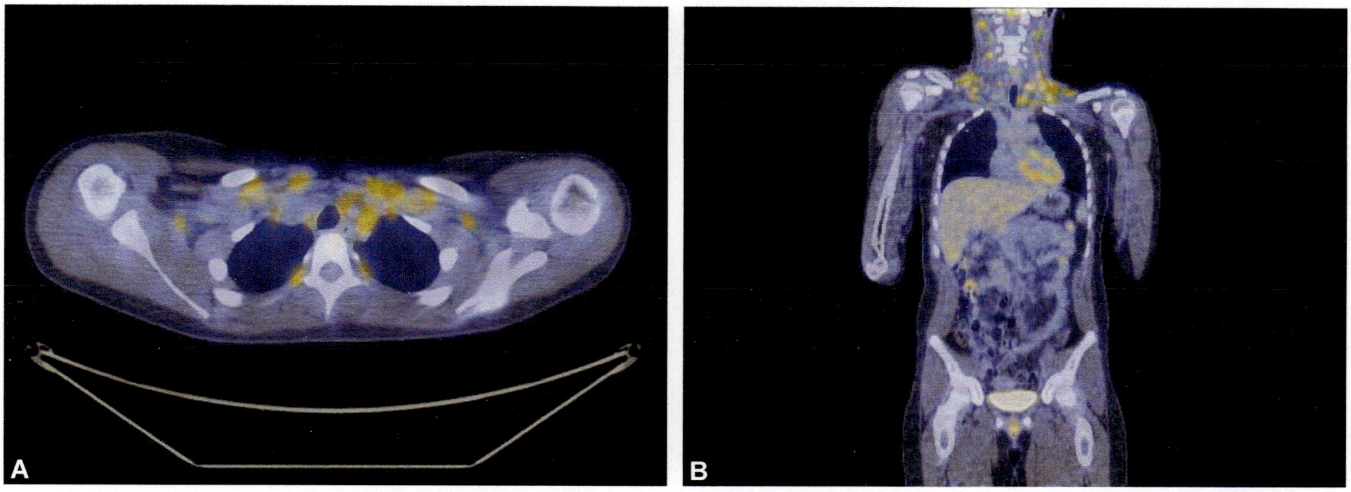

Figs. 4A and B: However, extensive brown fat activation is seen throughout the neck that presents as scattered FDG activity localizing within cervical adipose tissue. Other than the smaller persistent primary mass, no additional concerning foci were identified suspicious for progression of disease.

CASE 20: LYMPHOMA WITH SPLENIC INVOLVEMENT

Brief History

A 22-year-old male with Hodgkin's lymphoma presented for ^{18}F fluorodeoxyglucose (FDG) positron emission tomography/computed tomography (PET/CT) imaging for initial evaluation of his disease.

Findings

Findings are shown in Figures 1 and 2.

Main Teaching Points

- Focal or dramatically heterogenous FDG avidity of the spleen favors malignant involvement.
- Diffuse and homogenous splenic uptake can often be seen with aggressive chemotherapy regimens, especially after induction.
- Bone marrow rebound is a common finding in patients receiving aggressive chemotherapy regimens.

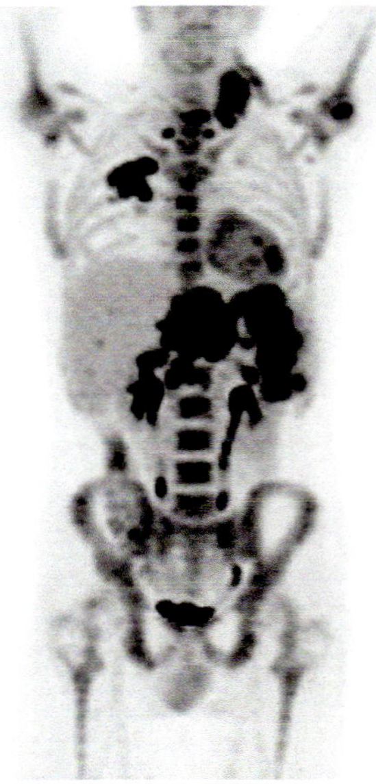

Fig. 1: Maximum intensity projection whole body image demonstrates numerous bulky hypermetabolic foci projecting over the chest and upper abdomen. Irregular focal uptake is noted in the left upper quadrant abdomen projecting over the spleen.

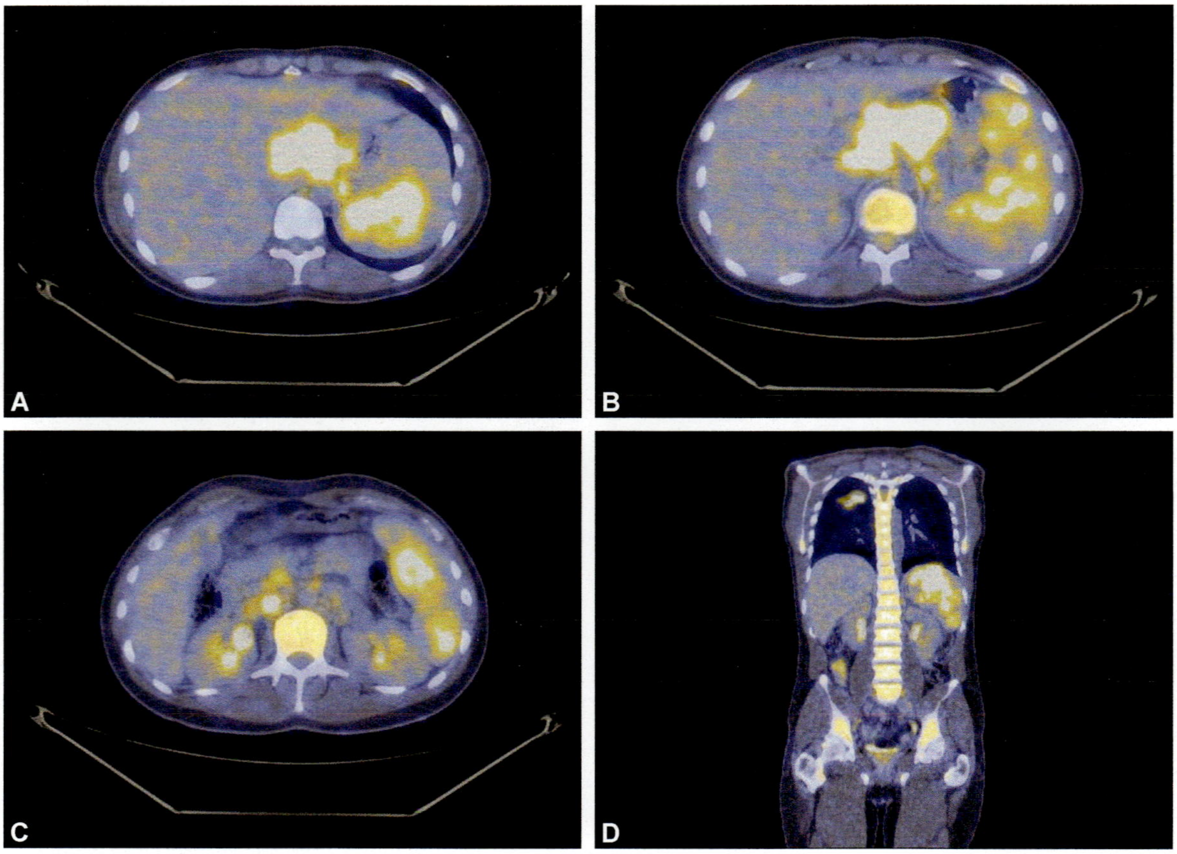

Figs. 2A to D: Multiple large areas of active disease are identified within the left neck, supraclavicular region, mediastinum, abdomen and pelvis. Prominent splenomegaly is seen with multiple hypermetabolic foci within the splenic parenchyma, representing diffuse splenic involvement of lymphoma. Incidental note is made of diffuse homogenous bone marrow activity, consistent with chemotherapy-related bone marrow rebound.

CASE 21: THYMIC REBOUND

Brief History

A 31-year-old male with history of non-small cell lung cancer status post left lower lobectomy and recent completion of chemotherapy underwent ^{18}F fluorodeoxyglucose (FDG) positron emission tomography/computed tomography (PET/CT) for reevaluation of his disease.

Findings

Findings are shown in Figures 1 and 2.

Main Teaching Points

- Thymic rebound is a hypertrophic glandular response that can be seen in patients with severe body surface burns, malignancy, or following chemotherapy. Most commonly, it is observed in young children or adolescents, and is relatively rare within the adult population.
- Increased hypermetabolic substernal soft tissue can be observed by FDG PET/CT due to active cell metabolism and glandular growth.
- Resolution of hypertrophy and hypermetabolism can take months to years to appreciate.

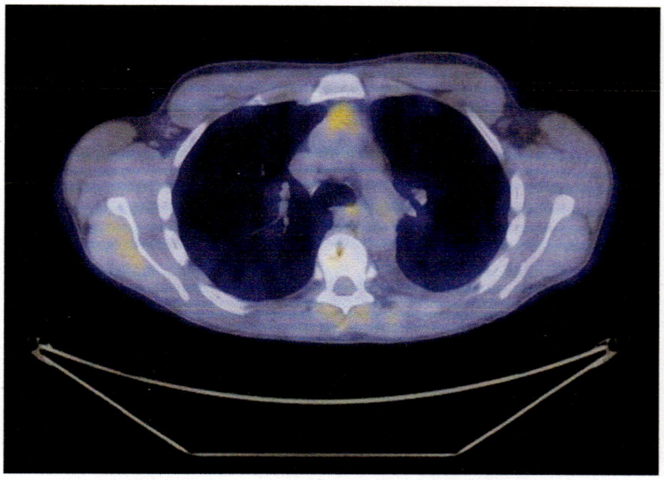

Fig. 1: Increased activity is seen within a hypertrophied thymus gland on images immediately following chemotherapy treatment.

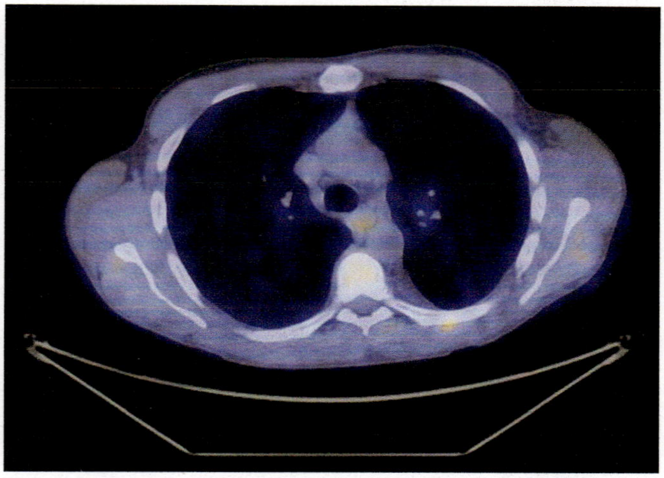

Fig. 2: Three months later, the finding has resolved.

CASE 22: LYMPHOMATOUS INVOLVEMENT OF BONE MARROW

Brief History

A 33-year-old male recently diagnosed with Hodgkin's lymphoma with computed tomography (CT) evidence of lytic osseous lesions underwent ^{18}F fluorodeoxyglucose (FDG) positron emission tomography/computed tomography (PET/CT) imaging to confirm malignant involvement.

Findings

Findings are shown in Figures 1 to 4.

Main Teaching Points

- ^{18}F fluorodeoxyglucose (FDG) PET/CT is a useful tool to confirm malignant involvement in a suspicious appearing lesion on CT and can also often unveil additional disease that has subtle or no anatomic correlate.
- Bone marrow rebound is increased hematopoietic metabolism secondary to increased demand from chemotherapy suppression. Rebound will often have the appearance of diffuse and homogenously intense FDG accumulation in all bone marrow of the axial and appendicular skeleton without evidence of lytic or sclerotic correlate. Heterogenous bone marrow uptake with anatomic distortion favors malignant involvement.

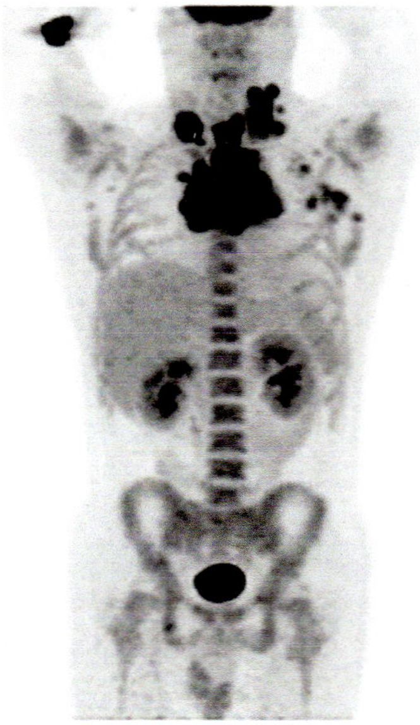

Fig. 1: Maximum intensity projection whole body image demonstrates extensive radiotracer uptake projecting over the mediastinum, lower neck, left chest and left axilla.

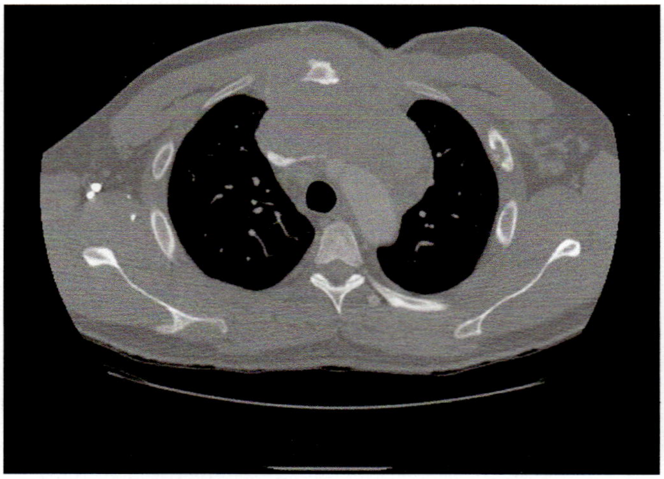

Fig. 2: In addition to bulky mediastinal lymphadenopathy, initial staging CT revealed a lytic lesion of the left third rib.

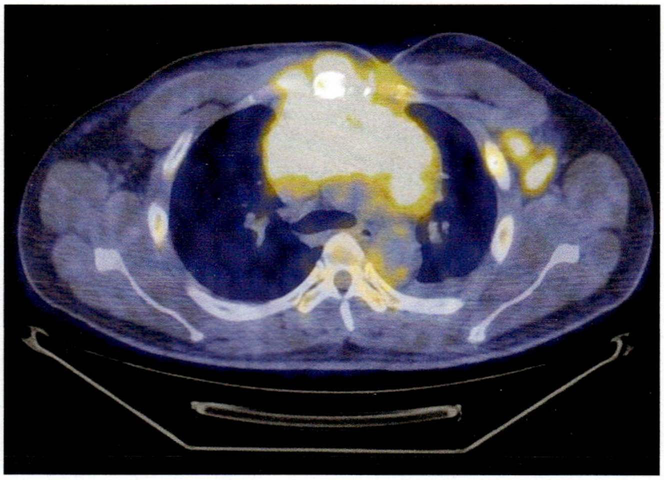

Fig. 3: Intense radiotracer accumulation is observed at this location on positron emission tomography/computed tomography (PET/CT) images, confirming lymphomatous involvement of bone marrow.

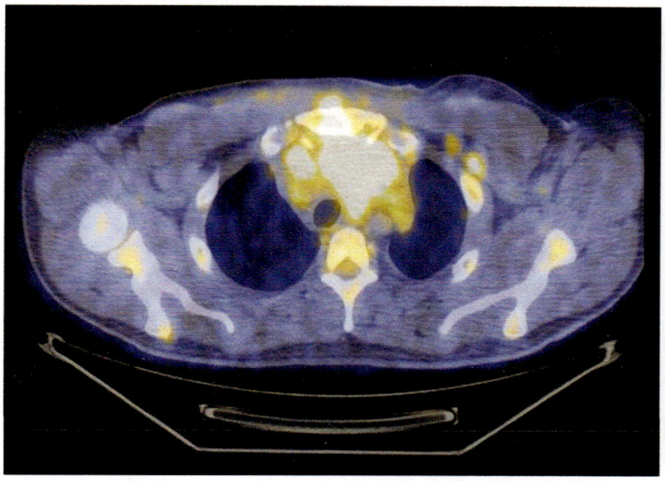

Fig. 4: Additional sites of patchy bone marrow involvement were identified within the scapulae and axial skeleton. No observable CT correlate was seen for these lesions.

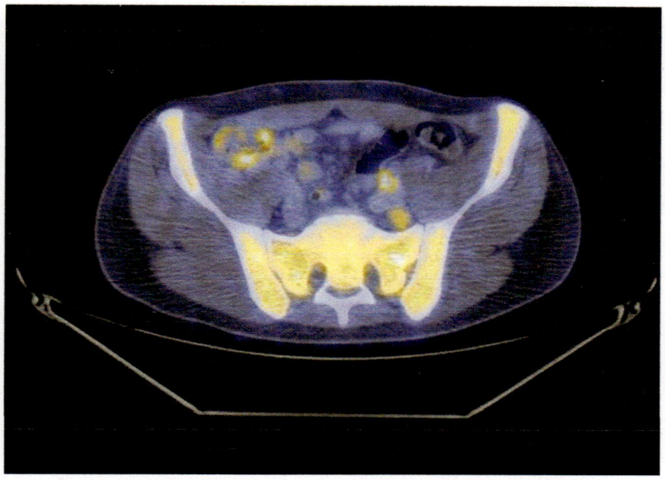

Fig. 5: In contrast to patchy, solitary or multifocal pattern of uptake seen with active lymphomatous involvement, marrow rebound secondary to chemotherapy or bone marrow stimulants is generally homogenous. For the latter pattern, diffuse bone marrow involvement with lymphoma will of course be in the differential diagnosis. Careful and detailed clinical history clearly will help in this differentiation.

CASE 23: MUSCULAR INVOLVEMENT OF LYMPHOMA

Brief History

A 55-year-old female presented with a pathologic fracture of the left tibia and was subsequently found to have diffuse metastatic lymphoma. She underwent ^{18}F fluorodeoxy-glucose (FDG) positron emission tomography (PET/CT) imaging for initial staging of her disease.

Findings

Findings are shown in Figures 1 and 2.

Main Teaching Points

- Primary muscular lymphoma is a rare condition that systemically metastasizes in the minority of patients. Most cases of lymphomatous muscular involvement are secondary to metastasis from a separate primary tumor.
- Adequate patient resting during the radiotracer uptake period will minimize physiologic muscle activity. This is particularly key to optimizing the sensitivity of detecting subtle lymphomatous musculature involvement.
- Sites of potential future pathologic fracture in weight-bearing bones are of orthopedic significance and should be clearly reported in the examination.

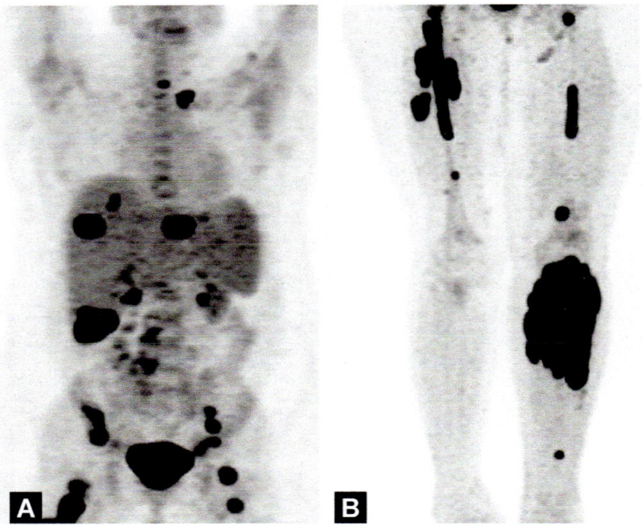

Figs. 1A and B: Maximum intensity projection whole body images demonstrate disseminated metastatic disease involving bone, liver and numerous lymph node stations. The most prominent area of uptake projects over the left proximal tibia.

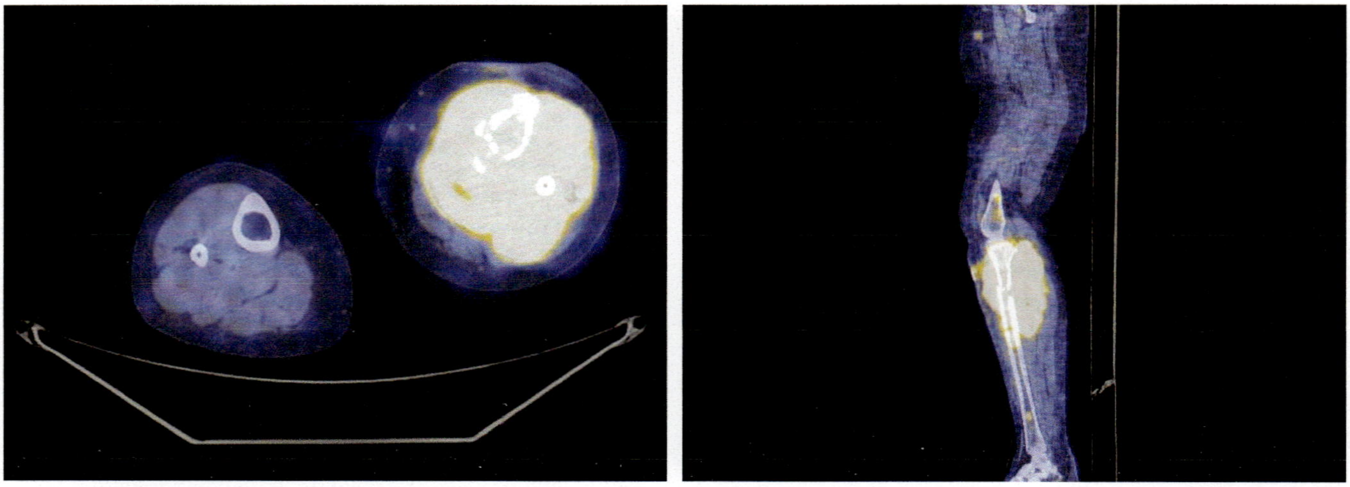

Fig. 2: A comminuted pathologic fracture is identified in the left proximal tibia, with extensive lymphomatous involvement of the adjacent musculature. Smaller bilateral femoral metastases are also present without evidence of cortical disruption, which are reported as sites at risk for future fractures.

CASE 24: PROGNOSTIC VALUE OF ^{18}F FLUORODEOXYGLUCOSE (FDG) POSITRON EMISSION TOMOGRAPHY/COMPUTED TOMOGRAPHY (PET/CT) AFTER A SINGLE CYCLE OF CHEMOTHERAPY

Brief History

A 59-year-old male with non-Hodgkin's lymphoma of the left neck status post a single cycle of CHOP-R chemotherapy underwent baseline FDG positron emission tomography (PET/CT) imaging to evaluate his disease.

Findings

Findings are shown in Figures 1 to 4.

Additional imaging was performed that followed the patient to complete remission after completion of chemotherapy.

Main Teaching Points

- Positron emission tomography/computed tomography (PET/CT) has been shown to have prognostic value to assess early metabolic response to a single cycle of standard chemotherapy in both breast cancer and lymphoma.
- Further research is currently underway to establish guidelines to alter management in cases where failure of early metabolic response to chemotherapy is observed.

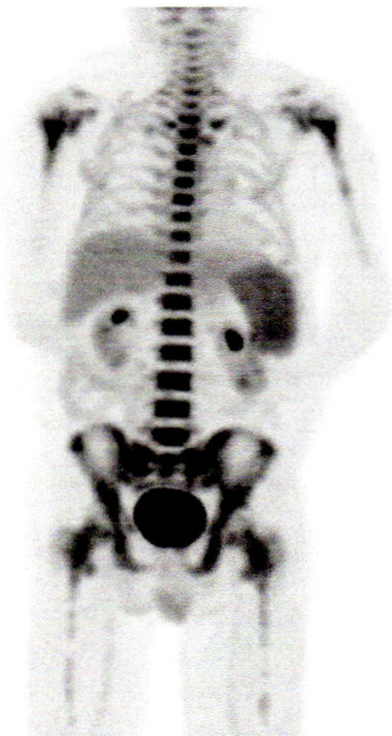

Fig. 1: Initial radiologic workup included computed tomography (CT) imaging of the neck, which demonstrates a large aggressive mass invading numerous left neck structures.

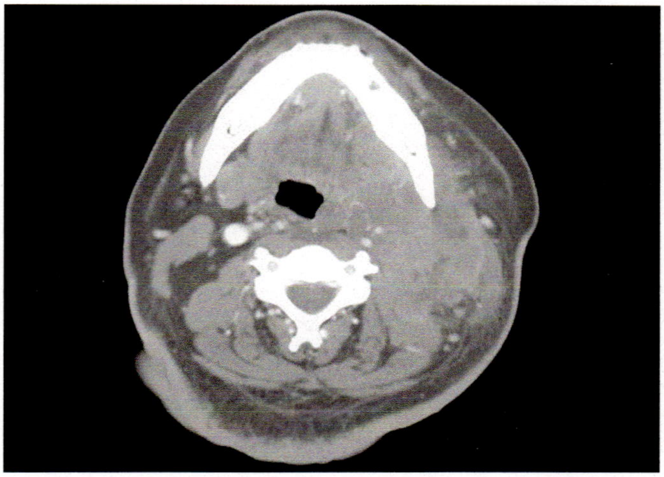

Fig. 2: Maximum intensity projection whole body image obtained after a single cycle of chemotherapy demonstrates hazy asymmetrical uptake over the left neck.

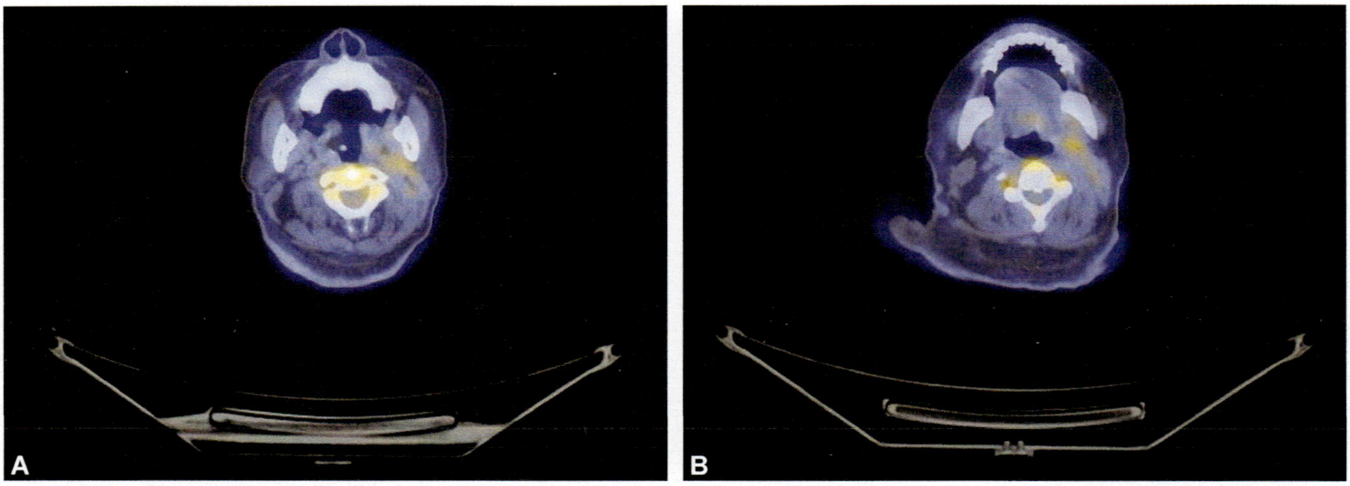

Figs. 3A and B: Transaxial positron emission tomography/computed tomography (PET/CT) images of the neck obtained after a single cycle of chemotherapy demonstrate significant regression of the left neck mass. Mildly increased radiotracer uptake is present within the remaining tumor volume, suggestive of residual active disease.

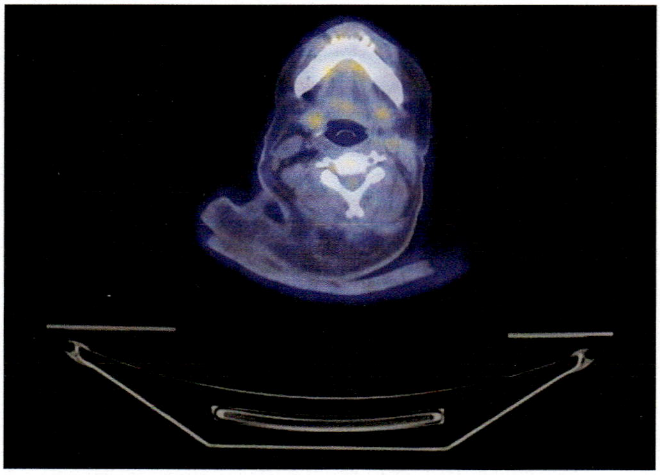

Fig. 4: Three months later, the patient has completed eight cycles of chemotherapy and is reimaged by positron emission tomography/computed tomography (PET/CT). Continued improvement of hypermetabolism is seen within the residual mass, consistent with favorable response to therapy. Additional serial imaging was subsequently obtained that followed the patient to complete remission after completion of chemotherapy.

CASE 25: RECURRENT MALIGNANT MELANOMA

Brief History

A 49-year-old male with malignant melanoma of the left back status post negative margin wide local excision and negative sentinel lymph node biopsy presents after 4 years of remission with subcutaneous nodularity over the surgical site. He subsequently underwent FDG positron emission tomography/computed tomography (PET/CT) imaging for evaluation of recurrent disease.

Findings

Findings are shown in Figures 1 and 2.

Main Teaching Points

- Local recurrence of malignant melanoma is a concerning event and is often associated with low 10-year survival and systemic metastases.
- When recurrent malignant melanoma is clinically suspected, PET/CT imaging is highly sensitive to confirm clinical suspicions and survey for systemic disease.

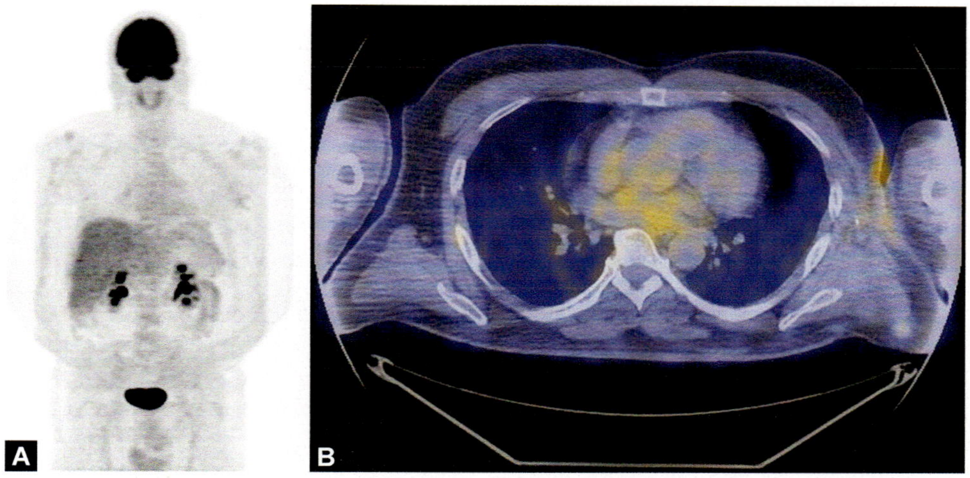

Figs. 1A and B: The immediate postoperative positron emission tomography/computed tomography (PET/CT) examination demonstrates expected postoperative changes in the left back and axilla consistent with recent surgery. No distant metastasis is identified.

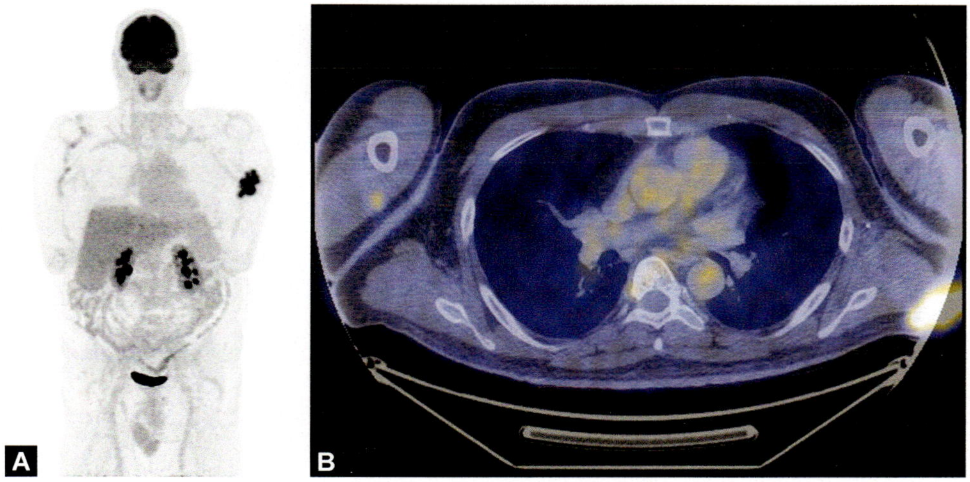

Figs. 2A and B: Four years later, follow-up positron emission tomography/computed tomography (PET/CT) demonstrates an intensely hypermetabolic soft tissue density in the postoperative bed, consistent with recurrent melanoma.

CASE 26: ADRENAL METASTASIS

Brief History

A 56-year-old female with non-small cell lung cancer status post left upper lobectomy underwent FDG positron emission tomography/computed tomography (PET/CT) for surveillance of her disease.

Findings

Findings are shown in Figures 1 and 2.

Main Teaching Points

- Unilateral adrenal uptake can be due to metastasis, benign adenoma, or adrenal primary malignancy.
- When the adrenal Standard Uptake Value (SUV) maximum measurement exceeds that of liver, primary malignancy or metastasis is a more likely concern.

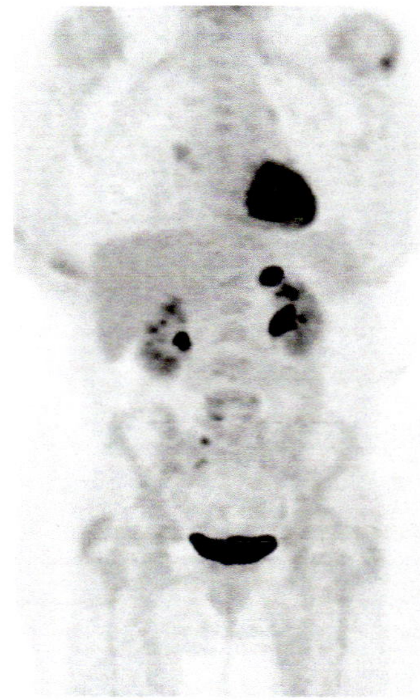

Fig. 1: Maximum intensity projection whole body image demonstrates focal radiotracer activity within the left adrenal gland.

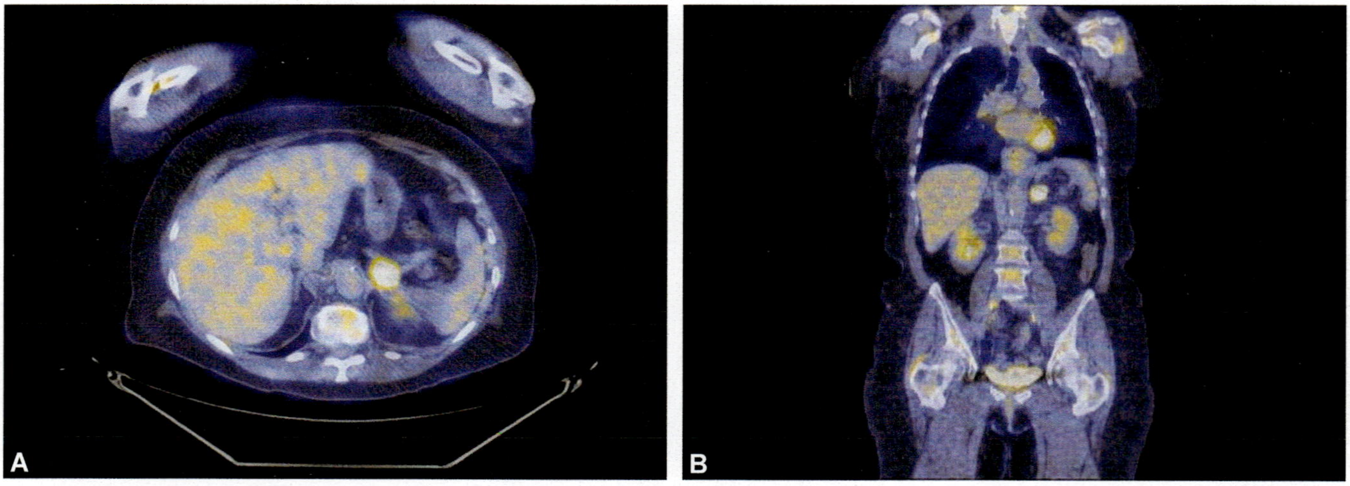

Figs. 2A and B: Intense focal radiotracer accumulation is identified in an enlarged left adrenal gland. This activity is visually greater than liver and is therefore worrisome for adrenal malignancy. Subsequent left adrenalectomy revealed recurrent non-small cell lung carcinoma.

CASE 27: PLEOMORPHIC SARCOMA

Brief History

A 53-year-old male with history of left neck pleomorphic sarcoma of unknown primary underwent excision and left extended radical neck dissection. Postoperatively, he underwent FDG positron emission tomography/computed tomography (PET/CT) for primary tumor localization and disease staging.

Findings

Findings are shown in Figures 1 to 3.

Main Teaching Points

- Due to local inflammatory changes, the sensitivity of PET/CT for evaluation of residual tumor in a recently postoperative bed is low.
- Positron emission tomography/computed tomography (PET/CT) imaging is useful for surveying for an unknown primary tumor and identifying foci of disease that have benign CT appearance.

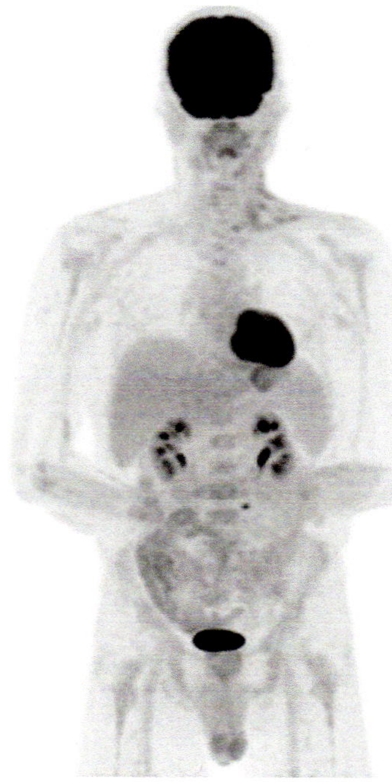

Fig. 1: Maximum intensity projection whole body image demonstrates mild asymmetrical radiotracer uptake projecting over the left neck. A tiny focus of activity is also seen within the left mid abdomen.

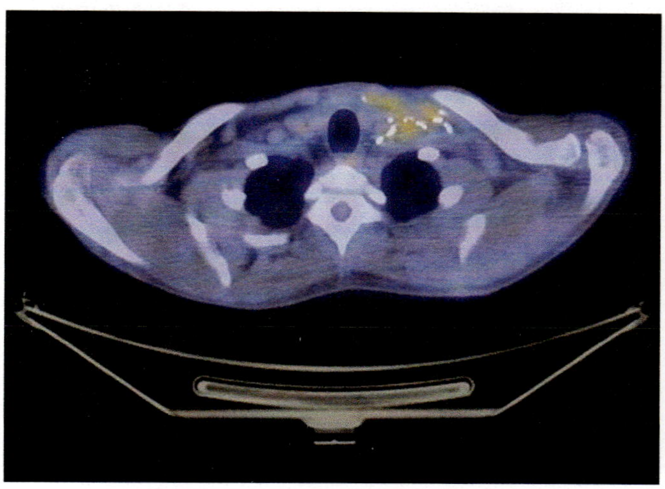

Fig. 2: Postsurgical changes and expected inflammatory FDG accumulation are observed in the postoperative bed in the left neck.

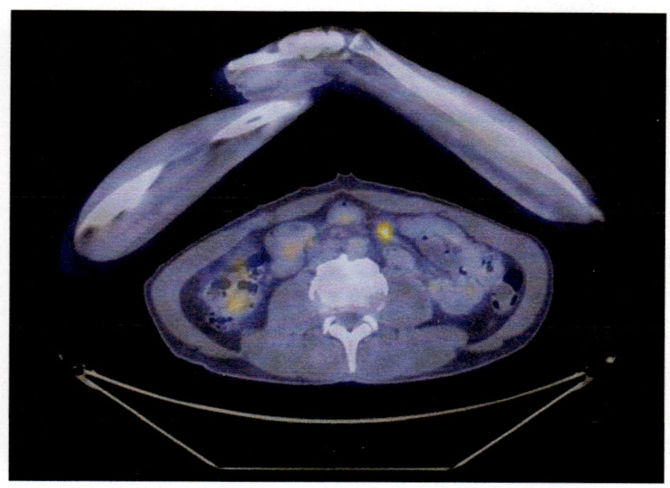

Fig. 3: The remainder of the examination is unremarkable except for a solitary focally intense hypermetabolic soft tissue deposit within the abdomen. The subcentimeter lesion is outside the gastrointestinal tract with fat planes separating it from adjacent structures. Due to its small size, it slightly favors metastasis over primary tumor.

CASE 28: BENIGN MUSCLE ACTIVITY

Brief History

A 48-year-old male presented with a large left neck mass that was subsequently biopsy proven as squamous cell carcinoma. Following chemoradiation therapy, there was incomplete clinical resolution of the mass, and he therefore underwent FDG positron emission tomography/computed tomography (PET/CT) imaging for evaluation of his disease.

Findings

Findings are shown in Figures 1 to 4.

Main Teaching Points

- Muscle uptake can be seen from either trauma or muscle strain, as well as from muscle use during the uptake period following dose administration.
- Adequate patient resting is critical because muscle uptake can decrease the sensitivity of the examination.

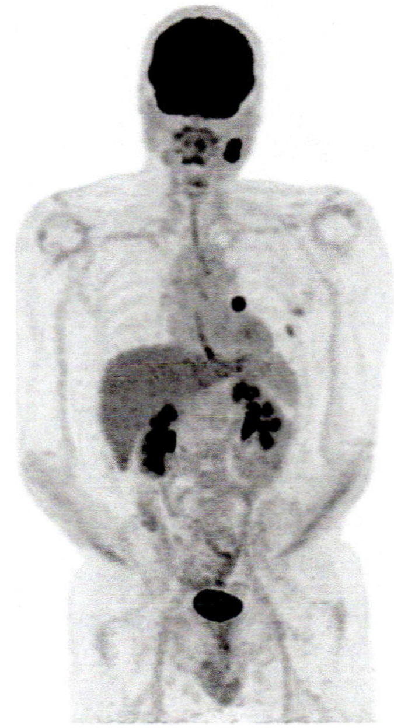

Fig. 1: Maximum intensity projection whole body image demonstrates hypermetabolic foci projecting over the left neck and chest. Diffuse radiotracer uptake is also noted within the bilateral forearms.

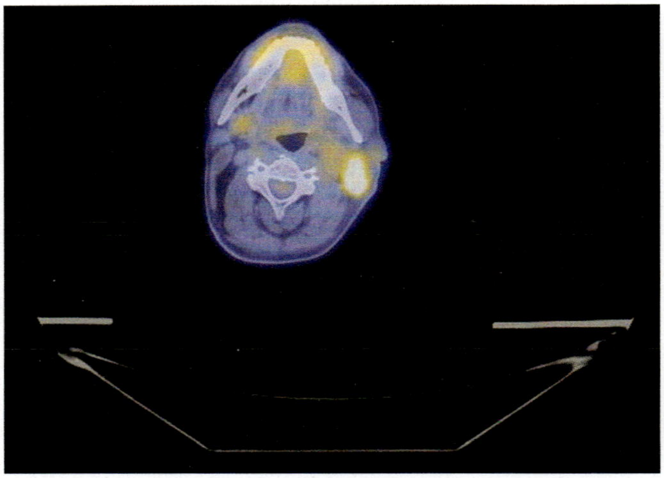

Fig. 2: The known primary malignancy is demonstrated in the left neck as an intensely hypermetabolic mass.

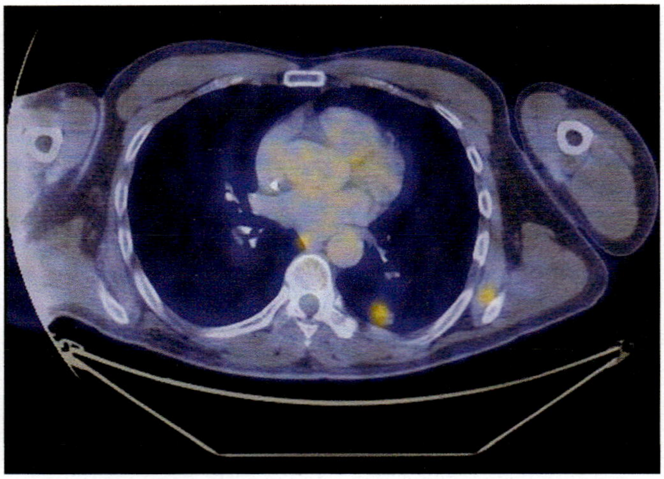

Fig. 3: A FDG avid soft tissue density in the left lower lung lobe is discovered that is concerning for either metastasis or synchronous malignancy. Also on this image, incidental note is made laterally of radiotracer uptake within the left serratus anterior muscle that likely represents muscle strain.

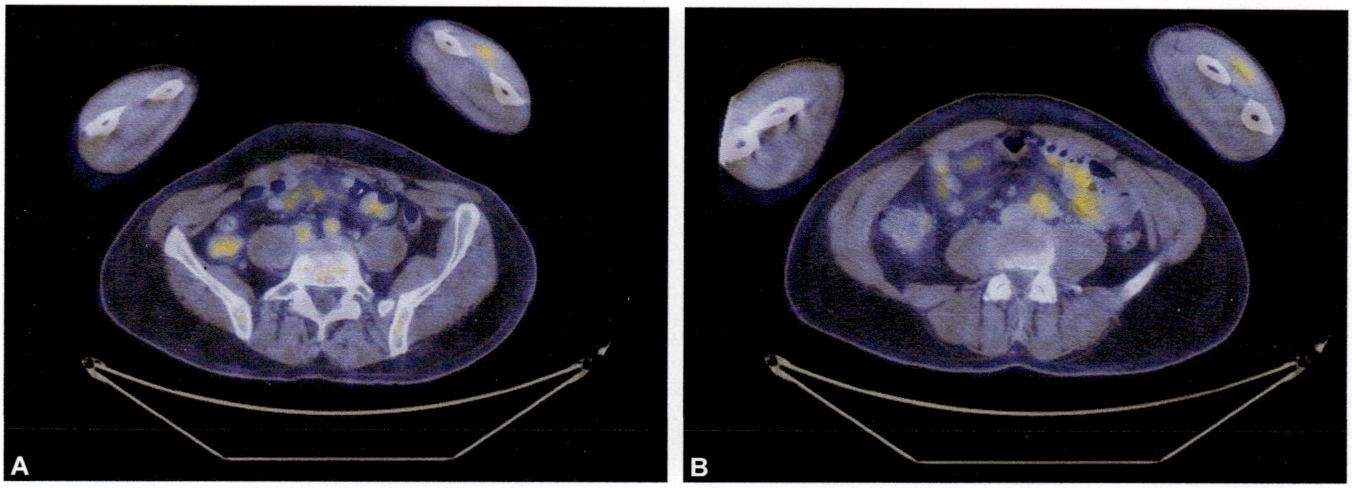

Figs. 4A and B: Diffuse radiotracer uptake is seen throughout the musculature of the bilateral forearms, likely from either prior muscle strain or muscle use during the uptake phase of the examination.

CASE 29: SENTINEL LYMPH NODE IDENTIFICATION FROM DOSE EXTRAVASATION

Brief History

A 41-year-old female with squamous cell carcinoma of the cervix status postchemotherapy and external beam radiation therapy underwent FDG positron emission tomography/computed tomography (PET/CT) imaging for surveillance of her disease. She experiences a minor dose extravasation in the right antecubital fossa at the time of dose injection.

Finding

Findings are shown in Figures 1 and 2.

The remainder of the examination was otherwise unremarkable.

Main Teaching Points

- Minor dose infiltration is a common problem encountered in PET imaging and can potentially lead to decreased Standard Uptake Value (SUV) measurements and sensitivity of the examination.
- When a dose extravasation occurs, it can often be outside the field of view due to antecubital fossa injection and standard imaging protocols requiring elevation of arms. In these cases, proper communication and reporting of injection complications is integral to preventing inaccurate interpretation of the examination to preventing inaccurate interpretation of the examination.

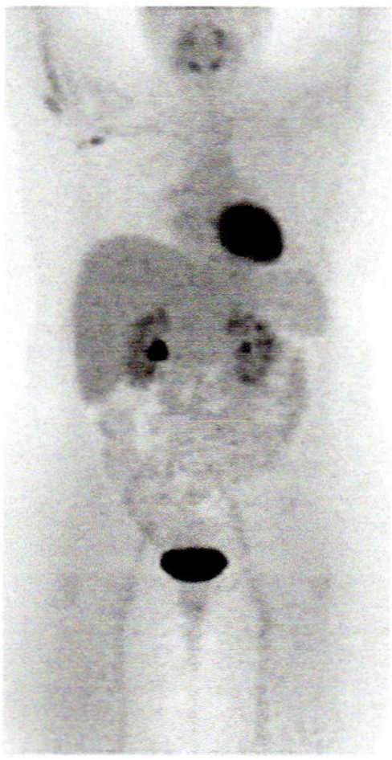

Fig. 1: Maximum intensity projection whole body image demonstrates radiotracer uptake within a right axillary lymph node and dose retention within the right brachial venous system. No other abnormal findings were identified to suggest recurrent malignancy.

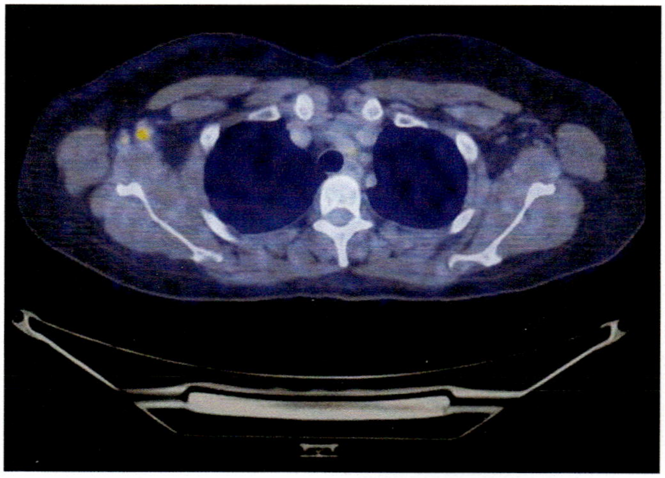

Fig. 2: Two FDG-avid lymph nodes are identified in the right axilla with mild radiotracer activity tracking down lymphatic channels of the right arm, demonstrating lymphoscintigraphy secondary to dose extravasation.

Abdomen and Pelvis Cases

CASE 1: COLORECTAL CANCER FOUND DURING STAGING OF ANOTHER PRIMARY SITE

Brief History

A 68-year-old male with known prostate carcinoma. However, he apparently has metastases to the lungs with no osseous involvement, which would be unusual for prostate cancer. PET/CT was ordered to evaluate for any other possible primary site.

Findings

Findings are shown in Figures 1 and 2.

A colonoscopy was subsequently performed and a biopsy of the circumferential rectal mass 10–15 cm from the anal verge demonstrated adenocarcinoma. A carcinoembryonic antigen (CEA) was also requested which turned out to be 23.5.

Main Teaching Points

- Colorectal carcinoma can often metastasize to the lungs and liver.
- It is the fourth most common cause of cancer death after lung, stomach and liver cancer.
- The most common colon cancer cell type is adenocarcinoma which accounts for 95% of cases.

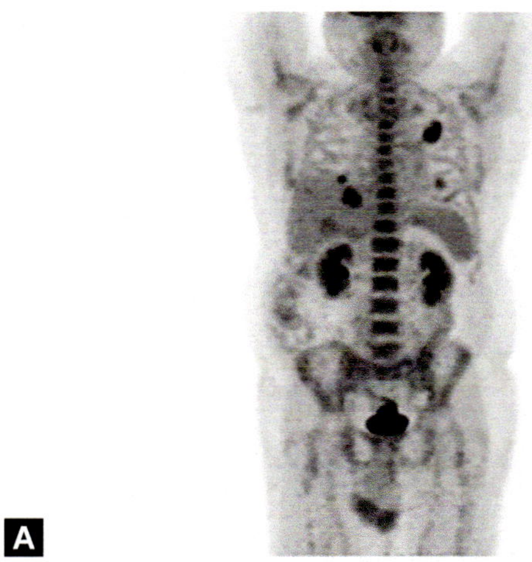

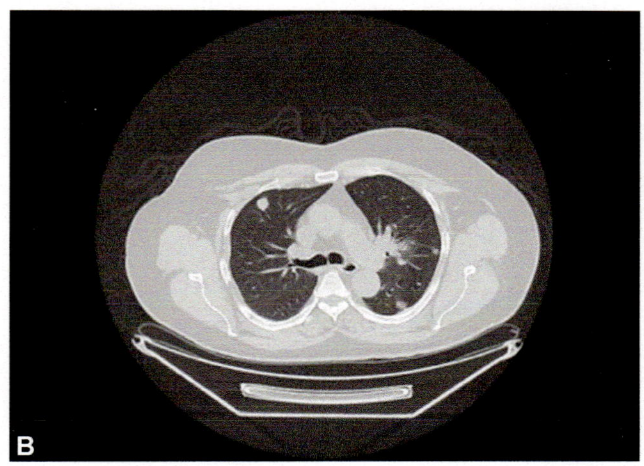

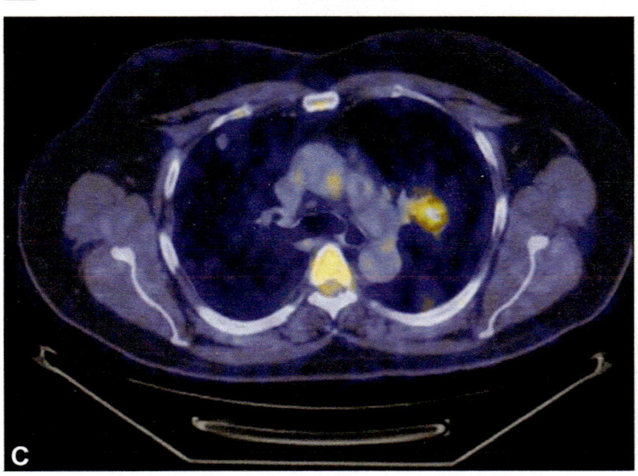

Figs. 1A to C: In the right upper lobe, there is a 1.5-cm pulmonary nodule with a SUVmax of 2.5. The posterior segment of the left lower lobe contains an 8-mm pulmonary nodule with a SUVmax of 2.6. The left hilum has a lymph node measuring 3.1 cm with a SUVmax of 10.3.

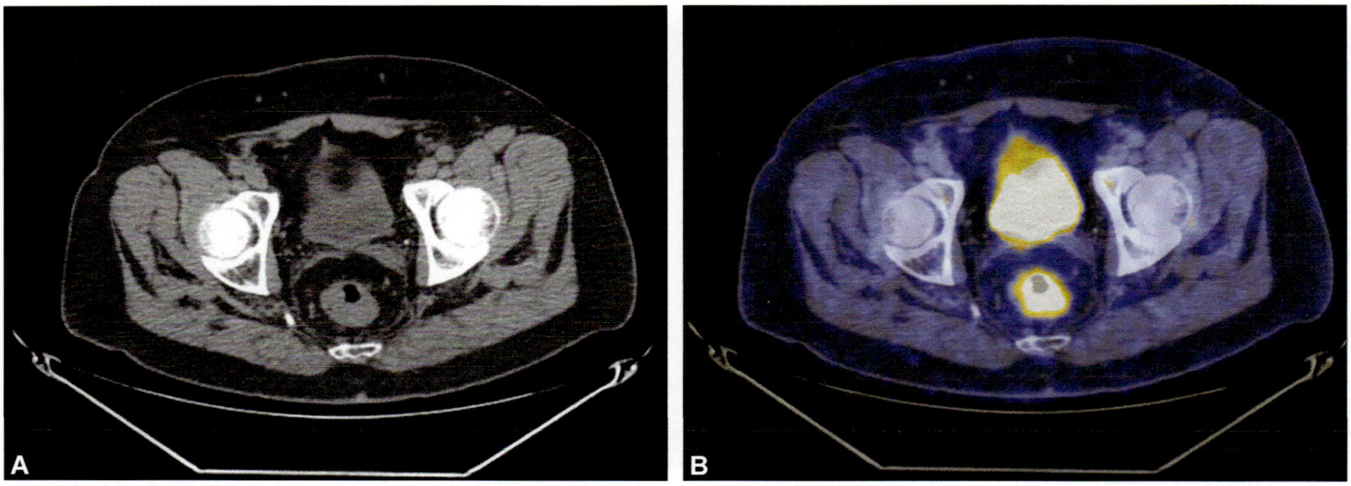

Figs. 2A and B: There is an area of increased uptake at the rectosigmoid junction on the PET/CT fusion and the MIP images. This is very unlikely to represent physiologic uptake. On the CT images, there appears to be an area of bowel wall thickening at this site. Taken together, this most likely represents colorectal carcinoma. Correlate with colonoscopy or other imaging as needed. No mesenteric lymphadenopathy to represent regional nodal spread is appreciated. No liver metastases.

CASE 2: LOCAL RECURRENCE AT ANASTOMOTIC SITE

Brief History

A 54-year-old male with known colon cancer status post hemicolectomy 2 years ago. PET/CT was ordered to evaluate for recurrence.

Findings

Findings are shown in Figures 1A to D.

Main Teaching Points

- Staple line recurrence showed perianastomotic/eccentric masses on CT and perianastomotic/eccentric FDG uptake.
- Background, diffuse, curvilinear and focal patterns of FDG uptake do not correlate with recurrence in the absence of a mass on CT.

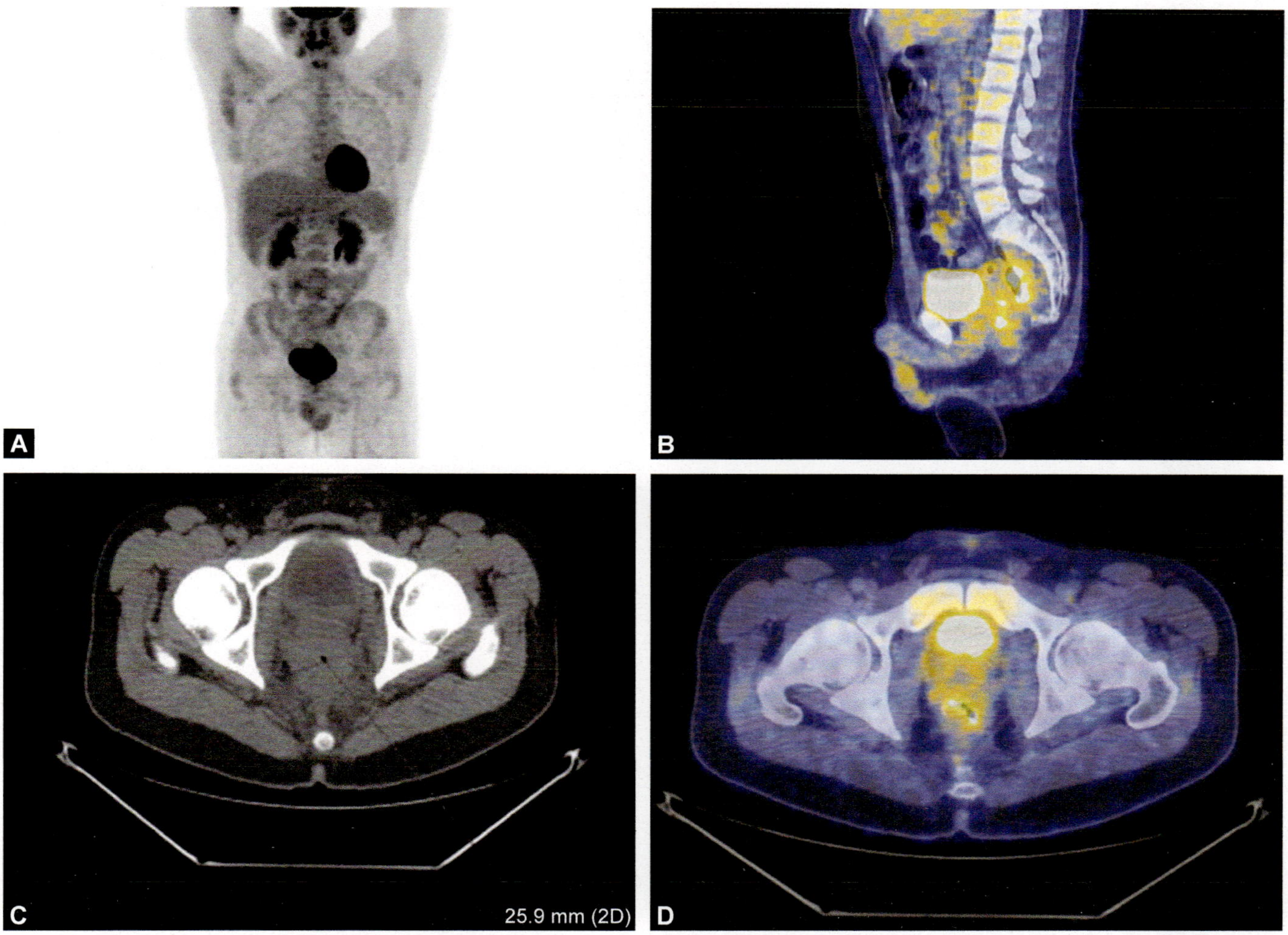

Figs. 1A to D: There are surgical changes in the pelvis compatible with a low anterior resection with marked soft tissue wall thickening about 2.6 cm just proximal to the anastomotic staple line and extending proximally for several centimeters. There is gradual tapering to normal thickness while still in the low pelvis. Notably, the luminal surface of this region shows intense FDG uptake with a SUVmax of 10.0 g/mL. Intense FDG-avidity centered at the mucosal surface is most likely inflammatory, but cannot exclude superimposed malignancy. Clinical correlation and direct visualization is recommended.

CASE 3: COLON CANCER POSTSURGICAL CHANGES AT ANASTOMOTIC SITE

Brief History

A 30-year-old female with history of metastatic colorectal carcinoma diagnosed in 2006 status post-neoadjuvant chemotherapy and concurrent radiation therapy. This was followed by a low anterior resection and wedge resection of solitary liver metastases.

Findings

Findings are shown in Figures 1A to C.

Main Teaching Points

- Anastomotic recurrences after colon cancer resection occur in 2–4% of patients. Anastomotic recurrences after rectal cancer resection occur in 10% of patients.
- Absence of a mass on the CT portion of the scan is very helpful in excluding staple line recurrences, given the broad overlap of SUVmax measurements at the staple line regions in patients with and without recurrence.

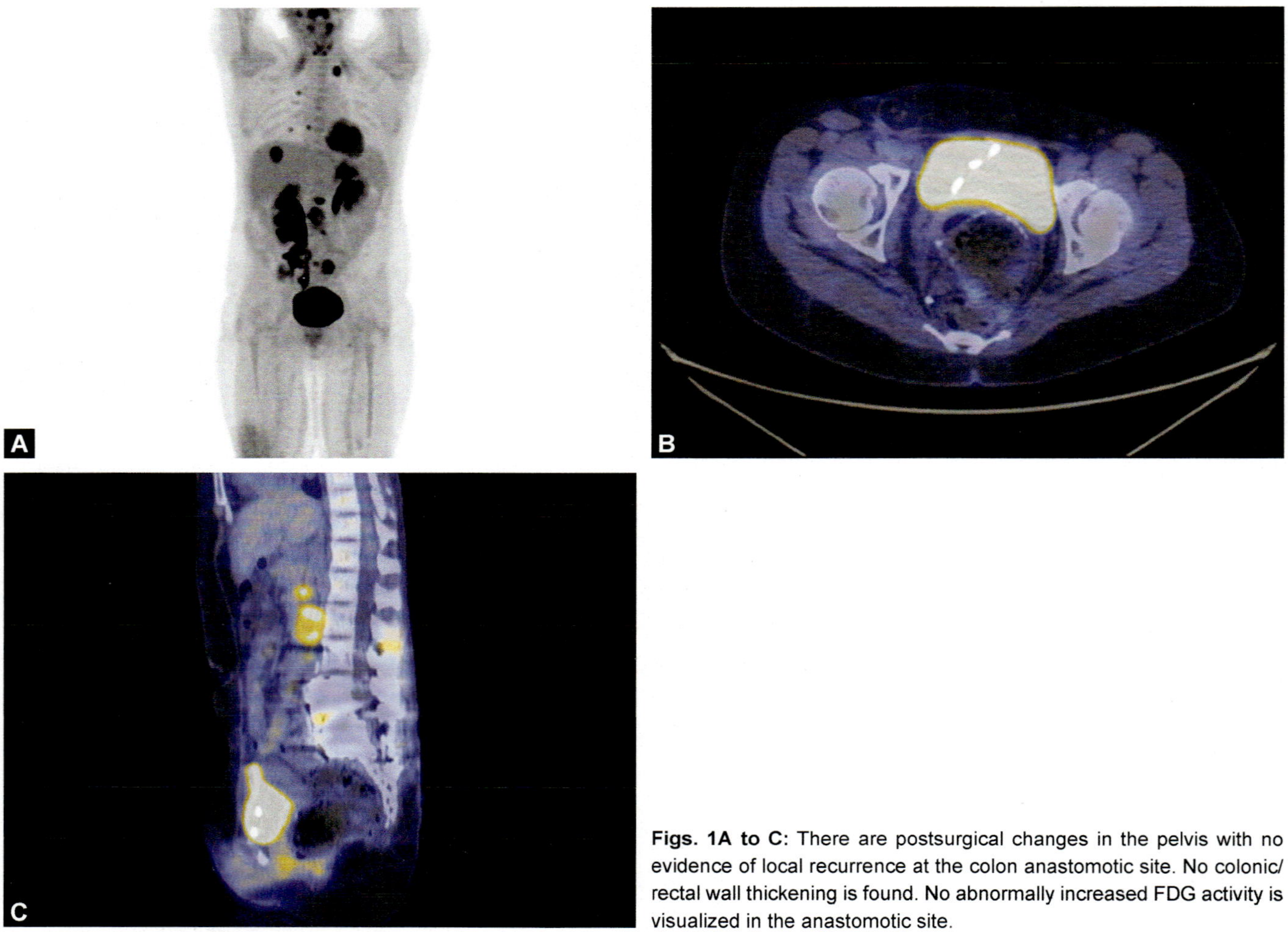

Figs. 1A to C: There are postsurgical changes in the pelvis with no evidence of local recurrence at the colon anastomotic site. No colonic/ rectal wall thickening is found. No abnormally increased FDG activity is visualized in the anastomotic site.

CASE 4: PERITONEAL CARCINOMATOSIS

Brief History

A 42-year-old male with primary rectal carcinoma status post-low anterior resection. PET/CT was ordered for surveillance of disease.

Findings

Findings are shown in Figures 1 to 4.

Main Teaching Points

- Peritoneal carcinomatosis from colorectal cancer has been associated with poor survival.
- Positron emission tomography/computed tomography is far superior to CT or MRI for detecting peritoneal carcinomatosis.

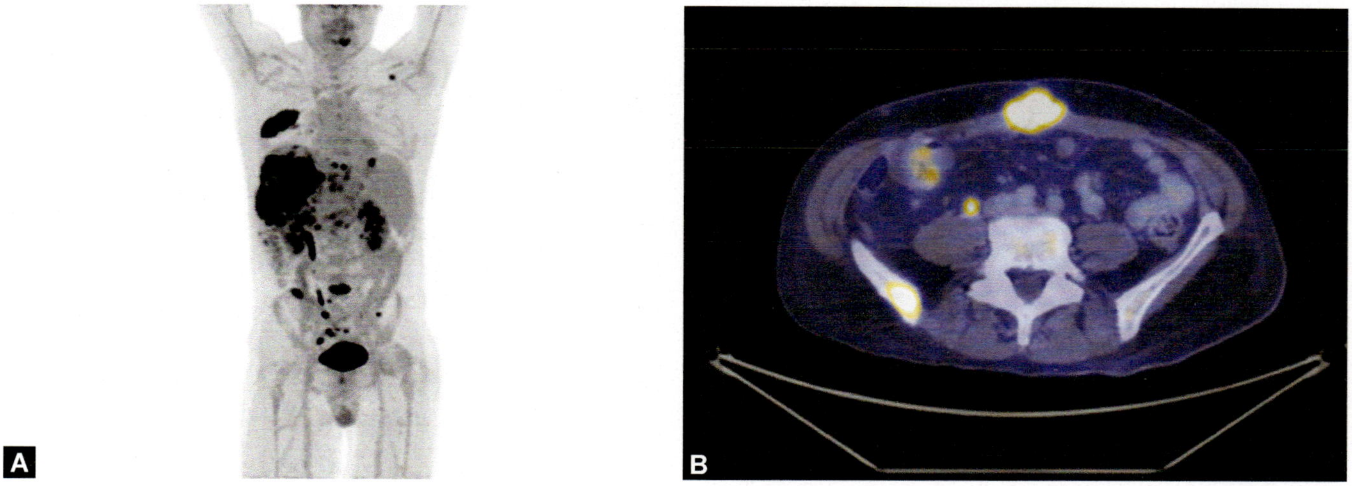

Figs. 1A and B: There is an FDG-avid soft tissue mass at the midline laparotomy site with a SUVmax of 10.5 g/mL. Note the heavy involvement of the liver and ribs.

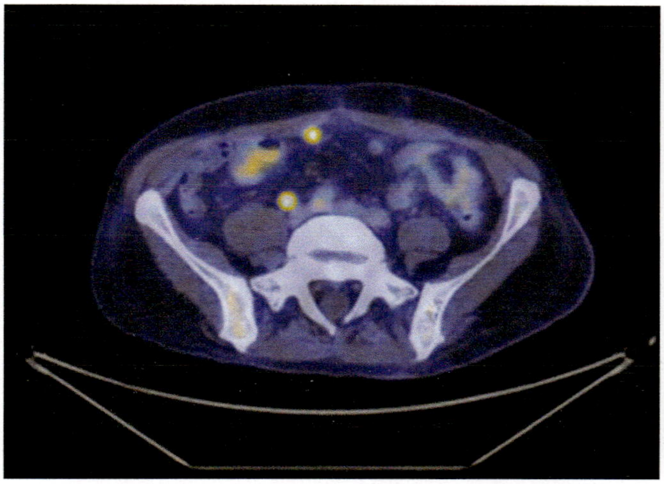

Fig. 2: The metastatic lesion in the right iliac bone has a SUVmax of 8.9.

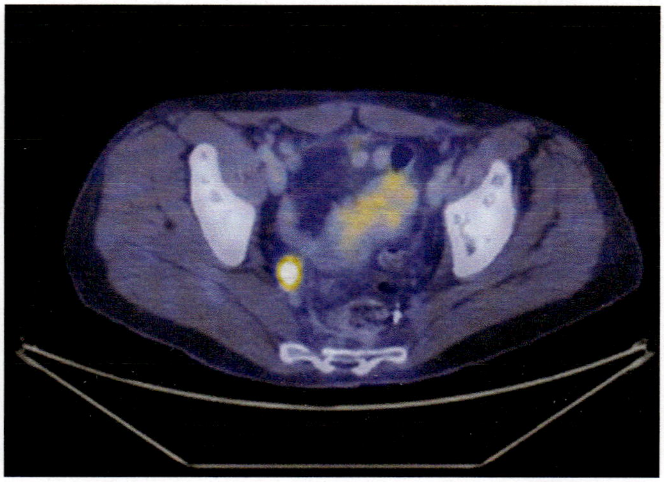

Fig. 3: The peritoneal focus adjacent to the descending colon measures has a SUVmax of 4.0. Another peritoneal focus is adjacent to the sigmoid colon with a SUVmax of 4.4.

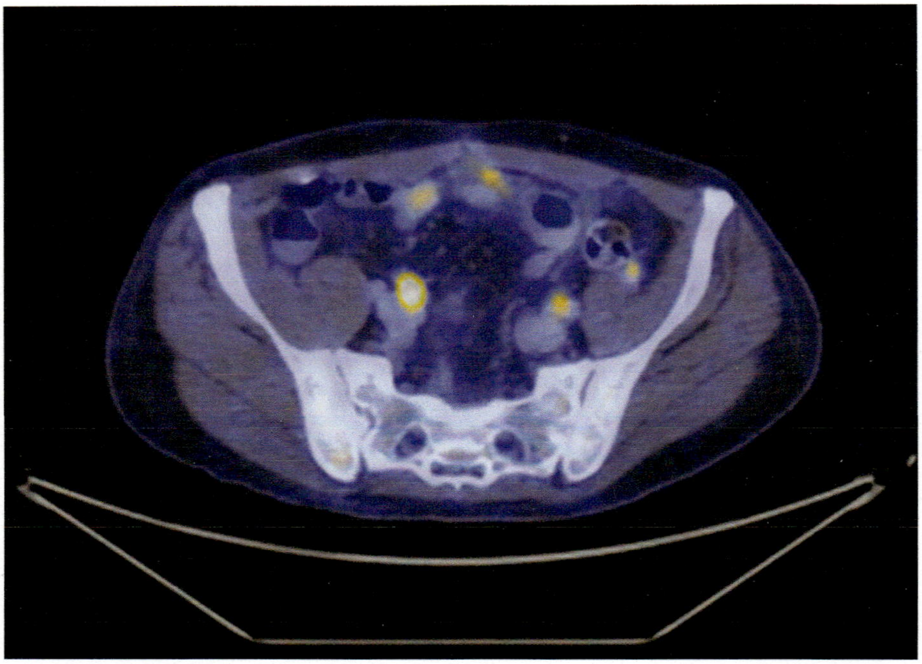

Fig. 4: Additionally, there is enlarged right posterior iliac chain lymph node with a SUVmax of 6.9. These findings are strongly suspicious for colon cancer metastasis to the bone, liver and peritoneum.

CASE 5: RESPONSE TO THERAPY

Brief History

A 45-year-old female with diagnosis of colorectal cancer status post-chemoradiation therapy. Primary team requests repeat PET/CT scan to evaluate for response to therapy

Findings

Findings are shown in Figures 1 to 4.

Main Teaching Points

- FDG PET/CT has an established role in staging colorectal cancer patients in the assessment of residual masses after treatment.
- Computed tomography has limitations in reliably distinguishing necrotic tumor or fibrotic scar from residual tumor tissue.
- FDG PET can change treatment management to prevent toxicity and reduce the costs of ineffective therapy without negatively affecting overall survival.

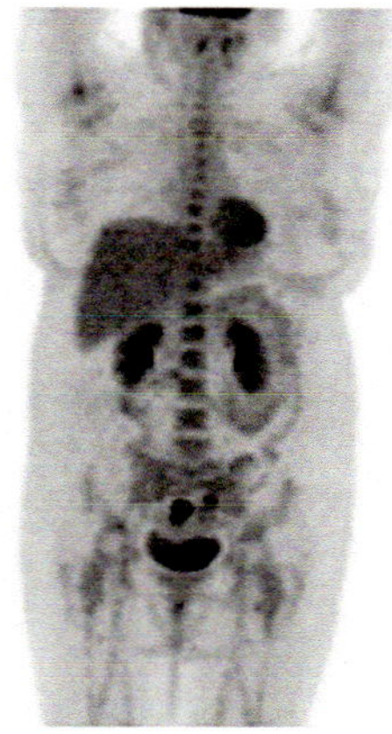

Fig. 1: This original MIP taken before treatment demonstrates a hypermetabolic rectal lesion which is compatible with the patient's known rectal cancer.

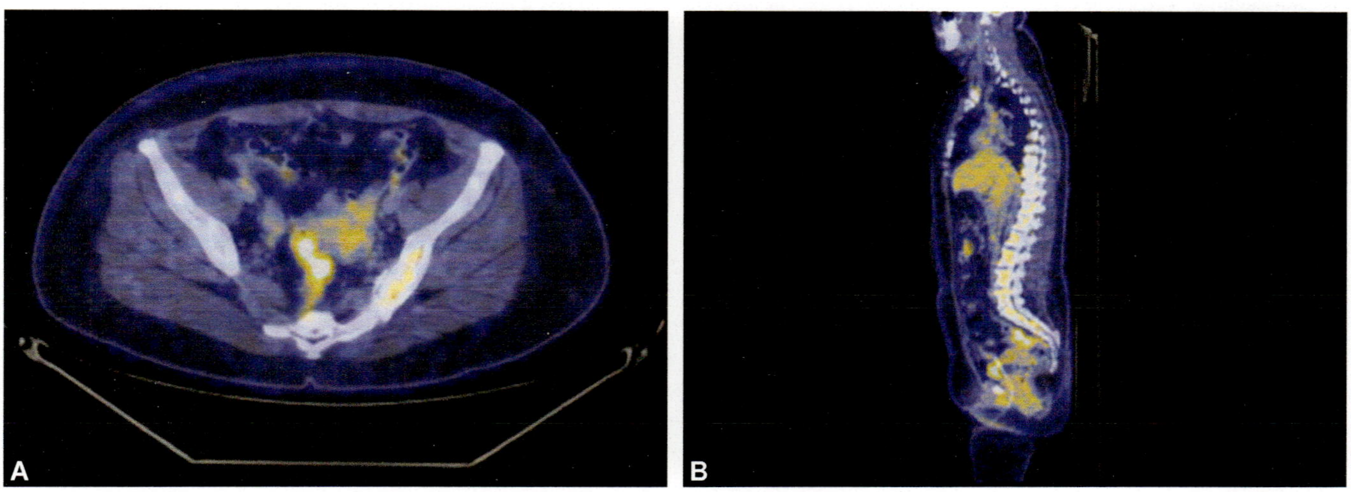

Figs. 2A and B: There is focal increased FDG activity within the rectum with a SUVmax of 7.9.

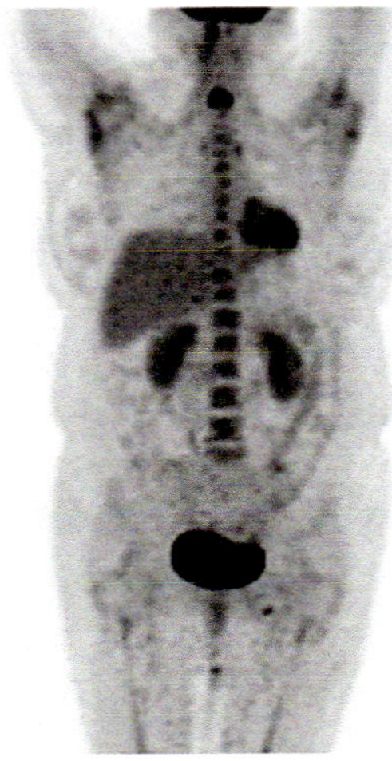

Fig. 3: After treatment, significant improvement is seen at the site of the primary rectal lesion compatible to response to therapy. This patient had chemotherapy with concurrent radiation treatment.

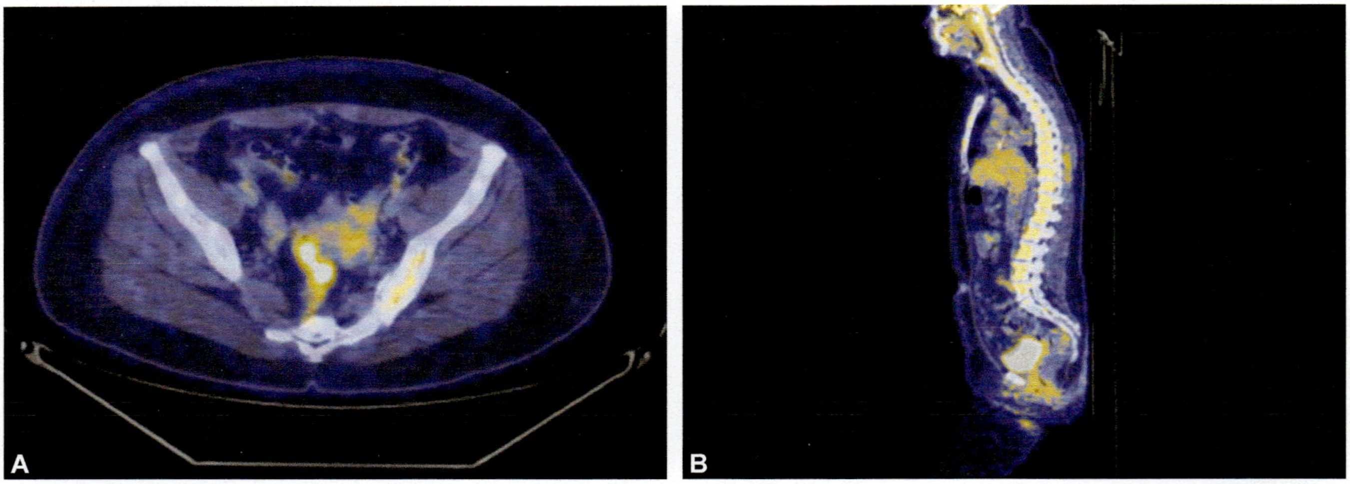

Figs. 4A and B: There is improved size and activity of the previously identified rectal lesion now with a SUVmax of 3.8, previously 7.9. Note the decreased marrow activity within the lower lumbosacral region due to radiation treatment.

CASE 6: POSITIVE RELAPSE WITH NEGATIVE CEA

Brief History

A 60-year-old man with a history of rectosigmoid adenocarcinoma status post-low anterior resection 5 years ago. He had chemotherapy with radiation treatment. His recent CEA level was normal at 2.0. A PET/CT was ordered to evaluate for recurrent tumor.

Findings

Findings are shown in Figures 1A to C.

Main Teaching Points

- CEA is a complex glycoprotein produced by 90% of colorectal cancers and contributes to the malignant characteristics of a tumor.
- In one study, FDG PET had a sensitivity 75% and a positive predictive value of 79% for detecting colorectal cancer recurrence when the CEA levels were positive. FDG PET can have a major impact on patients with an unexplained elevation in CEA levels.
- Sensitivity and specificity of CEA for detecting colorectal cancer recurrence was 0.64 [95% confidence interval (CI): 0.61–0.67] and 0.90 (95% CI: 0.89–0.91), respectively.

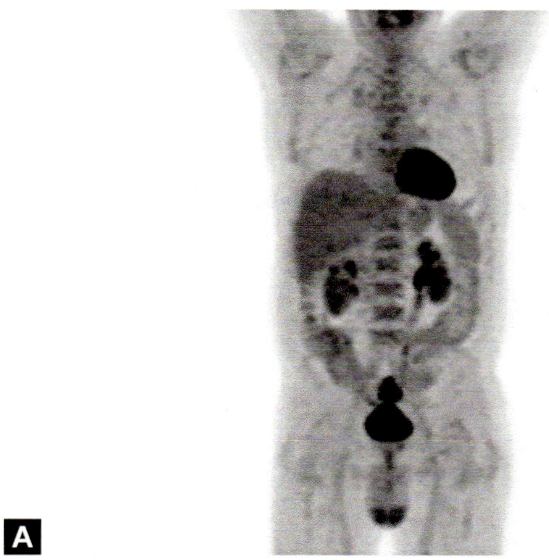

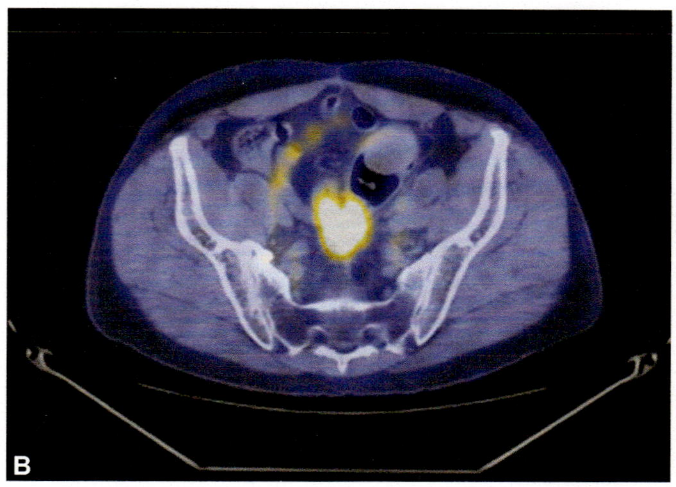

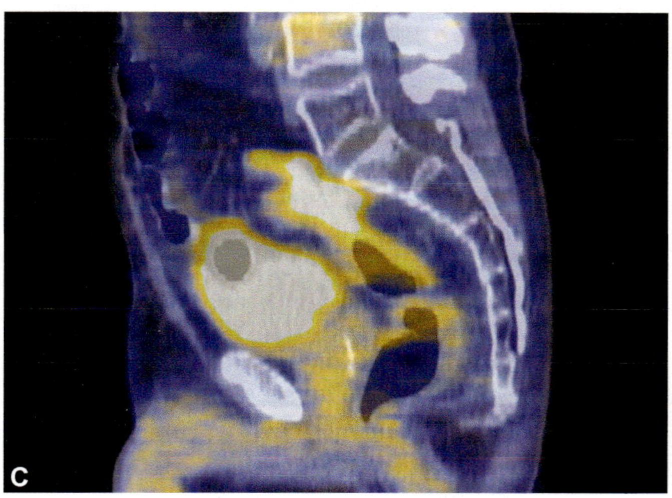

Figs. 1A to C: A large hypermetabolic soft tissue mass is at the rectosigmoid anastomotic site which measures 3.3 × 3.5 × 3.1 cm. The SUVmax at this site is 13.8 g/mL. This hypermetabolic soft tissue density extends into the pericolonic fat, into the mesentery, and into an adjacent portion of the distal ileum.

CASE 7: NEGATIVE FINDING WITH POSITIVE CEA

Brief History

A 55-year-old male with persistent right pleural effusion status post Video-assisted thoracoscopic surgery (VATS) with decortication. Aspiration of the pleural fluid revealed reactive mesothelial cells. Patient has continually lost weight despite improved nutrition. The CEA level was markedly elevated at 63. Cancer antigen-125 (CA-125) level was also elevated at 43. In addition, CT and colonoscopy showed no evidence of malignancy.

Findings

Findings are shown in Figures 1A to E.

Main Teaching Points

- FDG PET has an established role in staging colorectal cancer patients before surgical resection of metastases in the localization of recurrence in patients with an unexplained rise of serum CEA and in the assessment of residual masses after treatment.
- Serum CEA is a test with high specificity but insufficient sensitivity for detecting colorectal cancer recurrence in isolation. The suggested cut-off is 2.2 ng/mL for optimal balance of sensitivity and specificity.

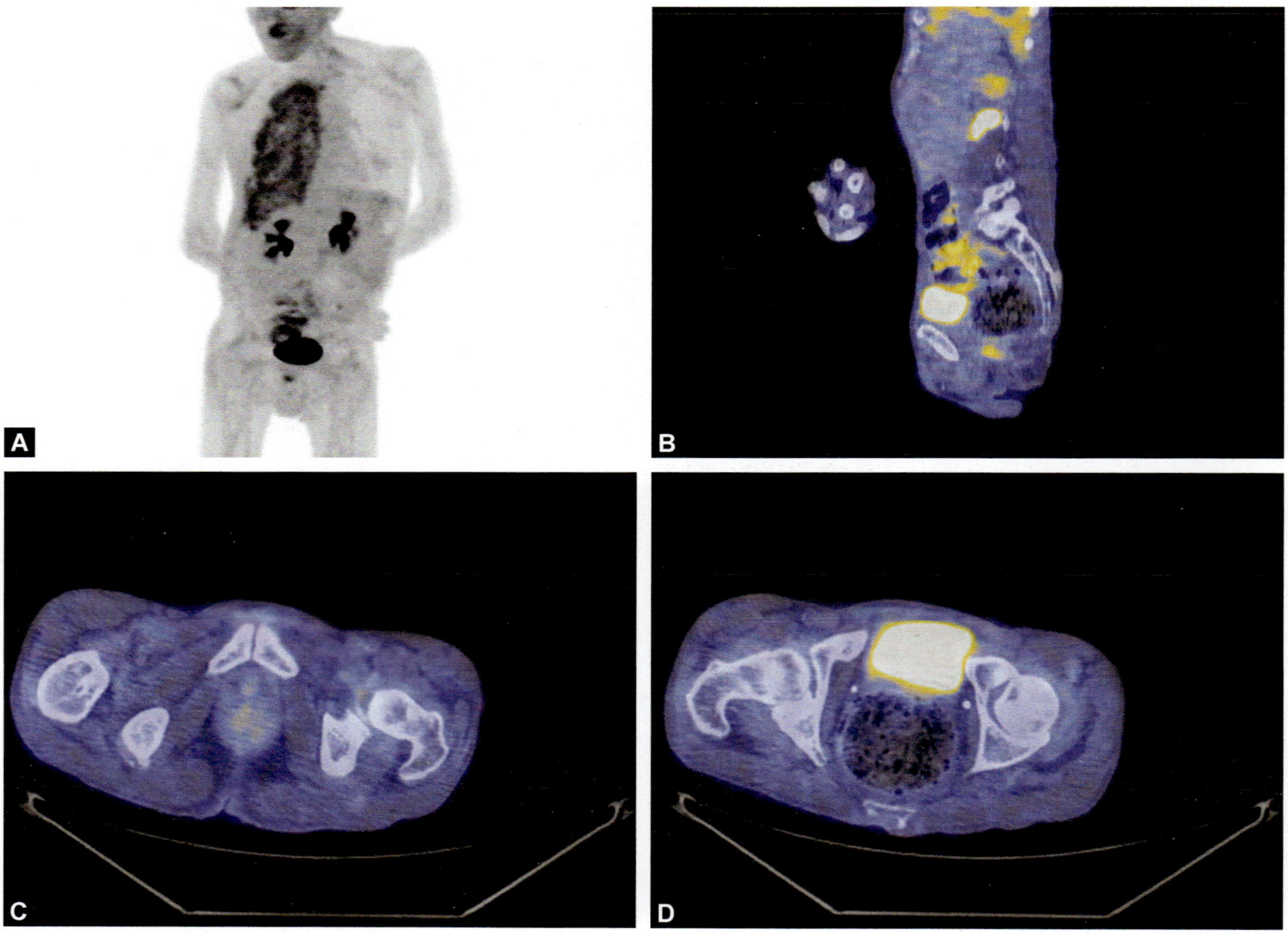

Figs. 1A to D

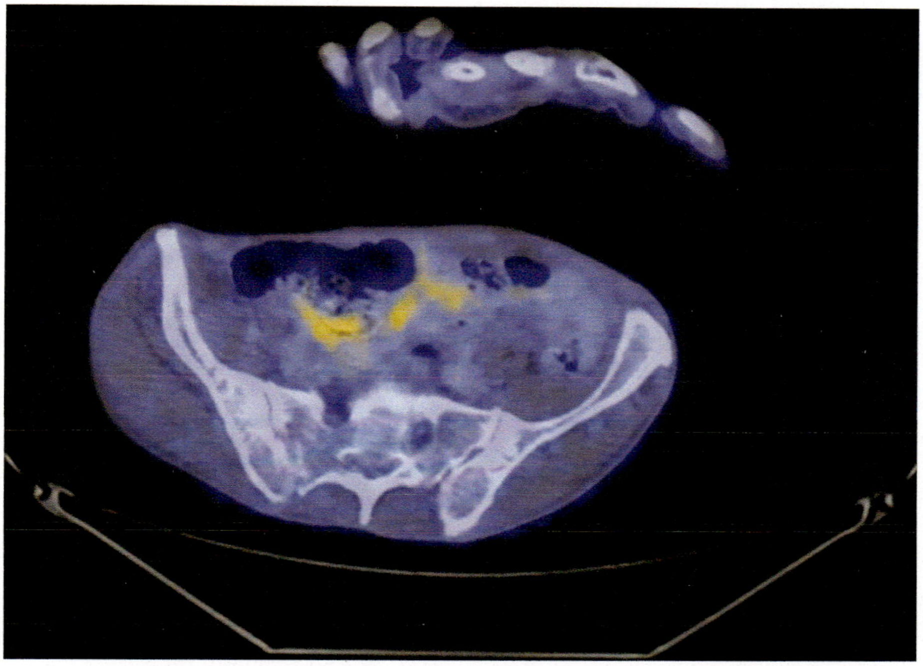

Figs. 1A to E: The colonic wall has a SUVmax of 7.1 g/mL and does not demonstrate any bowel wall thickening. At the rectum, the SUVmax is 4.2 which is likely physiologic. However, malignancy cannot completely be ruled out. Colonoscopy correlation is recommended.

CASE 8: COLORECTAL WITH HEPATIC METASTASIS

Brief History

A 41-year-old male with history of colorectal cancer status post-sigmoid colon resection, omental resection and liver wedge resection. Patient is experiencing a new right upper back pain and abdominal pain. A recent CT abdomen and pelvis demonstrated omental carcinomatosis.

Findings

Findings are shown in Figures 1 and 2.

Main Teaching Points

- For patients with colorectal cancer, FDG PET is a superior imaging modality for detecting liver metastases.
- Sensitivity estimates on a per-patient basis for a CT, MRI and FDG PET were 64.7%, 75.8% and 94.6%.
- FDG PET did not have a higher sensitivity on a per-lesion basis.

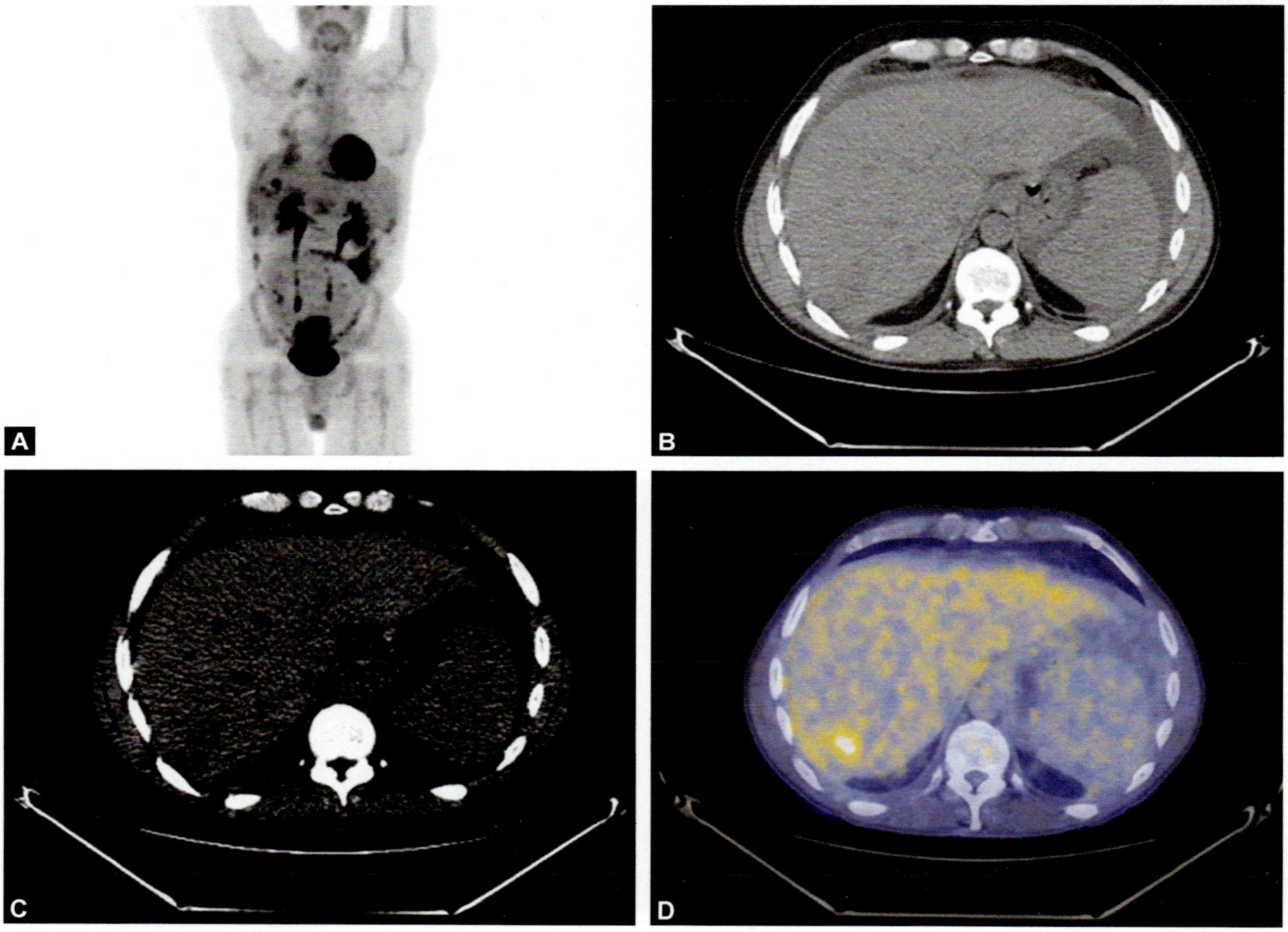

Figs. 1A to D: The CT demonstrates perihepatic ascites. On abdominal windowing, there is no apparent hepatic lesion. However, on liver windowing, a nonspecific hypodense lesion is revealed. The 1.5 × 1.5 cm increased focal activity overlying the hypodensity confirms the liver metastasis with a SUVmax of 8.4.

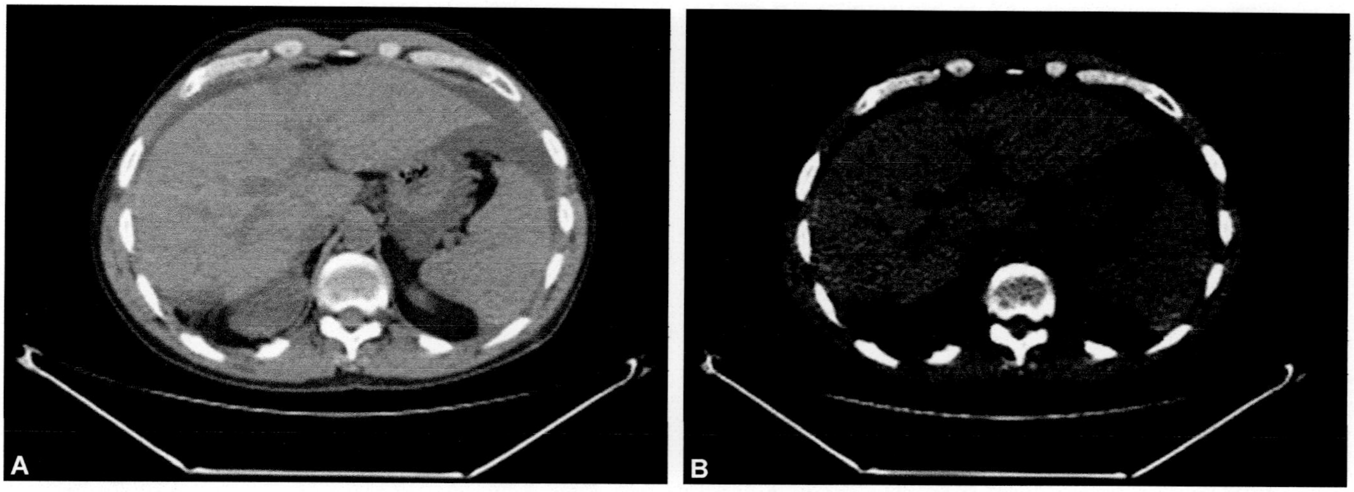

Figs. 2A and B: The anterior surface of the liver shows another hypermetabolic metastasis with a SUVmax of 7.3.

CASE 9: CERVICAL CANCER WITH METASTASIS

Brief History

A 54-year-old female with newly diagnosed cervical cancer. PET/CT was ordered to evaluate for metastasis.

Findings

Findings are shown in Figures 1 to 3.

Main Teaching Points

- Human papillomavirus infections are found in 90% of cervical cancers.
- The most common cell type of cervical cancer is squamous.
- Cervical cancer most commonly spreads to the bladder, intestines, lungs and liver.

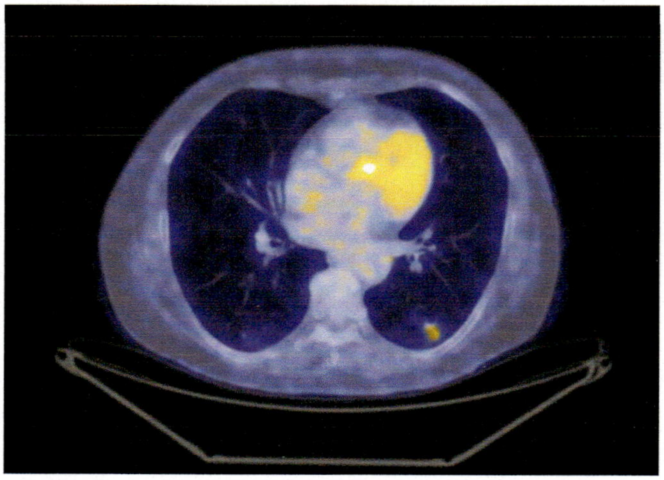

Fig. 1: There is a nodule in the left lower lobe with a maximum standard uptake value (SUVmax) of 3.1 g/mL which may represent a metastatic site. Biopsy of this nodule is recommended for confirmation.

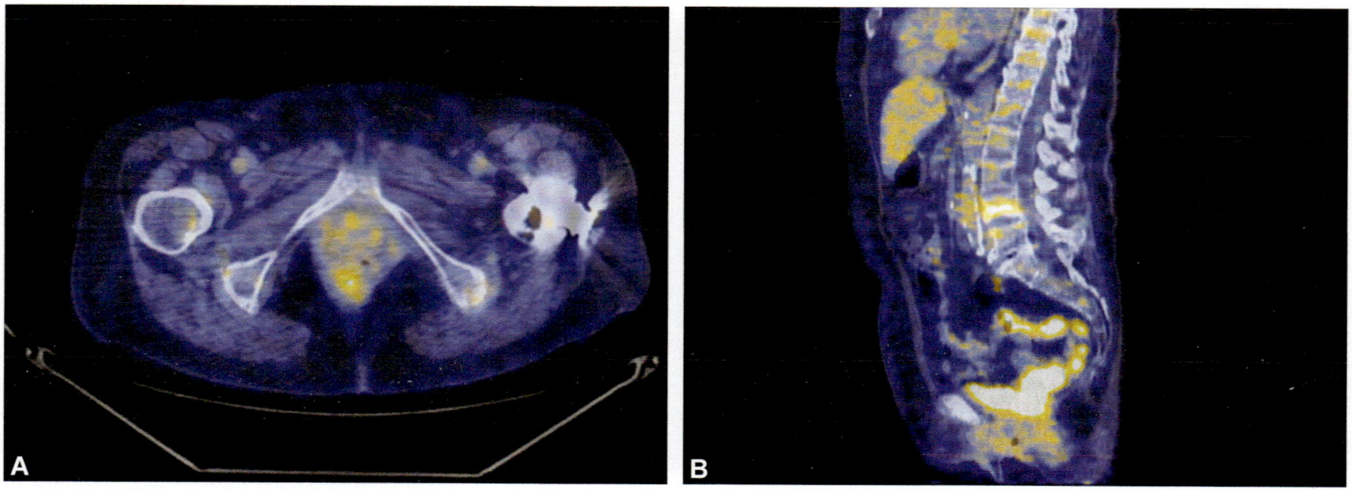

Figs. 2A and B

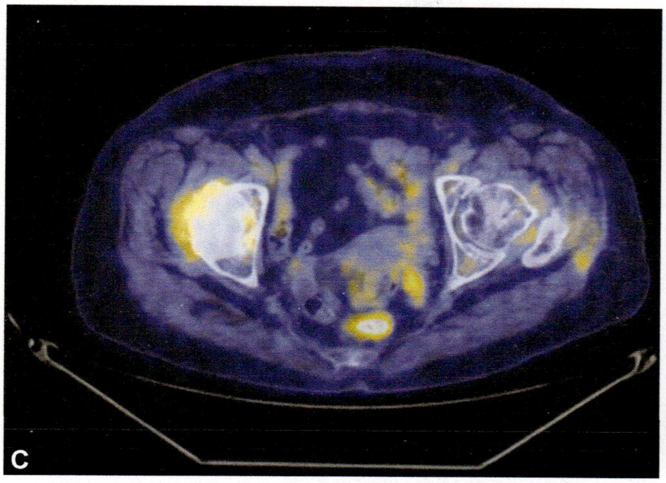

Figs. 2A to C: However, the rectum, uterus and vagina demonstrate physiological FDG activity.

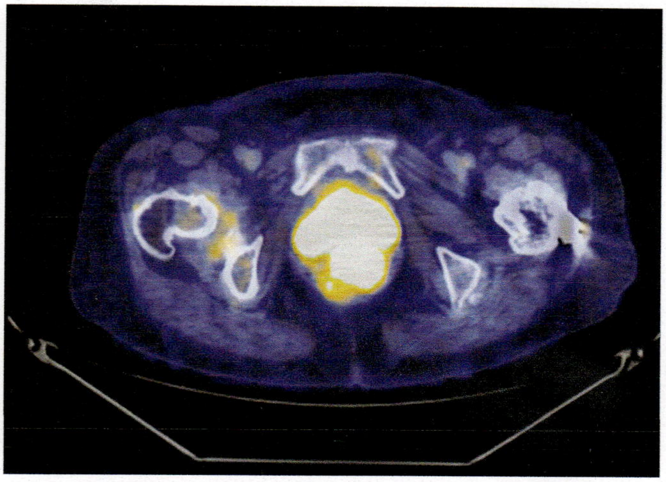

Fig. 3: Superior and posterior to the bladder, a large cervical mass has intense FDG activity with a SUVmax of 19.6 g/mL. Otherwise, there is no regional or distant hypermetabolic lymph node metastasis.

CASE 10: CERVICAL CANCER WITH RESPONSE TO THERAPY

Brief History

A 72-year-old female with adenocarcinoma of the cervix. This PET/CT is to establish the baseline.

Findings

Findings are shown in Figures 1 and 2.

Main Teaching Points

- Survival improves when radiotherapy is combined with cisplatin-based chemotherapy.
- Thirty five percent of patients with invasive cervical cancer have persistent or recurrent disease after treatment.
- FDG PET is useful for staging extrapelvic cervical metastases or optimally detecting a recurrence. MRI is better for evaluating the locoregional area for possible disease.

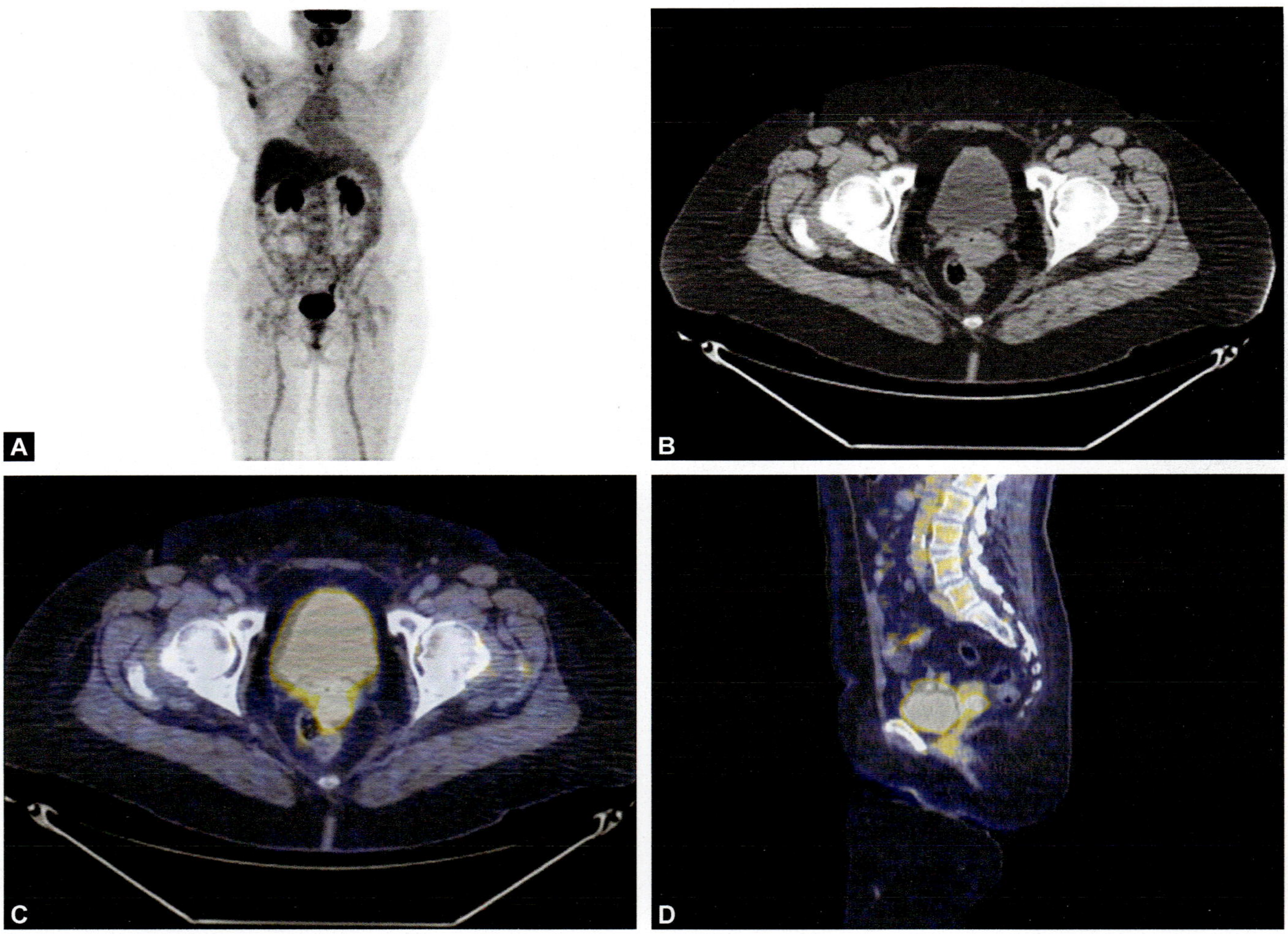

Figs. 1A to D: This baseline PET/CT demonstrates a focus of markedly increased FDG activity at the expected location of the cervix and vaginal cuff. The SUVmax is 28 g/mL.

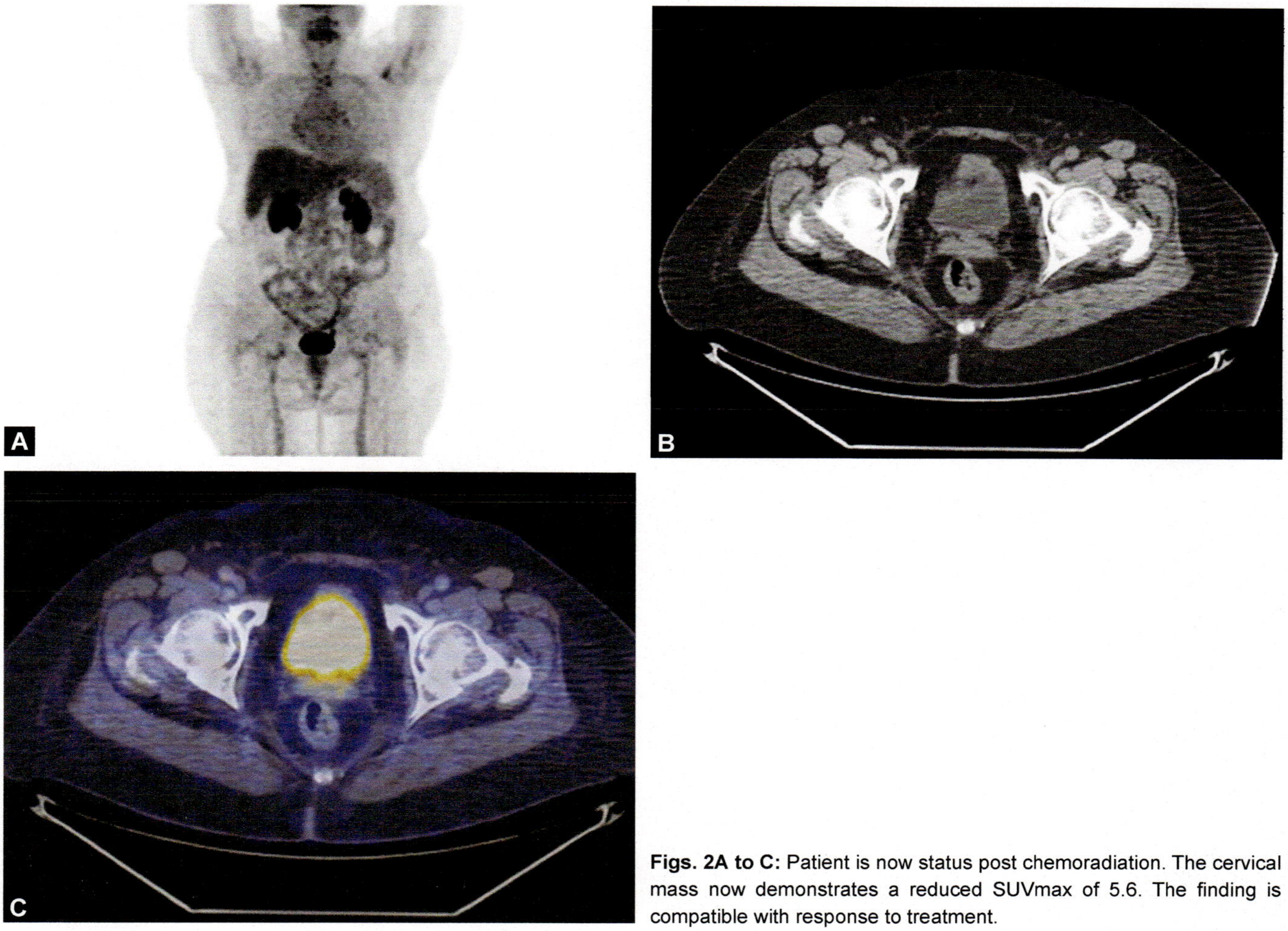

Figs. 2A to C: Patient is now status post chemoradiation. The cervical mass now demonstrates a reduced SUVmax of 5.6. The finding is compatible with response to treatment.

CASE 11: OVARIAN CANCER SPREAD

Brief History

A 68-year-old female with ovarian adenocarcinoma status post completion of chemotherapy. The CA-125 has been worsening and was at 120 at the time of this PET/CT acquisition.

Findings

Findings are shown in Figures 1 to 5.

In summary, multiple hypermetabolic peritoneal implants are seen in the right colic region, left splenic bed, superior aspect of uterus, and on the surface of the liver consistent with metastatic ovarian cancer. A hypermetabolic thickened stomach body wall may have ovarian cancer involvement.

Main Teaching Points

- Krukenberg tumors are metastases from a primary site, classically the gastrointestinal tract, that have spread to the ovaries. This example is not a Krukenberg tumor.
- Ovarian metastasis appears to have mild to moderate FDG uptake with a mean SUVmax of 4.6.
- Small, necrotic, mucinous, cystic, or low-grade tumors are difficult to detect on PET/CT and may contribute to false negatives.

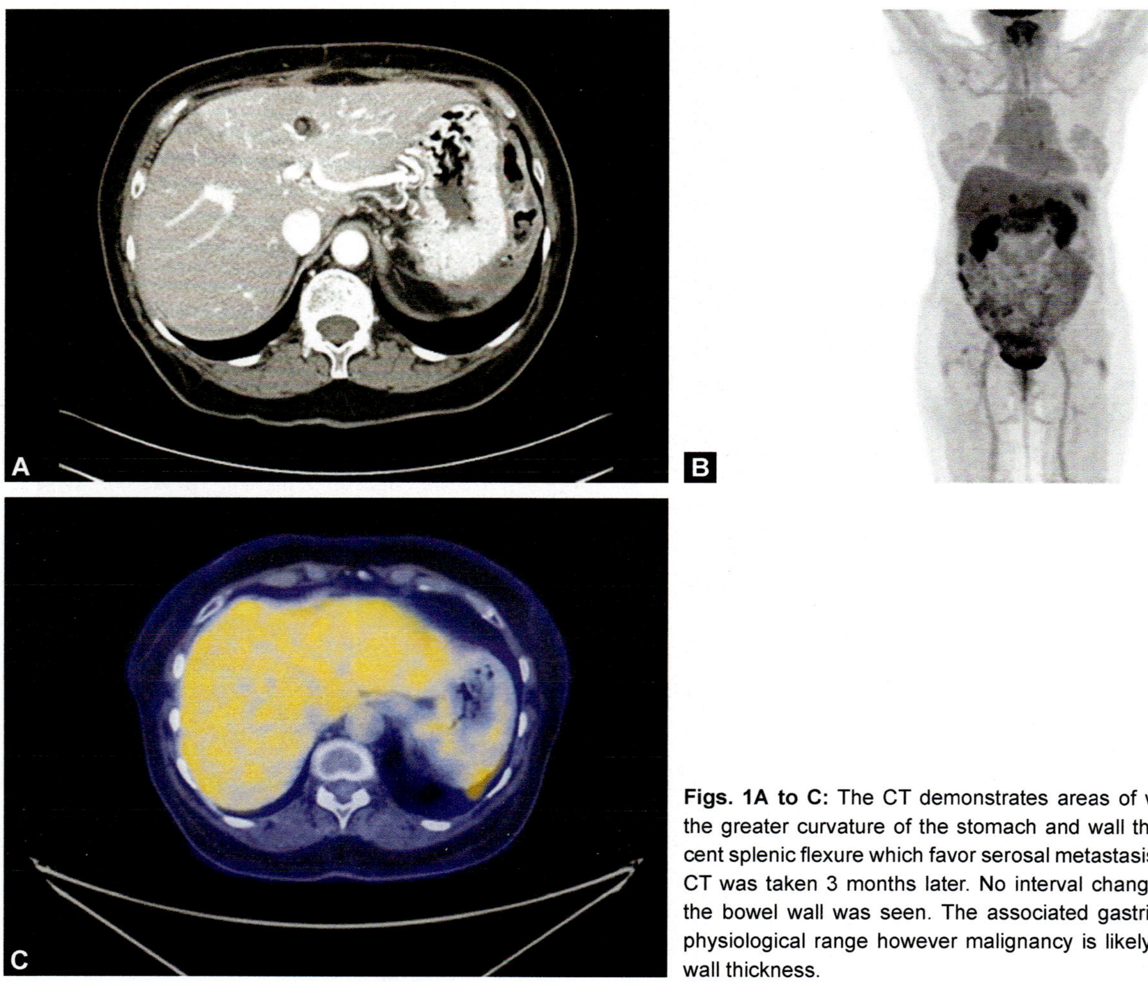

Figs. 1A to C: The CT demonstrates areas of wall thickening along the greater curvature of the stomach and wall thickening of the adjacent splenic flexure which favor serosal metastasis. A subsequent PET/CT was taken 3 months later. No interval change in the thickness of the bowel wall was seen. The associated gastric/bowel activity is in physiological range however malignancy is likely given the abnormal wall thickness.

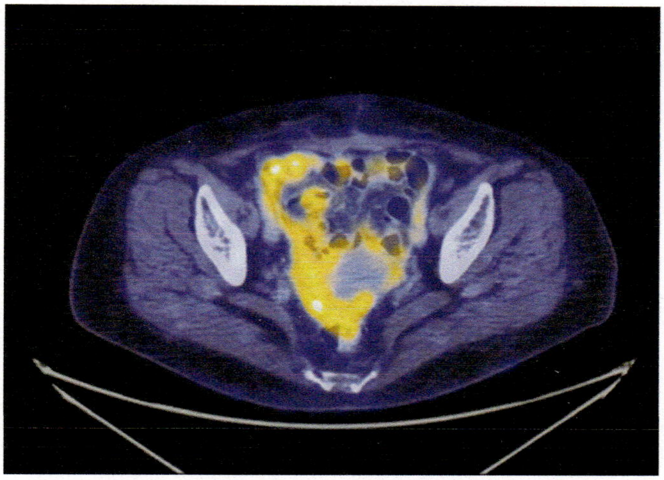

Fig. 2: In the pelvis, a low density rim is seen around the superior aspect of the uterus that enhances with a SUVmax of 5.8. The uterus itself contains multiple degenerating fibroids.

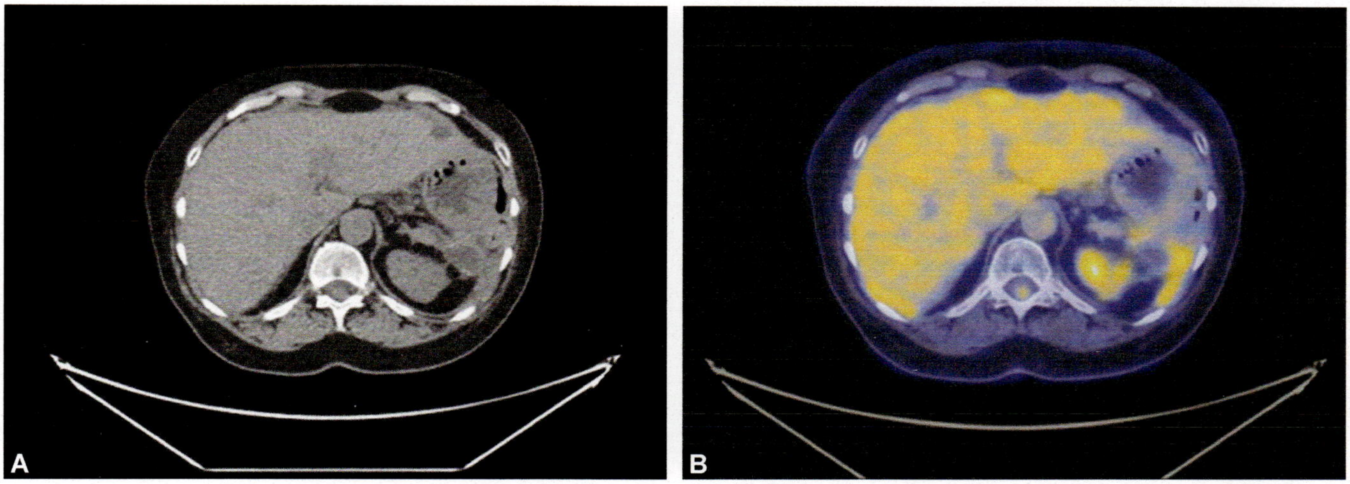

Figs. 3A and B: There are several peritoneal implants seen on the surface of the liver. The largest one demonstrates a SUVmax of 5.3.

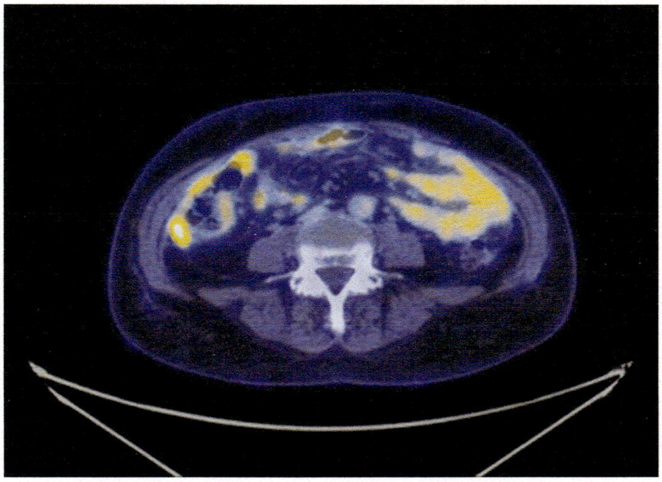

Fig. 4: This slice demonstrates a peritoneal implant with a SUVmax of 4.2 g/mL at the right lower quadrant anteriorly. It is adjacent to the bowel.

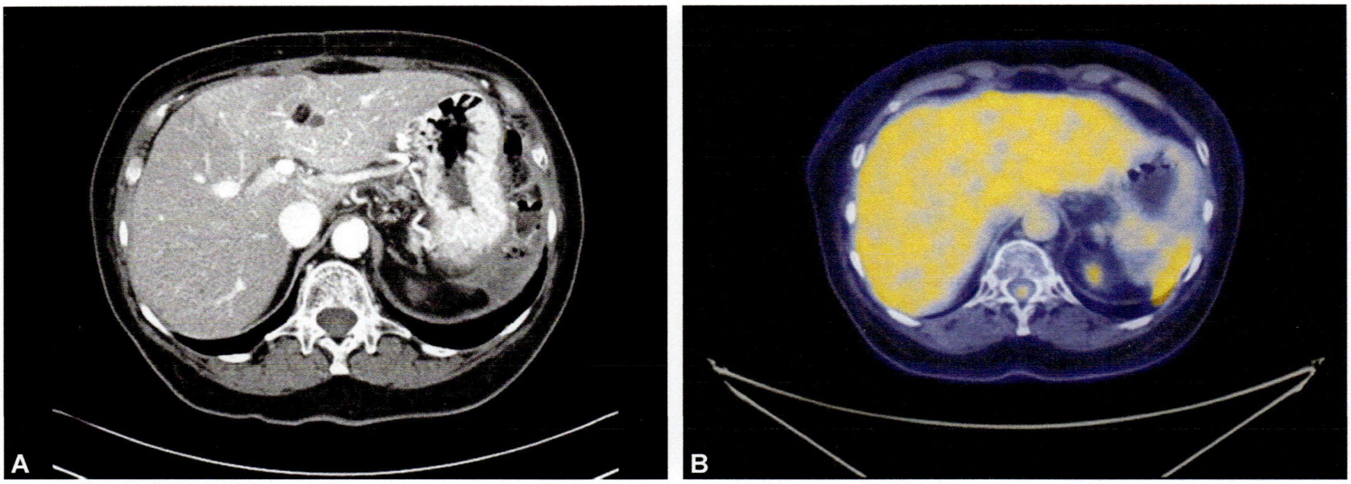

Figs. 5A and B: Just lateral to the perisplenic, seroma is a hypermetabolic peritoneal implant with a SUVmax of 3.9.

CASE 12: OVARIAN CANCER WITH POOR RESPONSE TO THERAPY

Brief History

A 56-year-old female with ovarian cancer status post chemotherapy. The CA-125 has not normalized but clinically, patient shows no signs of recurrent disease. PET/CT is requested to evaluate for any focal or diffuse residual disease.

Findings

Findings are shown in Figures 1 to 5.

In summary, there is a large heterogeneous hypermetabolic pelvic mass, multiple hypermetabolic retroperitoneal and mediastinal lymph nodes, and a small hypermetabolic pleural effusion all worrisome for metastatic disease.

Main Teaching Points[1]

- In the post-therapy setting, PET/CT is most useful for evaluation of patients with rising serum CA-125 levels. PET/CT is also able to determine disease recurrence in the absence of elevated CA-125 levels.
- When Standard Uptake Value (SUV) has dropped by 20% after chemotherapy, there is a significantly increased correlation with overall survival. No such correlation has been reported between clinical or CA-125 response criteria and overall survival.

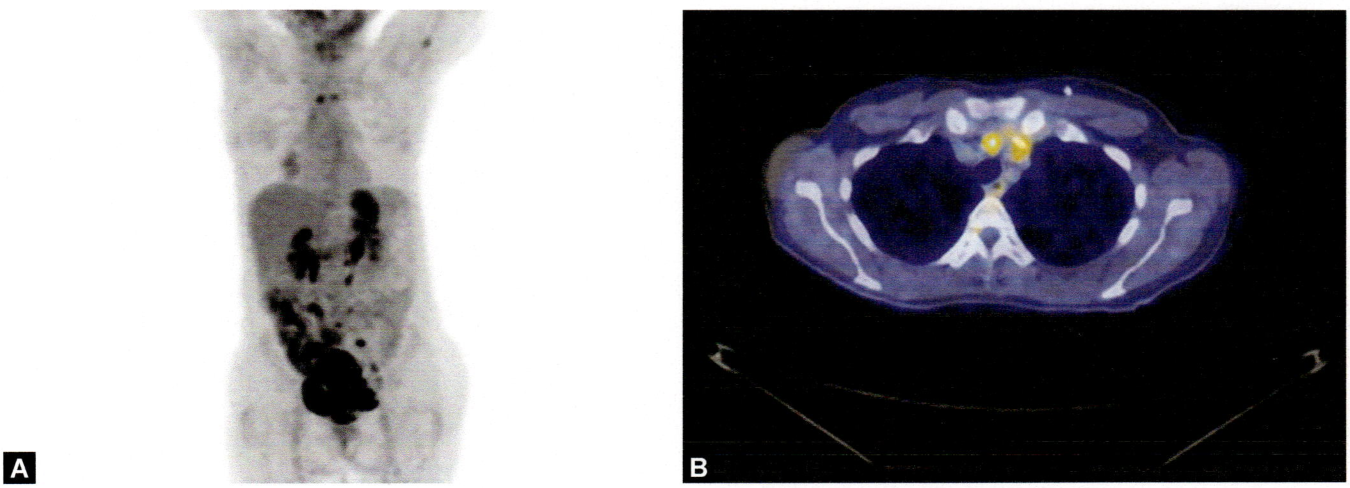

Figs. 1A and B: There is a 7-mm left paratracheal lymph node located in superior mediastinum with a SUVmax of 3.9.

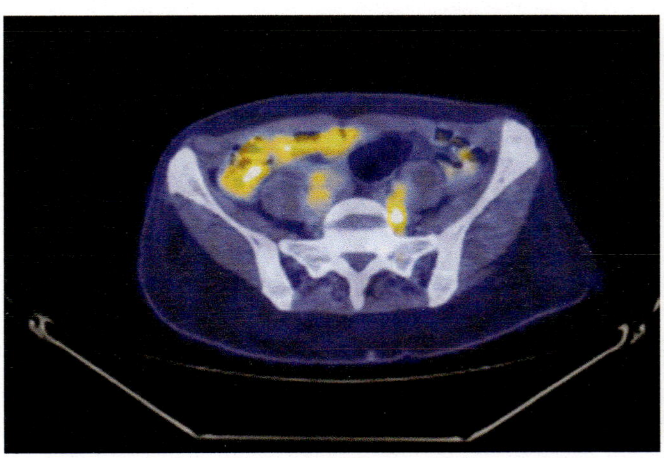

Fig. 2: There is a left iliac lymph node that measures 1.0 × 0.8 cm with a SUVmax of 6.7.

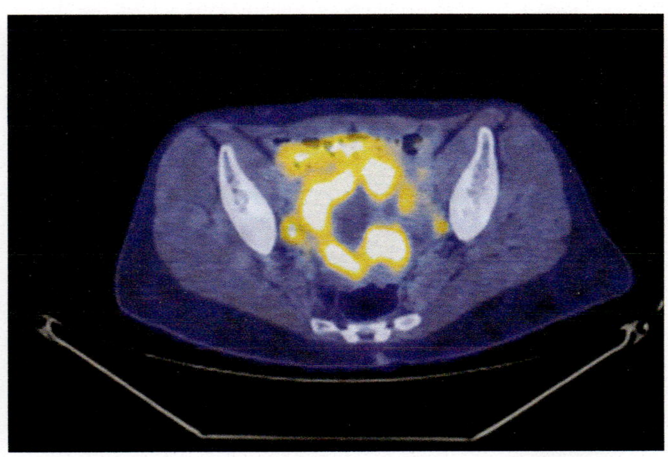

Fig. 3: A very large pelvic mass is seen in the anterior portion of the pelvis. It is multiloculated with cold areas of FDG uptake and a SUVmax of 14.1.

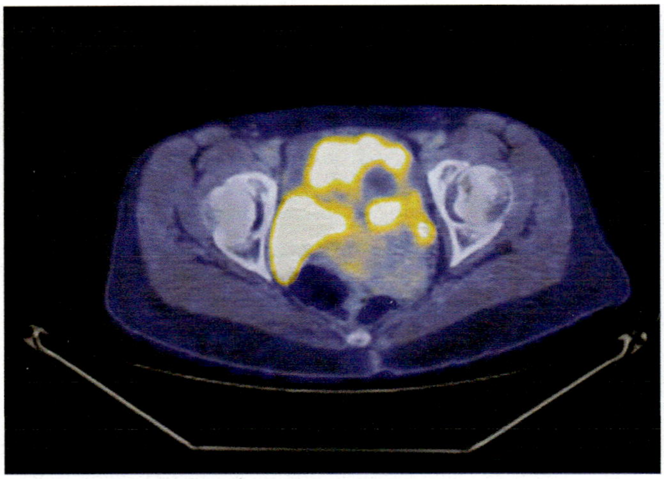

Fig. 4: The mass effect of the pelvic mass has displaced the bladder to the right pelvis.

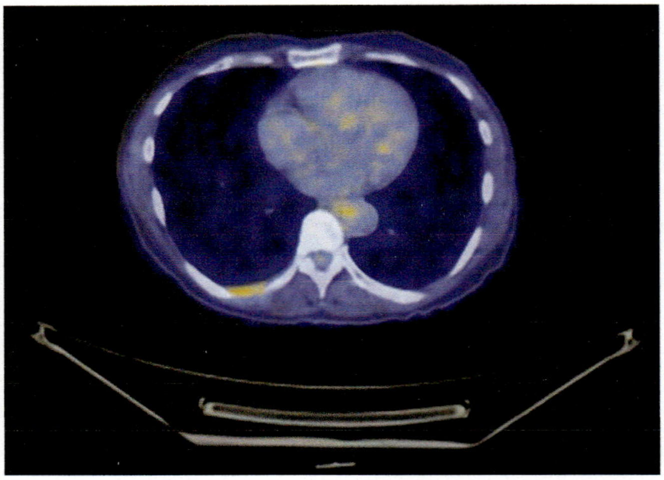

Fig. 5: There is a right pleural effusion posterior to the lung with a SUVmax of 3.5.

CASE 13: MENSES

Brief History

A 22-year-old female with history of Hodgkin's lymphoma status post chemotherapy.

Findings

Findings are shown in Figures 1 and 2.

Main Teaching Points[1]

- In premenopausal women, the endometrial FDG uptake changes cyclically, increasing during ovulation and menstruation.
- Postmenopausal endometrial uptake is abnormal.

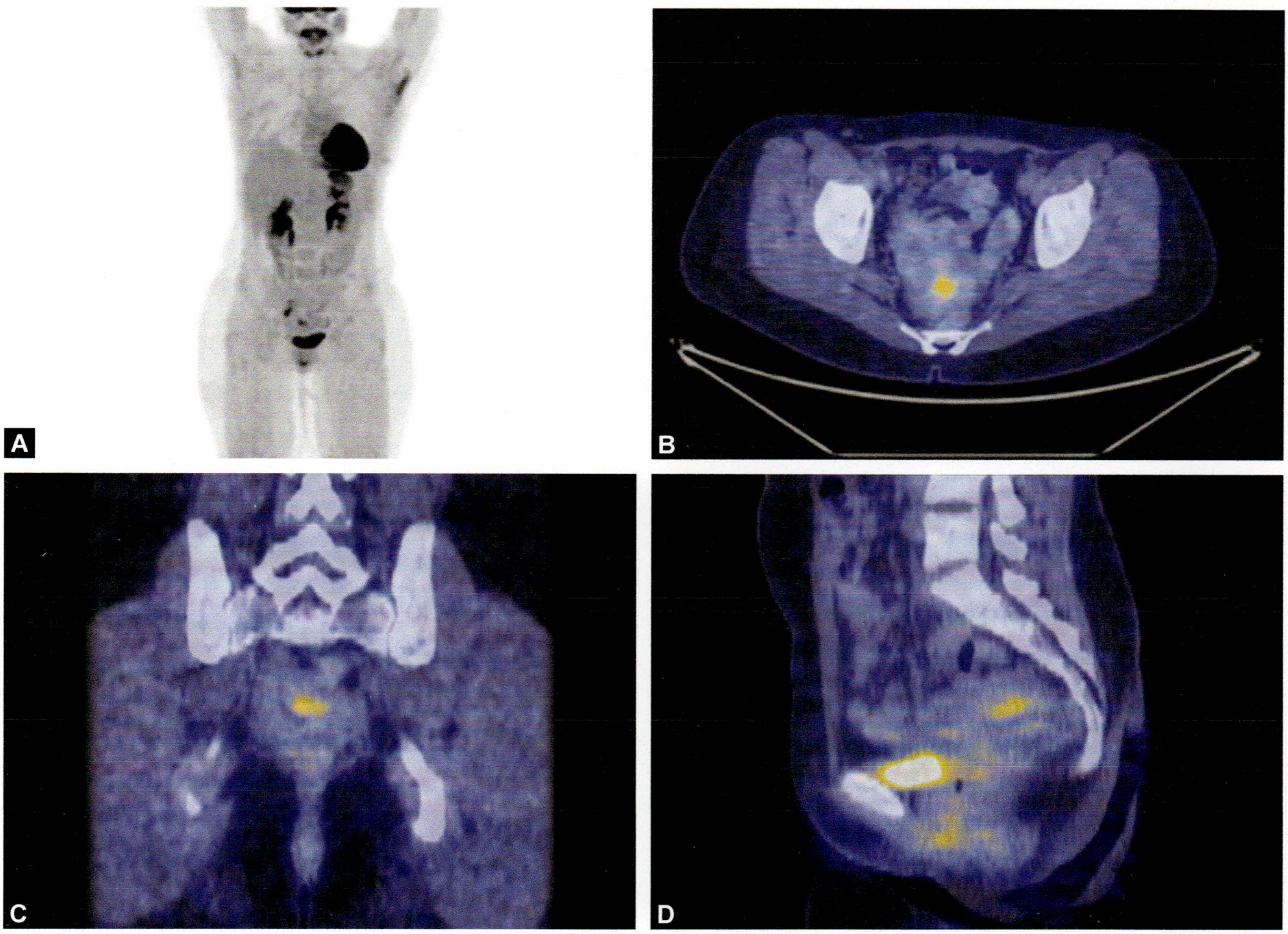

Figs. 1A to D: Focal FDG activity seen within the uterine fundus is physiologic and related to menses. Also, hypermetabolic focus in the right adnexa associated with cystic structure is most likely related to corpus luteal cyst physiologic activity.

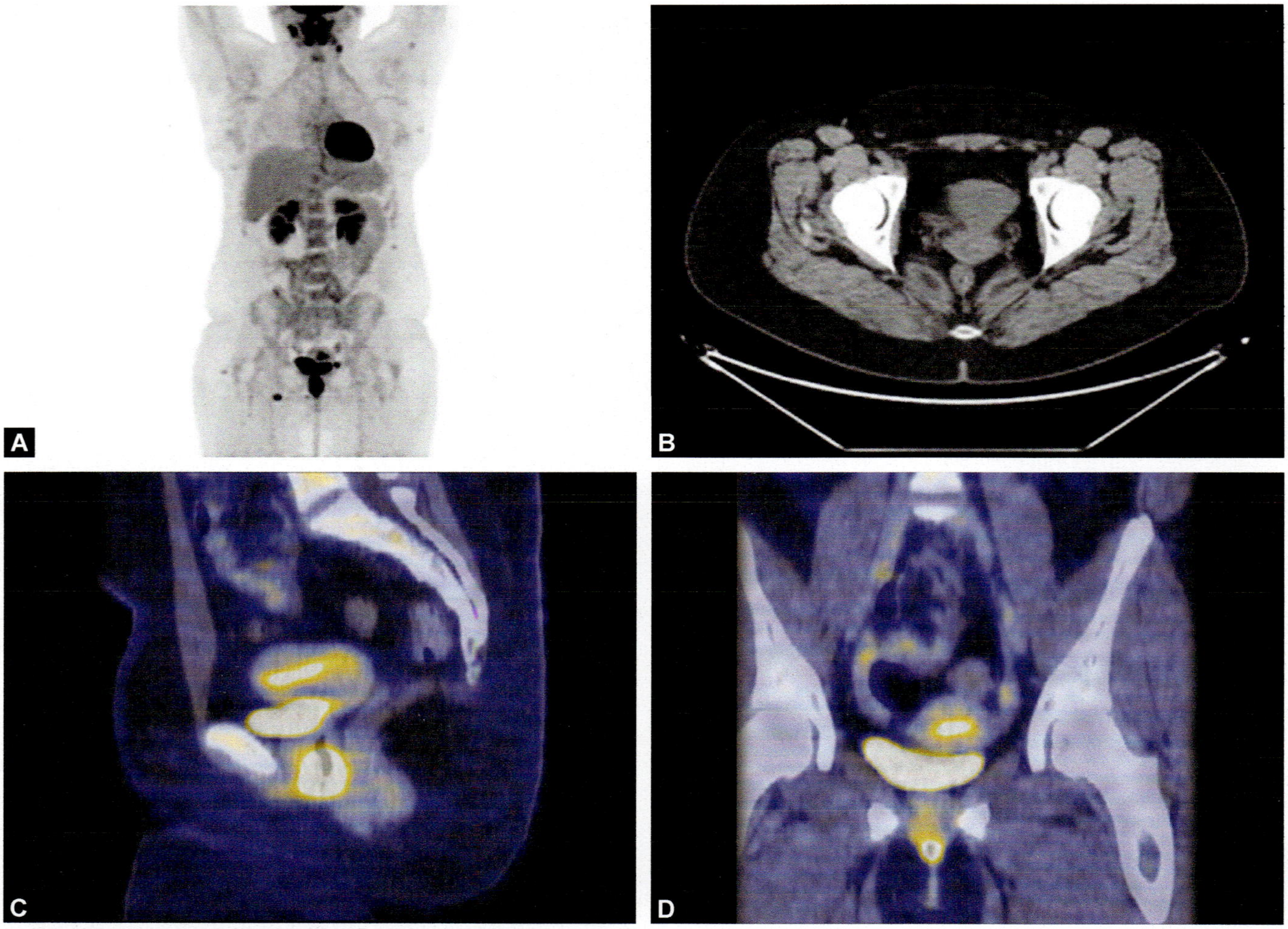

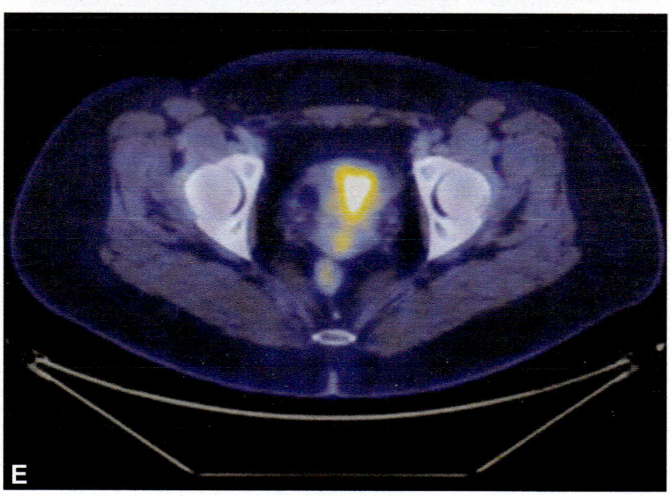

Figs. 2A to E: Another patient with physiologic FDG activity in the uterus and ovaries, most likely due to menses.

CASE 14: ENDOMETRIAL CARCINOMA WITH RESPONSE TO TREATMENT

Brief History

An 89-year-old with uterine papillary serous carcinoma status post-exploratory laparotomy, hysterectomy, left salpingo-oophorectomy and bilateral pelvic/periaortic lymph node dissection. The patient completed chemotherapy and vaginal brachytherapy shortly thereafter.

Findings

Findings are shown in Figures 1, 2 and 3.

Note the nonspecific uptake in the midline abdominal scar associated with postoperative changes, also resolved.

Main Teaching Points

- Positron emission tomography/computed tomography is very useful for detecting recurrence in endometrial carcinoma. The sensitivity and specificity of FDG PET imaging in the post-therapy surveillance of endometrial carcinomas is reported to be 96% and 78%.
- In endometrial carcinoma, 50% of the recurrences can occur both above and below the diaphragm, while 15% occur only above the diaphragm.
- Cancer antigen 125 (CA125) is often obtained after initial treatment to monitor for recurrence. It is highly specific and when elevated, PET/CT can further localize the recurrence.

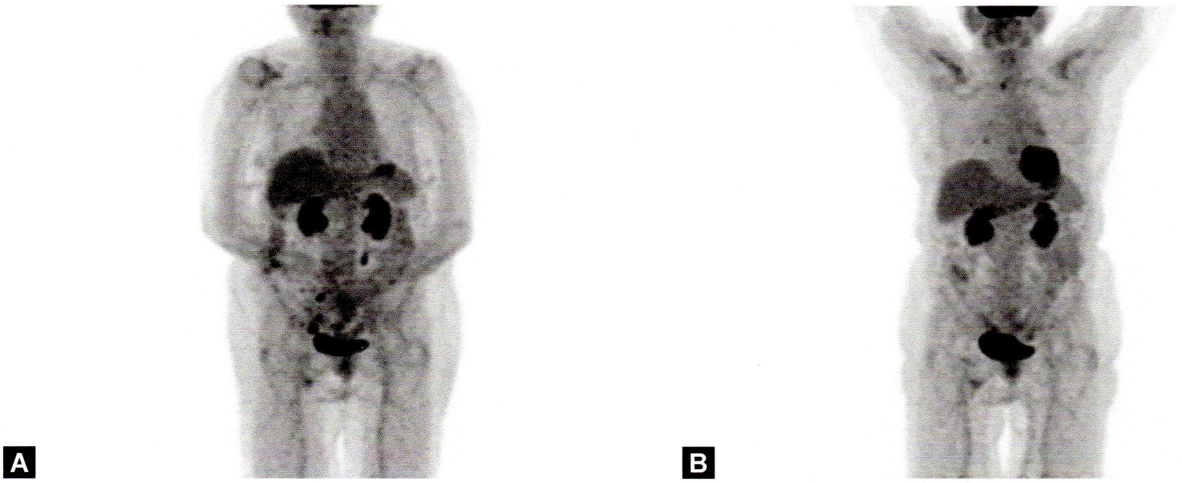

Figs. 1A and B: Pre and post chemoradiation therapy maximum intensity projection (MIP) whole body images demonstrate hypermetabolic right inguinal and iliac lymph nodes on pre-therapy Image (A) which are resolved on post-therapy image (B).

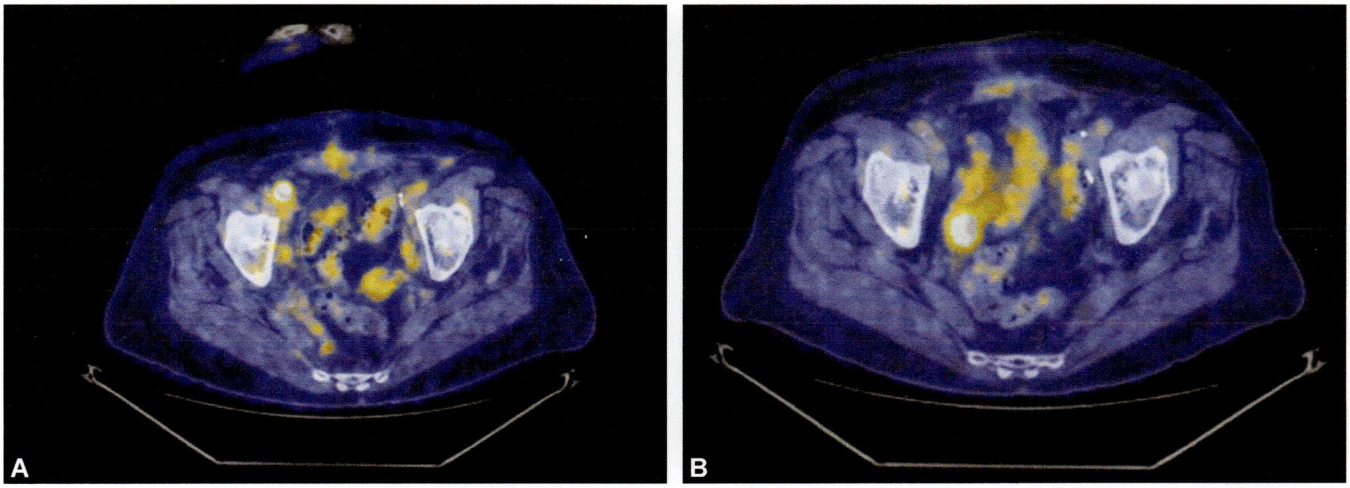

Figs. 2A and B: A hypermetabolic 1.3-cm right inguinal lymph node had a SUVmax of 16.2. It has subsequently resolved on Figure B. There is also a hypermetabolic 1.2-cm right common iliac lymph node which had a SUVmax of 9.5, resolved.

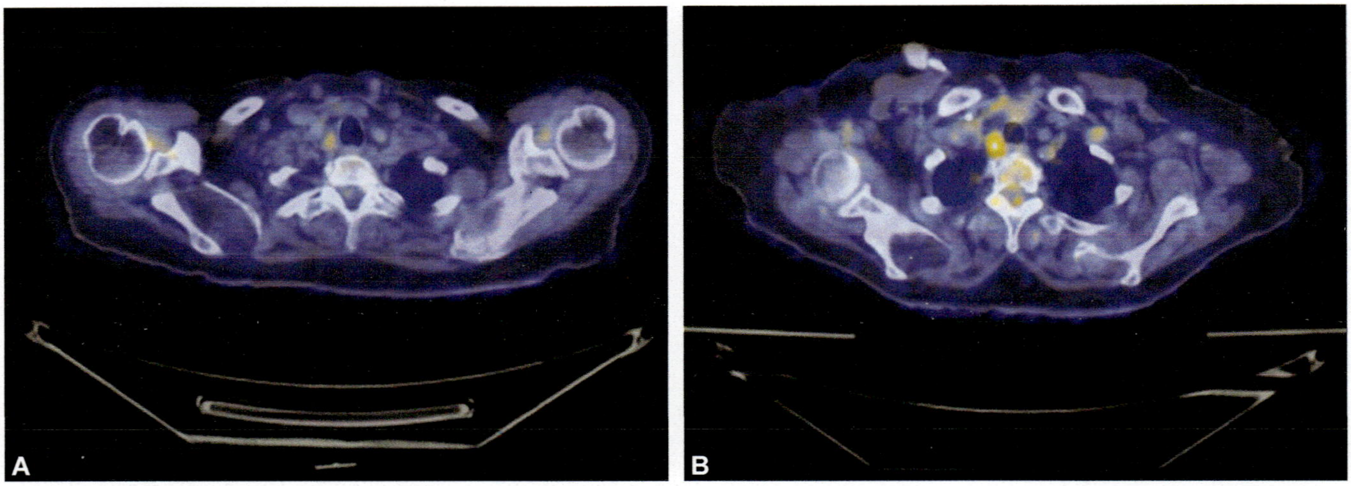

Figs. 3A and B: There has been interval increased FDG activity within a previously seen right paratracheal lymph node, now demonstrates SUVmax of 5.9 g/ml. It is stable in size, measuring 1.3-cm. Differential considerations include metastatic versus reactive inflammatory lymph node.

CASE 15: ENDOMETRIAL CANCER—INITIAL EVALUATION

Brief History

A 64-year-old female with biopsy-proven endometrial cancer with myometrial invasion. PET/CT ordered to detect metastatic disease.

Findings

Findings are shown in Figures 1 and 2.

Main Teaching Points

- Adenocarcinoma of the endometrium is the most frequent and most curable gynecological cancer in postmenopausal women.
- The subtype of endometrial carcinoma known as papillary serous carcinoma is extremely malignant.
- The incidence of lymph node metastasis increases from 3% with superficial myometrial invasion to more than 40% with deep myometrial invasion.

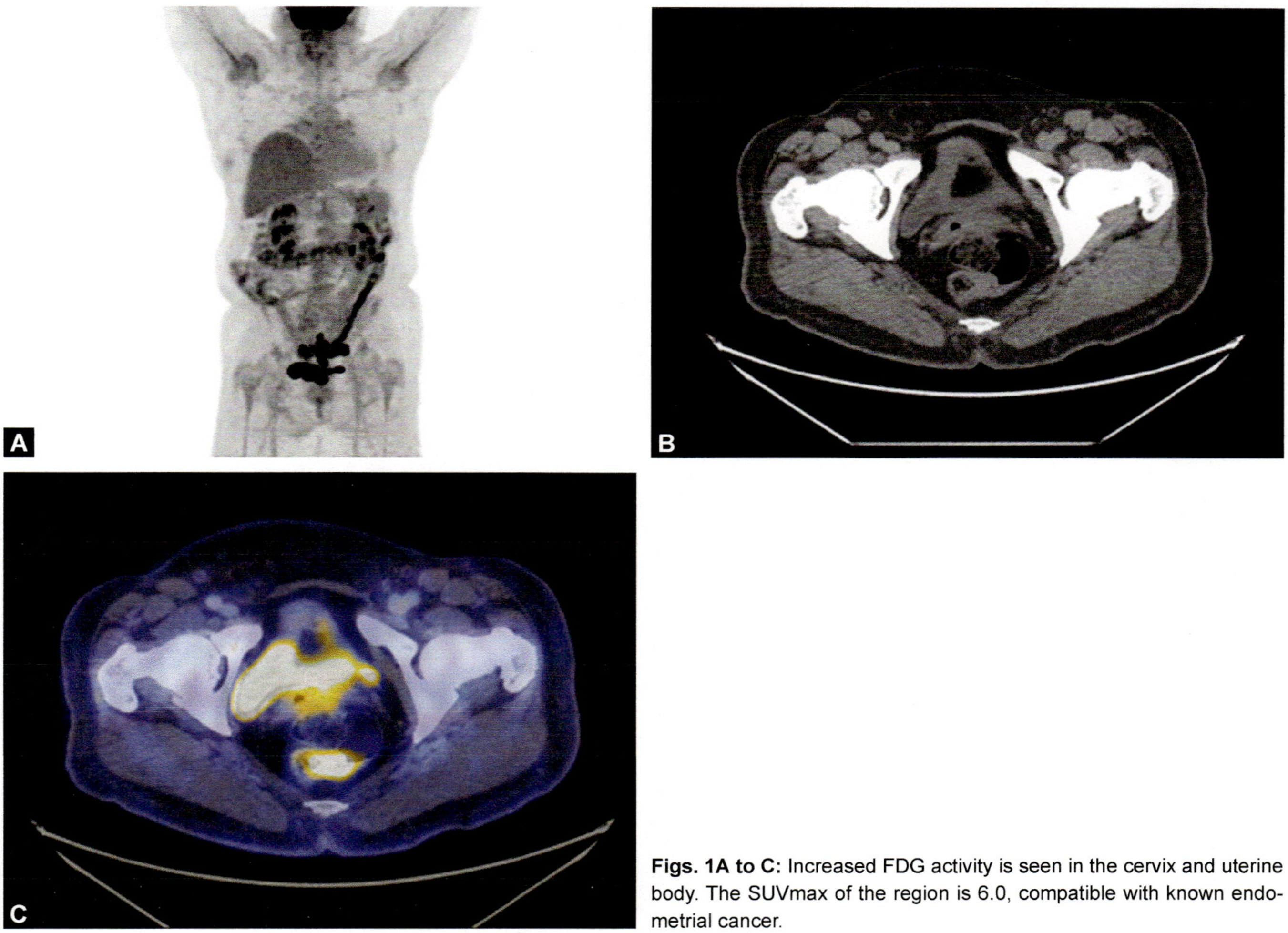

Figs. 1A to C: Increased FDG activity is seen in the cervix and uterine body. The SUVmax of the region is 6.0, compatible with known endometrial cancer.

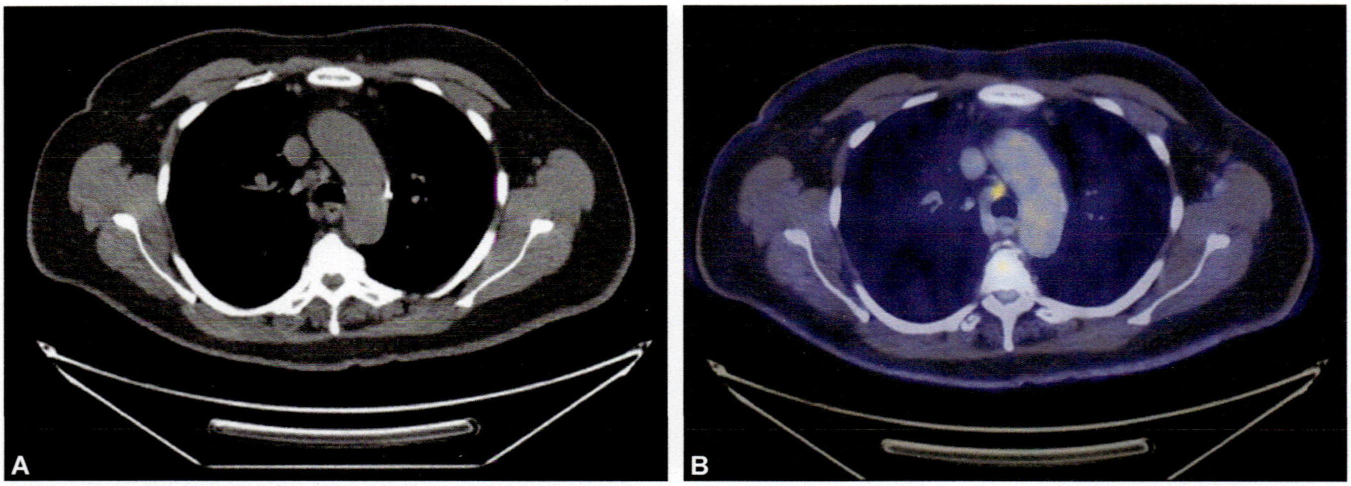

Figs. 2A and B: A hypermetabolic precarinal lymph node measures 0.7-cm with a SUVmax of 2.5. Other shotty mediastinal lymph nodes are visualized but demonstrate no abnormal FDG activity. The mild FDG activity of only one mediastinal lymph node would favor reactive inflammatory change rather than metastasis. Clinicians should correlate with any prior recent history of respiratory infection.

CASE 16: UTERINE LEIOMYOMA

Brief History

A 40-year-old female with nodular sclerosing Hodgkin's disease status post six cycles of chemotherapy.

Findings

Findings are shown in Figures 1 to 3.

Main Teaching Points

- Eighteen percent of fibroids can be hypermetabolic. Therefore, the most common pattern of FDG uptake in fibroids is actually one demonstrating a lack of uptake.
- On CT, most uterine fibroids are hypometabolic or isometabolic relative to the myometrium.
- The average SUVmax of a hypermetabolic fibroid is 2.34.
- Calcified fibroids or degenerated leiomyoma develop when the fibroid tumor outgrows its own blood supply. A degenerated leiomyoma has significantly higher uptake than a non-degenerated leiomyoma.

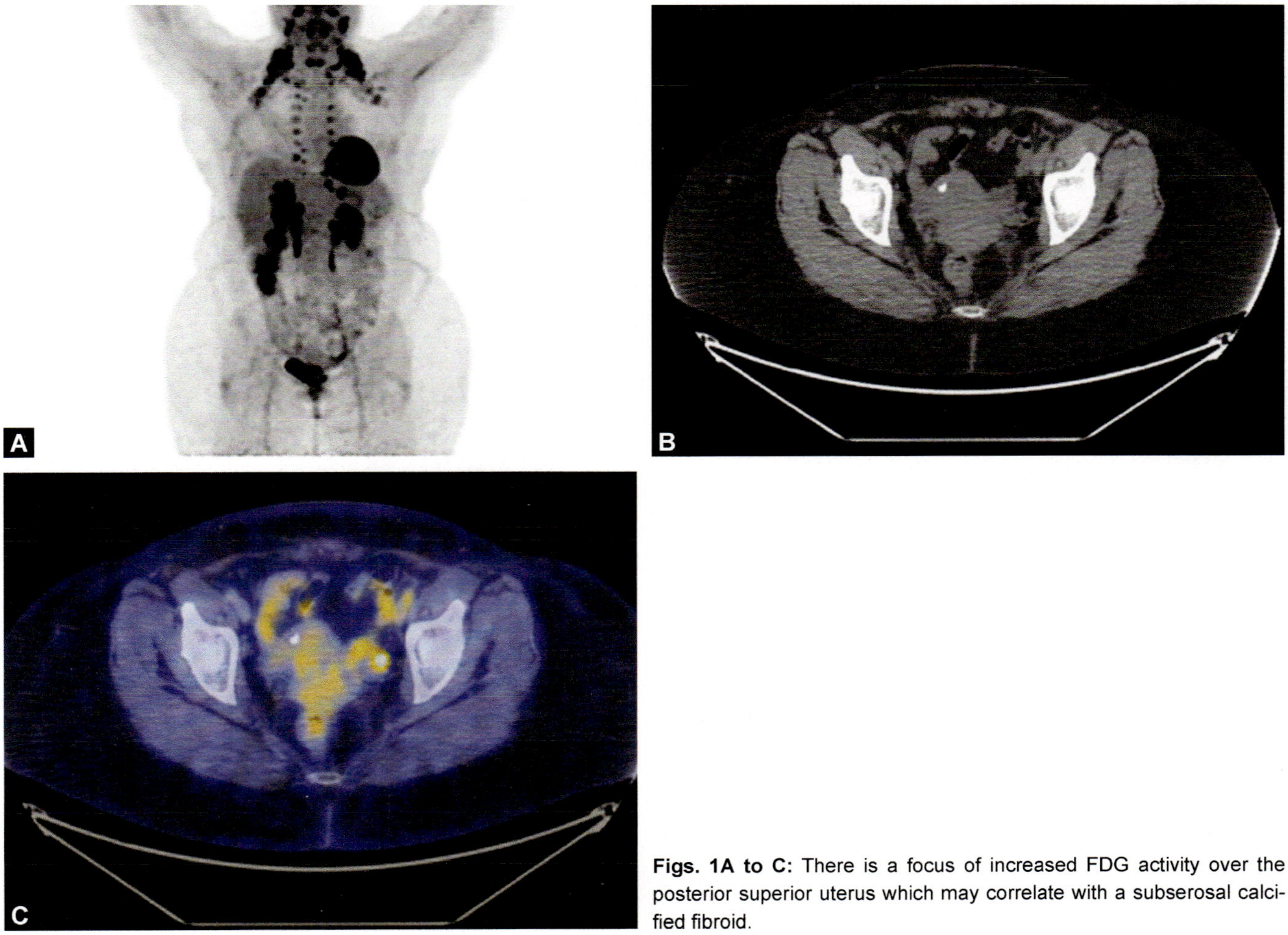

Figs. 1A to C: There is a focus of increased FDG activity over the posterior superior uterus which may correlate with a subserosal calcified fibroid.

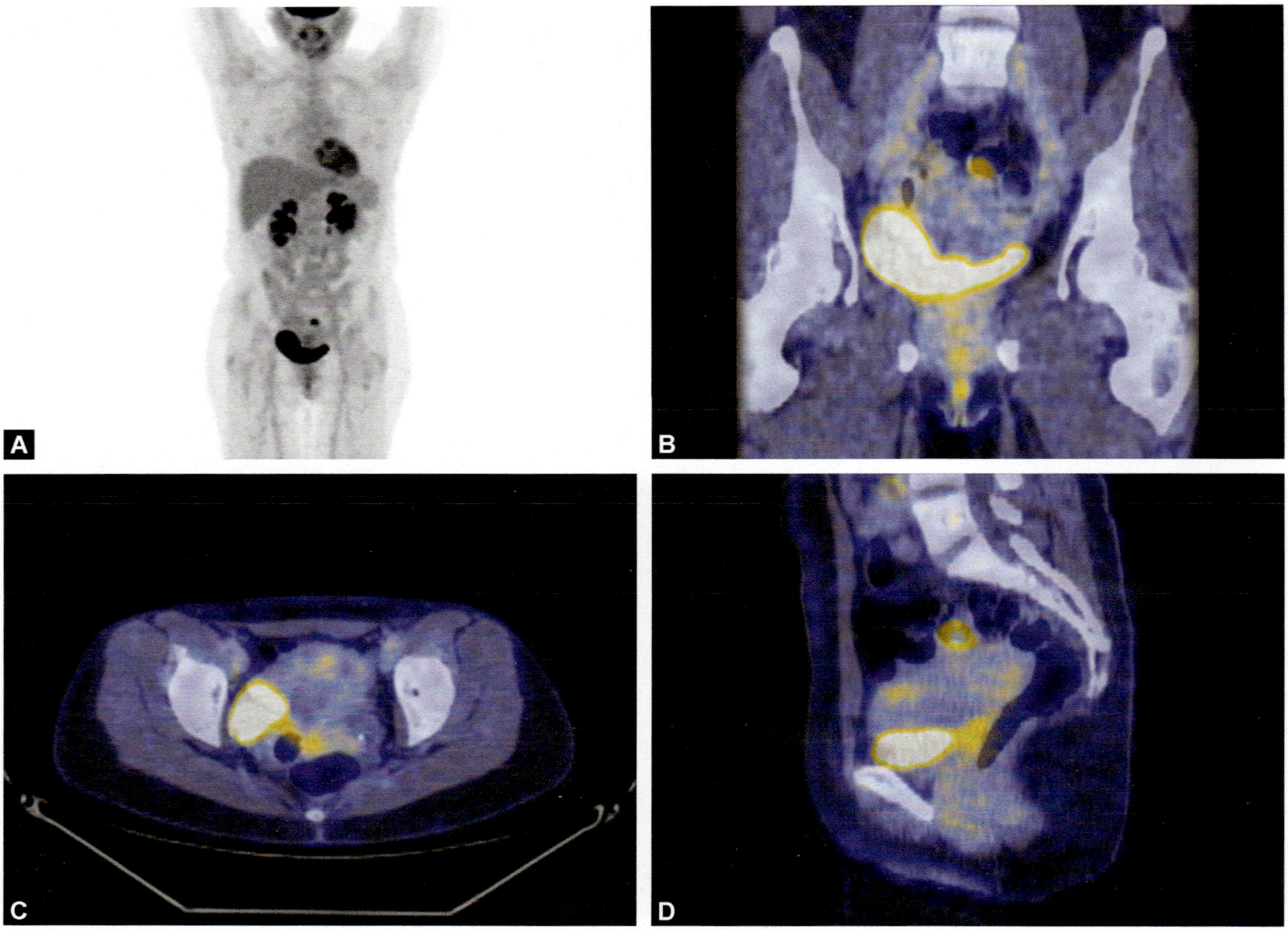

Figs. 2A to D: A subsequent PET/CT shows that the uterine focus has a SUVmax of 6 g/mL, and remains unchanged in size over a year.

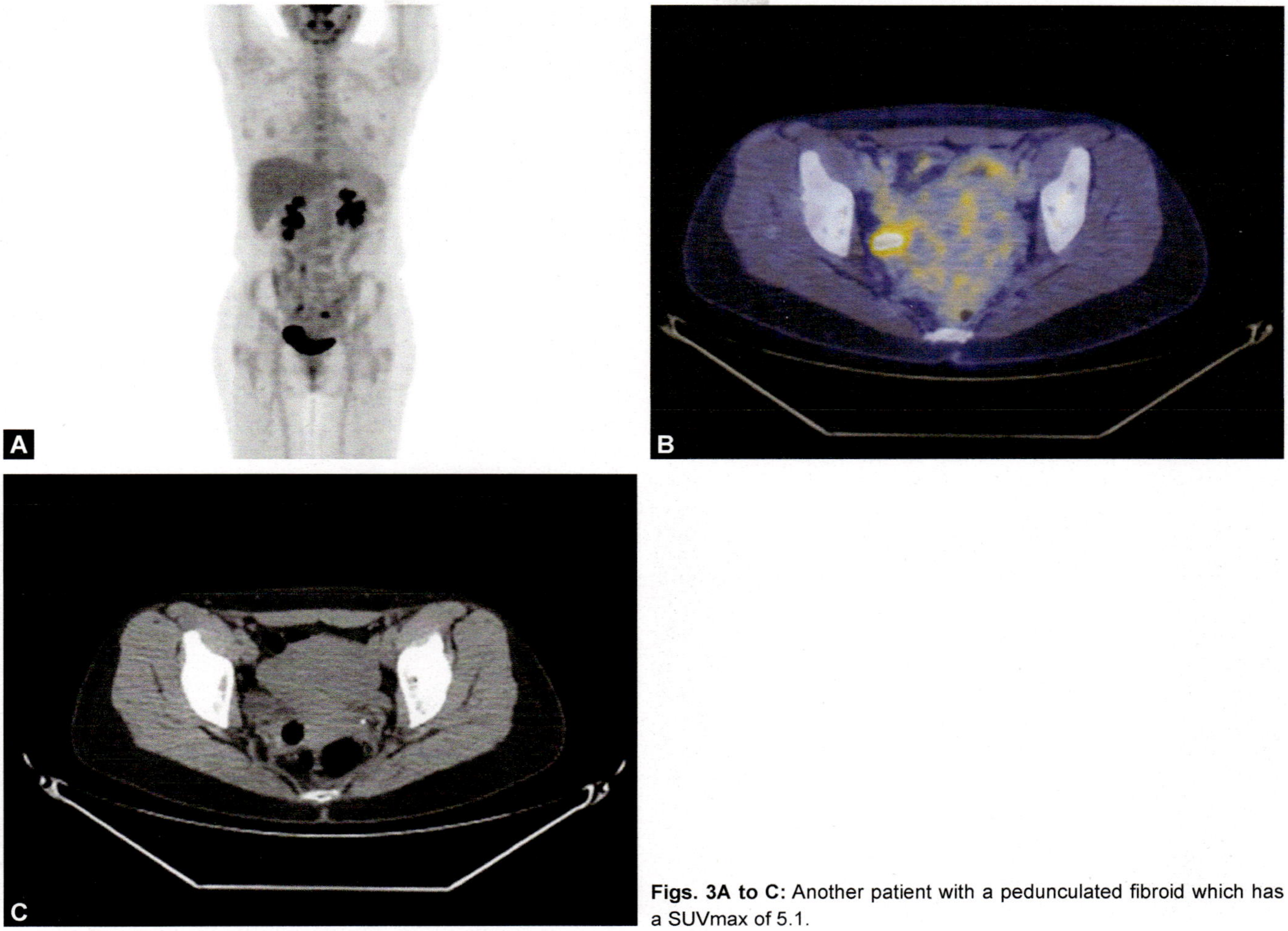

Figs. 3A to C: Another patient with a pedunculated fibroid which has a SUVmax of 5.1.

CASE 17: LARGE UTERINE LEIOMYOMA

Brief History

A 60-year-old female with newly diagnosed right breast cancer in June 2009, status post lumpectomy and right axillary dissection. A PET/CT study has been requested to evaluate for staging of the disease.

Findings

Findings are shown in Figures 1A to D.

Main Teaching Points

- Endogenous estrogen and hormone replacement therapy increase the FDG uptake of fibroids. Therefore, fibroids can also demonstrate variability of FDG uptake.
- Leiomyomas with focal FDG uptake can be seen in both pre- and postmenopausal women with a higher incidence in premenopausal women.

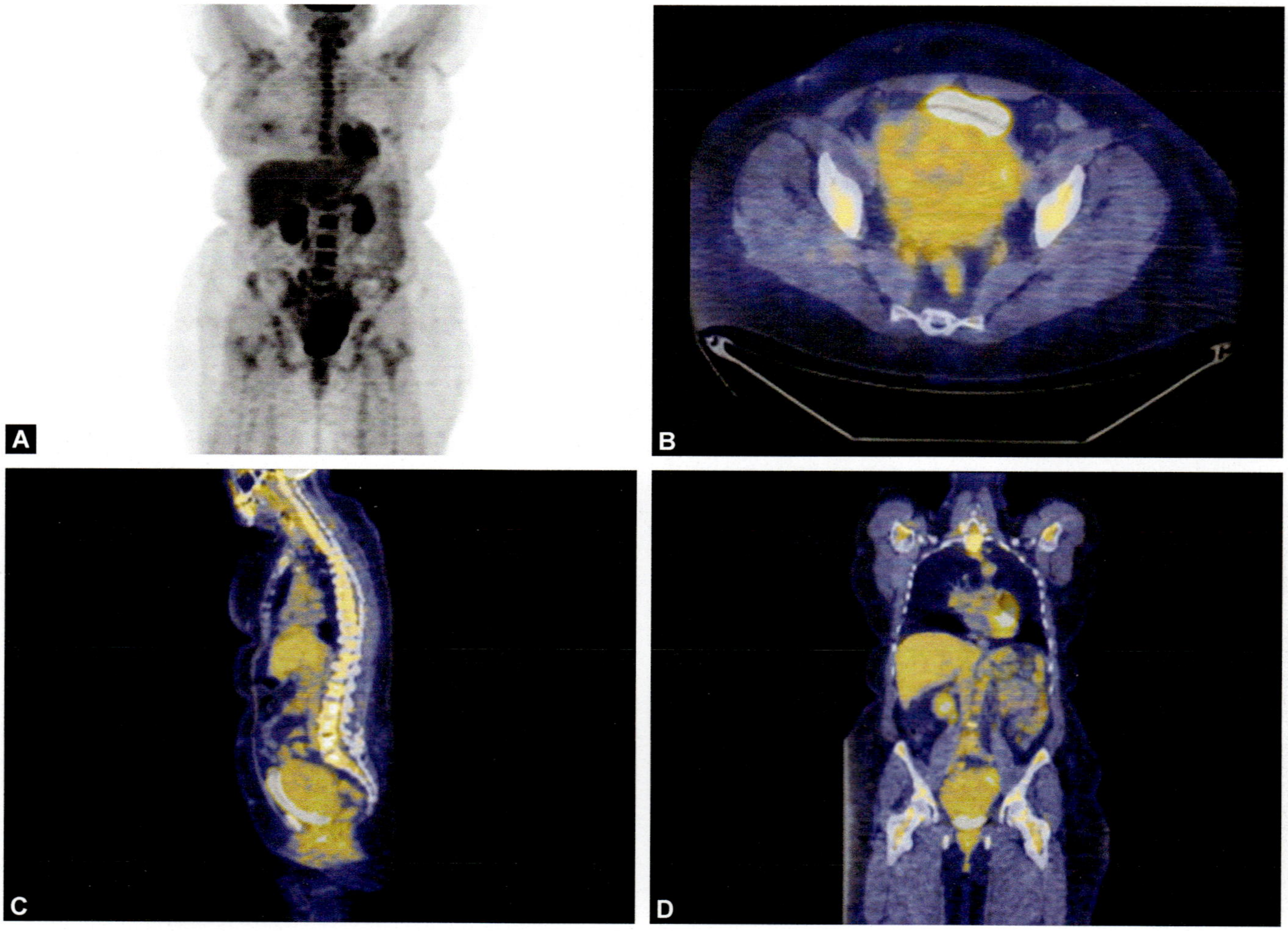

Figs. 1A to D: Nonspecific FDG uptake within a large fibroid uterus, with mass effect on the urinary bladder.

Head and Neck Cases

CASE 1: OCULAR MELANOMA

Brief History

A 55-year-old male with left-sided ocular melanoma status post-laser therapy and radiation. Patient was referred to evaluate for metastatic disease.

Findings

Findings are shown in Figures 1 and 2.

Main Teaching Point

- The activity of choroidal melanomas is not completely dependent upon tumor size.[1]

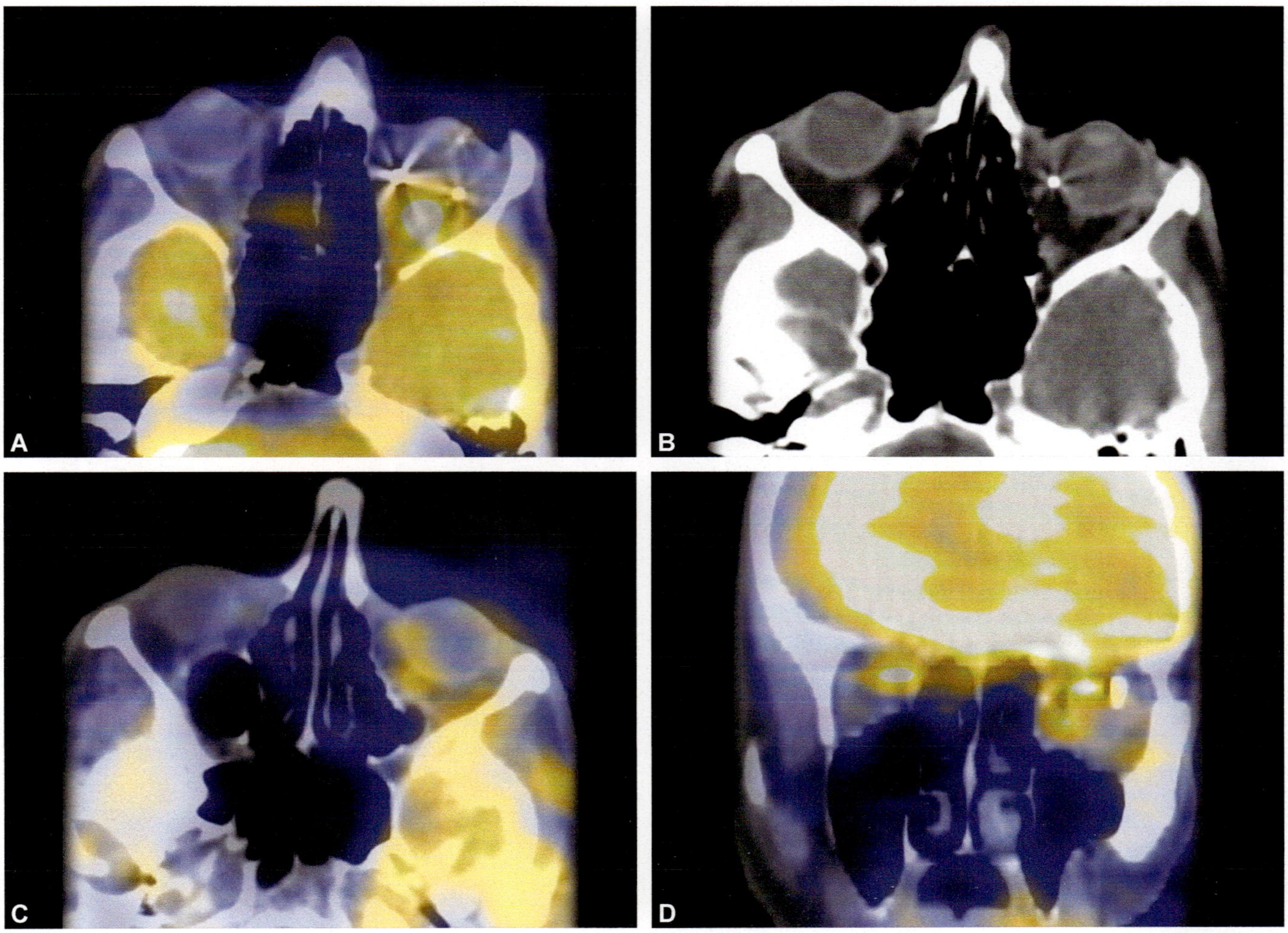

Figs. 1A to D: The FDG positron emission tomography/computed tomography shows postsurgical change involving the left orbit. There are several radiotherapy markers which cause the beam-hardening artifact. Although more activity can be seen on the posterior aspect of the left orbit than the right, this is considered inflammatory due the radiation therapy.

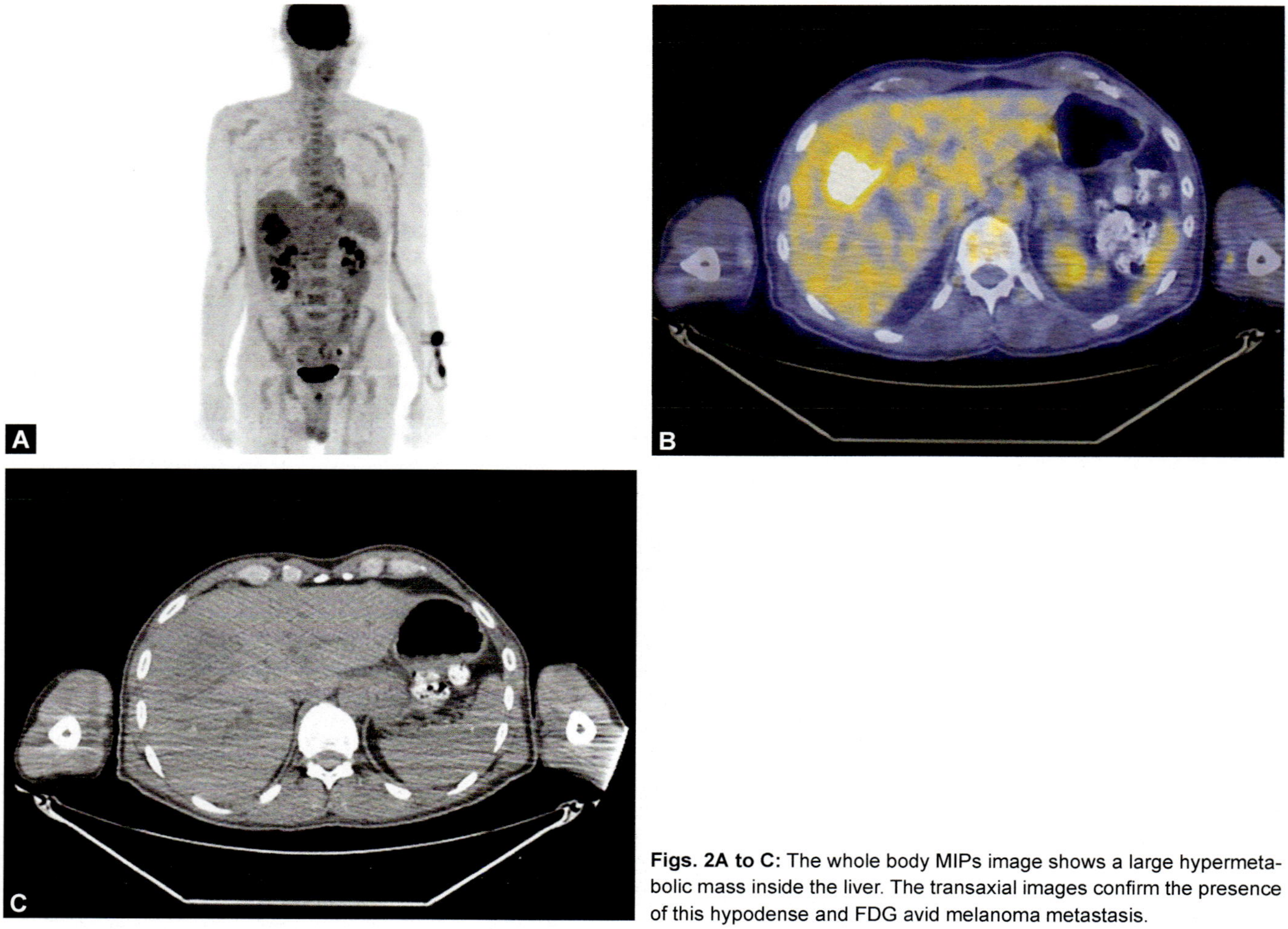

Figs. 2A to C: The whole body MIPs image shows a large hypermetabolic mass inside the liver. The transaxial images confirm the presence of this hypodense and FDG avid melanoma metastasis.

- A small study of ocular melanomas showed a false positive rate of 5.7% when further evaluated by histopathology and/or additional imaging.[2]
- There is a tendency of uveal melanoma to metastasize to the liver, and FDG positron emission tomography (PET) is a valuable investigation for the detection of these liver metastases.[3]

REFERENCES

1. Available from http://bjo.bmj.com/content/89/10/1265.short
2. Available from http://bjo.bmj.com/content/89/10/1270.short
3. Available from http://www.sciencedirect.com/science/article/pii/S0748798306001752

CASE 2: MELANOMA WITH DISTANT METASTASES

Brief History

Evaluate for metastatic disease in this patient who was recently diagnosed with subcutaneous melanoma of the right ankle.

Findings

Findings are shown in Figures 1 to 3.

Main Teaching Points

- Positron emission tomography/computed tomography detects significantly more visceral and nonvisceral metastases than PET or computed tomography

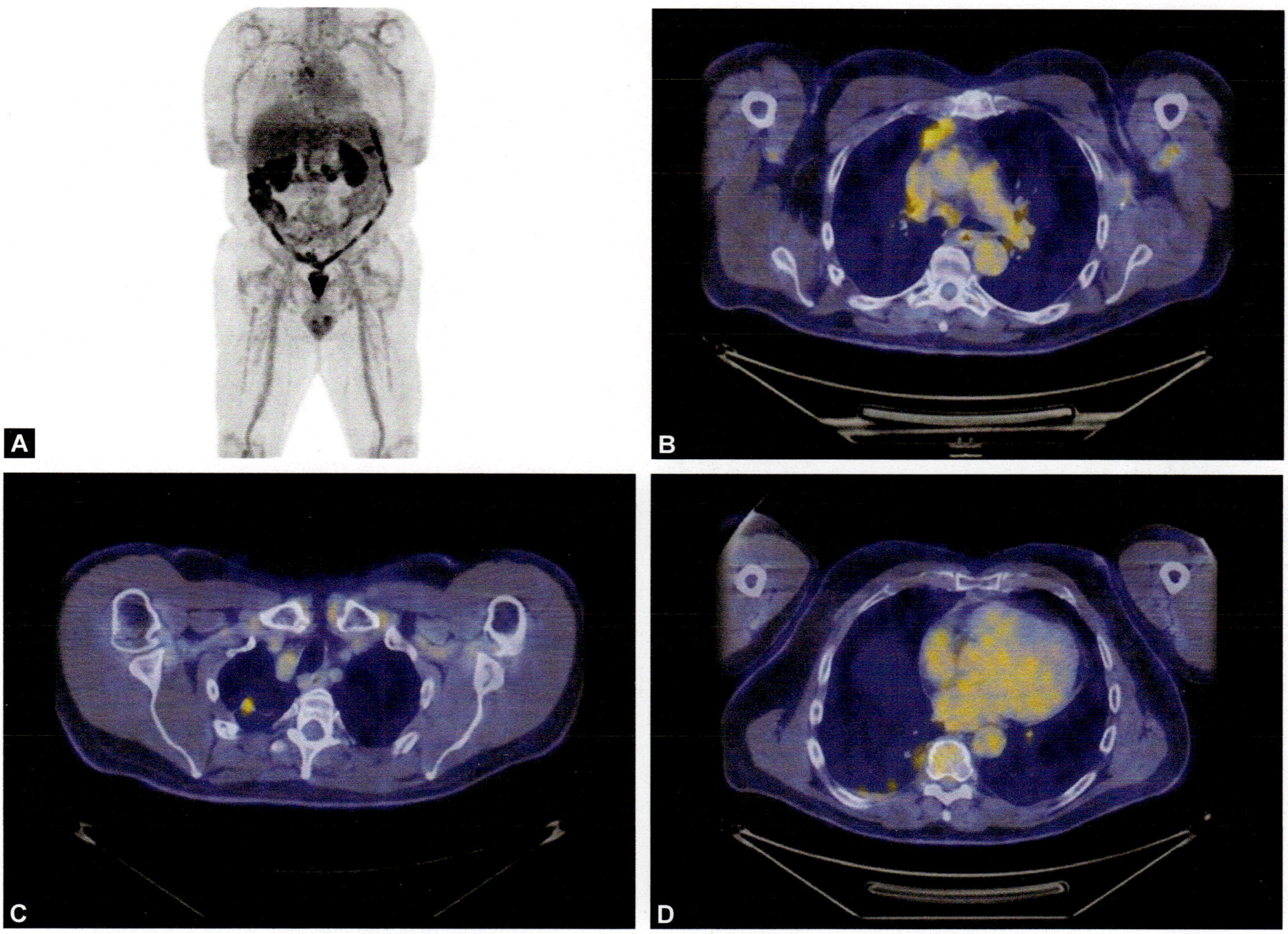

Figs. 1A to D: Widespread metastatic disease is seen involving the bilateral lungs, hilum, pleural wall and mediastinum.

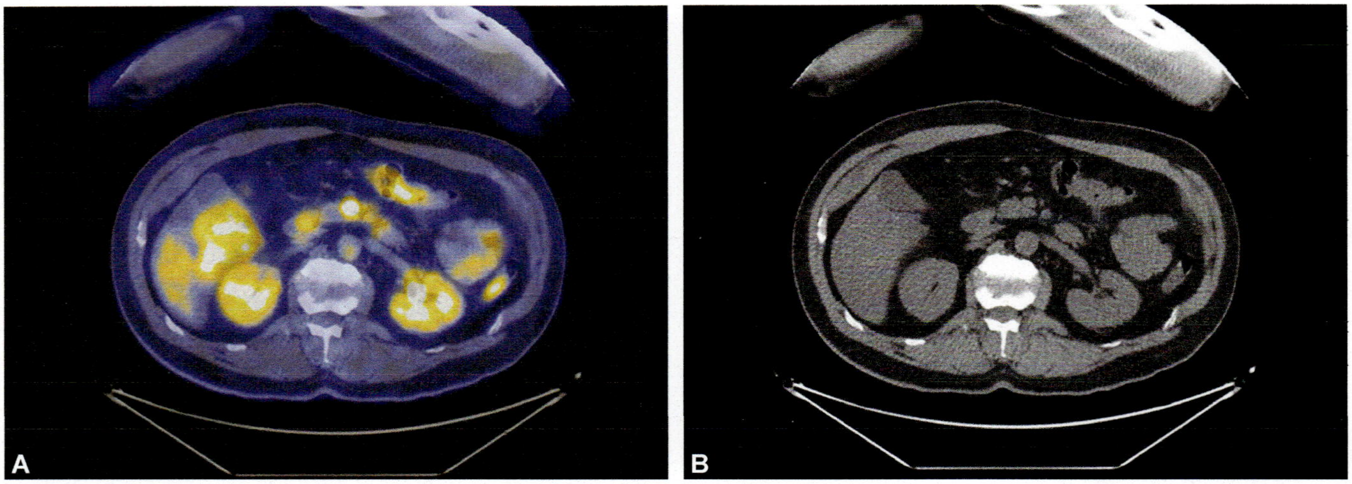

Figs. 2A and B: There is a pancreatic focus of high FDG activity but no computed tomography correlate. This is highly suspicious for a melanoma involvement of the body of the pancreas.

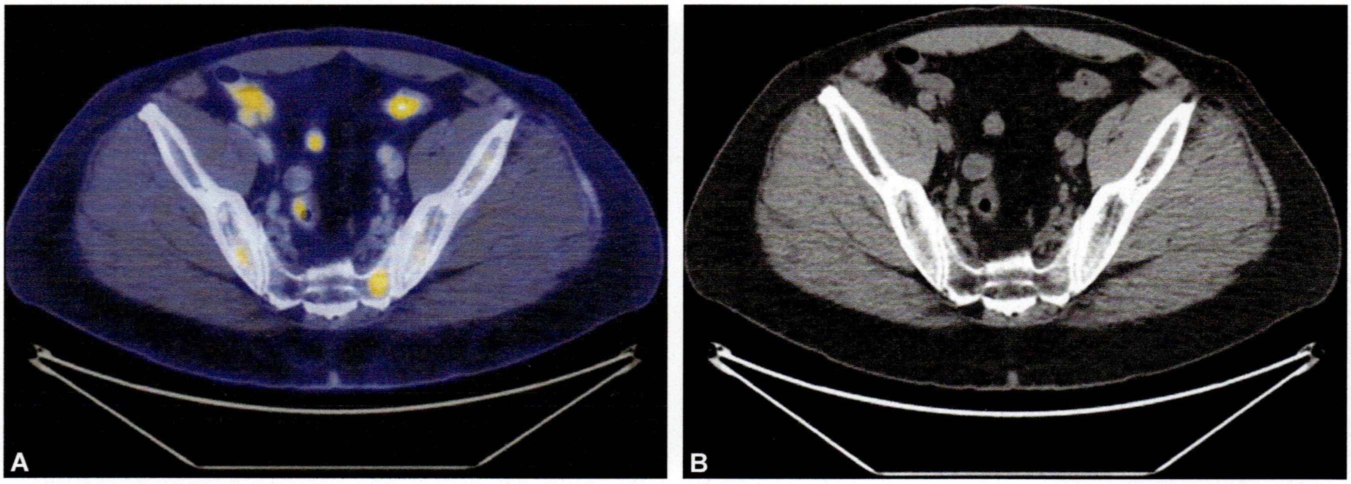

Figs. 3A and B: In addition, a sclerotic focus of FDG activity is also seen in the sacrum, which is also suspicious for metastasis.

(CT) alone. PET/CT was 98% sensitive for melanoma metastasis.[1]

- Cutaneous melanoma frequently metastasizes and is difficult to treat.[2] The most common organs involved were the lymph nodes followed by lungs, liver, brain, bone, heart and adrenal glands.
- A meta-analysis suggests that FDG PET is not useful for the initial diagnosis of melanoma, or in patients with thin primary lesions less than 1 mm and no evidence of metastases.[3]

REFERENCES

1. Available from http://jco.ascopubs.org/content/24/7/1178.short
2. Available from http://www.sciencedirect.com/science/article/pii/S000129980400039X
3. Available from http://onlinelibrary.wiley.com/doi/10.1002/1097-0142%2820010415%2991:8%3C1530::AID-CNCR1162%3E3.0.CO;2-%23/full

CASE 3: PET/CT OF EPILEPSY

Brief History

Evaluate for a seizure focus in a patient with epilepsy resistant to medical management.

Findings

Findings are shown in Figures 1 to 4.

Main Teaching Points

- If imaging is acquired during the immediate post-ictal period, there may actually be hypoperfusion of the seizure focus.[1]
- Interictal imaging is much less sensitive than either ictal or post-ictal scanning, as perfusion to the seizure focus has often normalized.
- Interictal PET and ictal subtraction single-photon emission computed tomography studies can provide complementary information to more accurately evaluate medically intractable epilepsy preoperatively.[2]

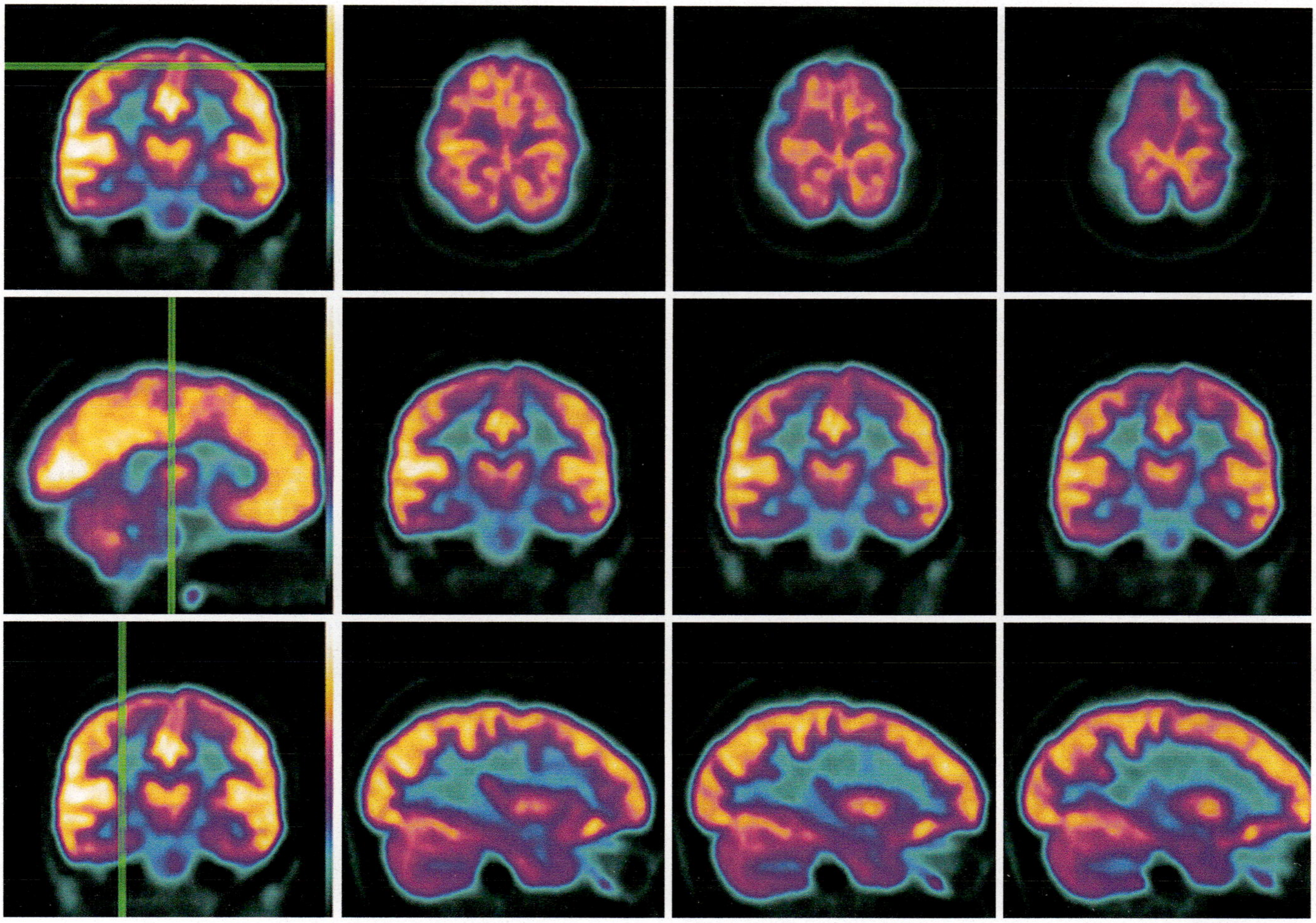

Fig. 1: This interictal FDG-positron emission tomography study demonstrates decreased metabolism at the frontal paramedial region. This may represent a seizure focus site and is best visualized in the middle row on the coronal view.

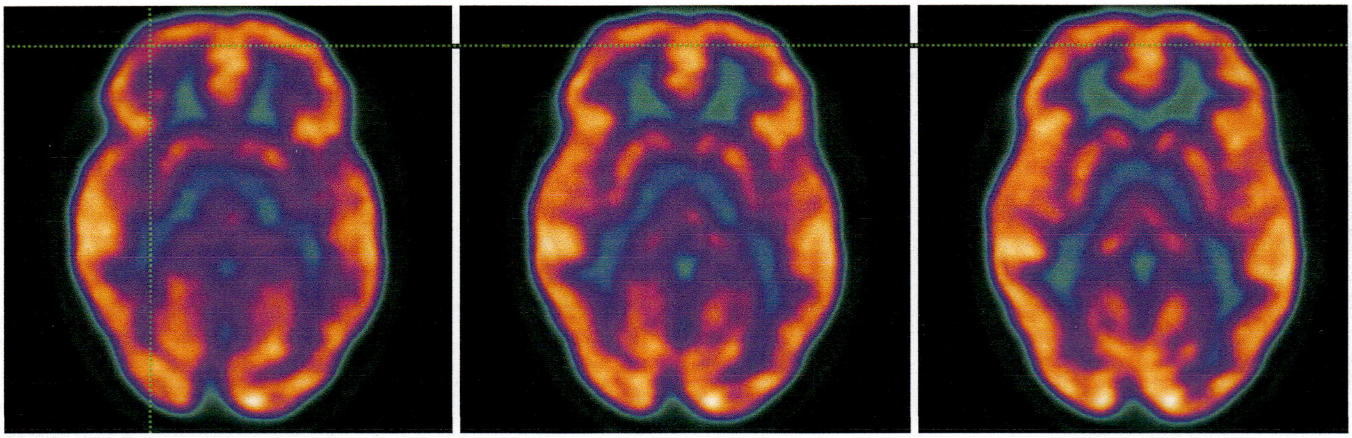

Fig. 2: On the same study, there is a small focus of decreased activity at the right frontal lobe.

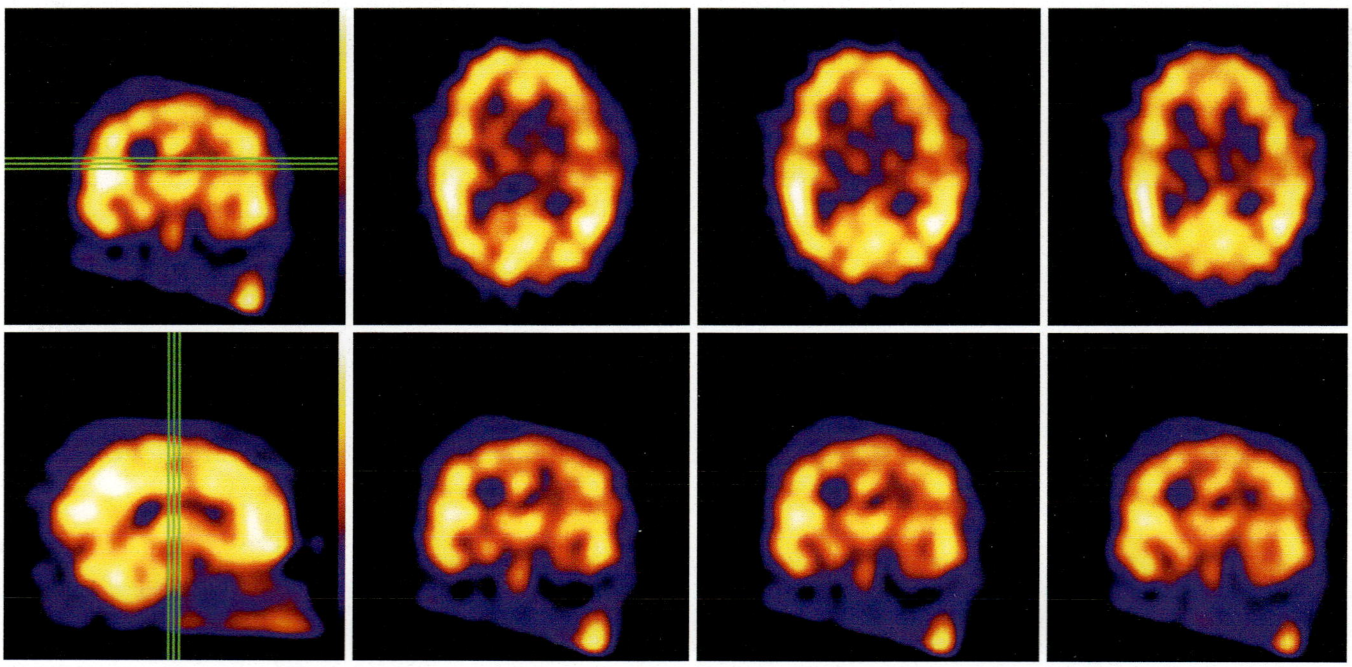

Fig. 3: This interictal brain Tc-99m-hexamethylpropyleneamine oxime-single-photon emission computed tomography (HMPAO-SPECT) of the same patient demonstrates a small area of asymmetrically decreased perfusion in the left frontoparietal region. This defect could not be correlated with other examinations and may represent noise.

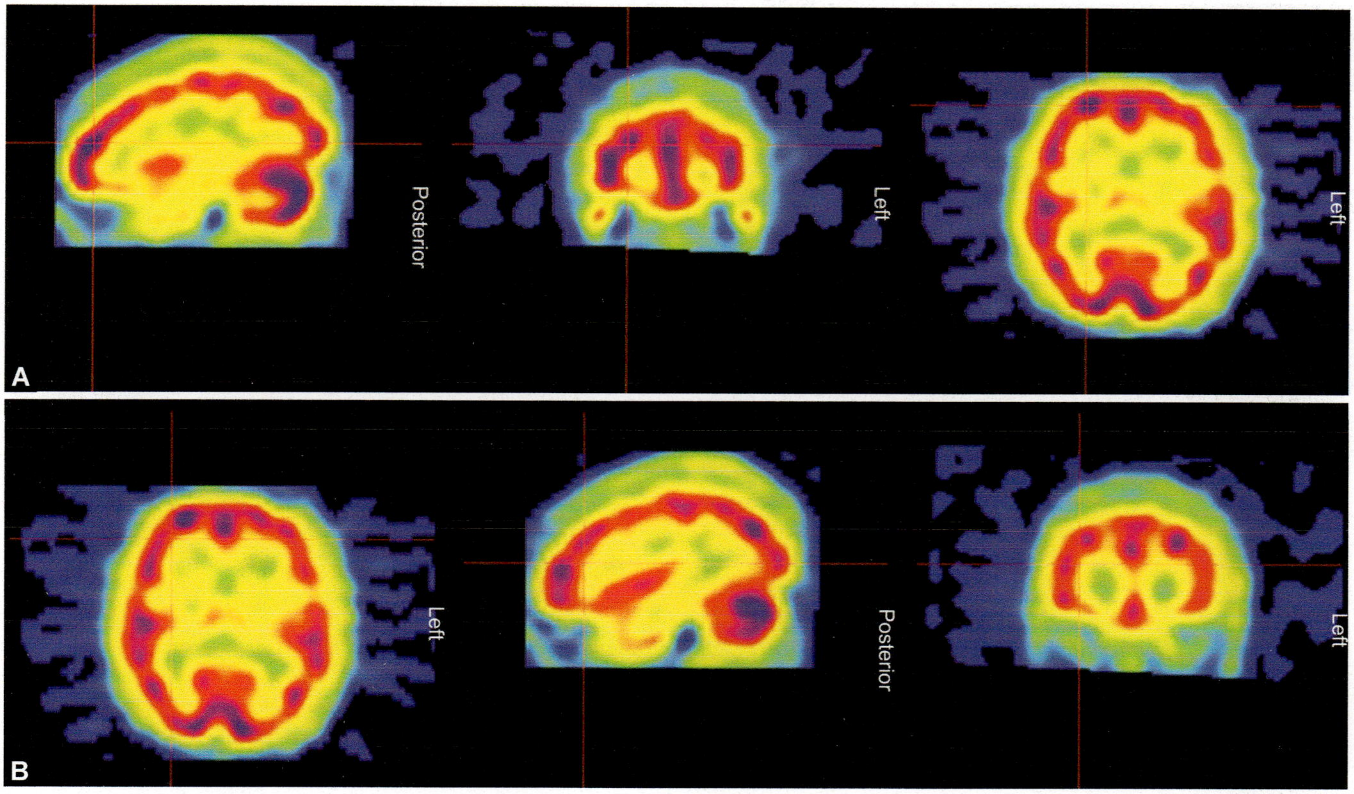

Figs. 4A and B: Subtraction images were processed using a new ictal single-photon emission computed tomography (SPECT) minus the previously mentioned interictal SPECT. Review of the images demonstrates mild increased perfusion in the right frontal region. This same region matches the area of mild hypoperfusion on the interictal FDG PET/CT mentioned above. This right frontal focus is suspicious for seizure activity.

REFERENCES

1. Available from https://www.urmc.rochester.edu/smd/rad/neurocases/Neurocase484.htm
2. Available from http://www.ncbi.nlm.nih.gov/pubmed/23030361

CASE 4: FDG PET OF TEMPORAL LOBE EPILEPSY

Brief History

A 52-year-old male with olfactory aura and episodes of staring, resistant to medications.

Findings

Findings are shown in Figures 1 and 2.

Main Teaching Points

- A common pathological abnormality found in temporal lobe epilepsy is medial temporal sclerosis whereby the hippocampal neurons have atrophied.[1]
- FDG PET is the best modality for determining post-surgical outcome. However, magnetic resonance imaging (MRI) is most influential for determining surgical candidacy.[2]
- FDG PET is 85–90% sensitive for detecting medial temporal lobe epileptic foci.[3]

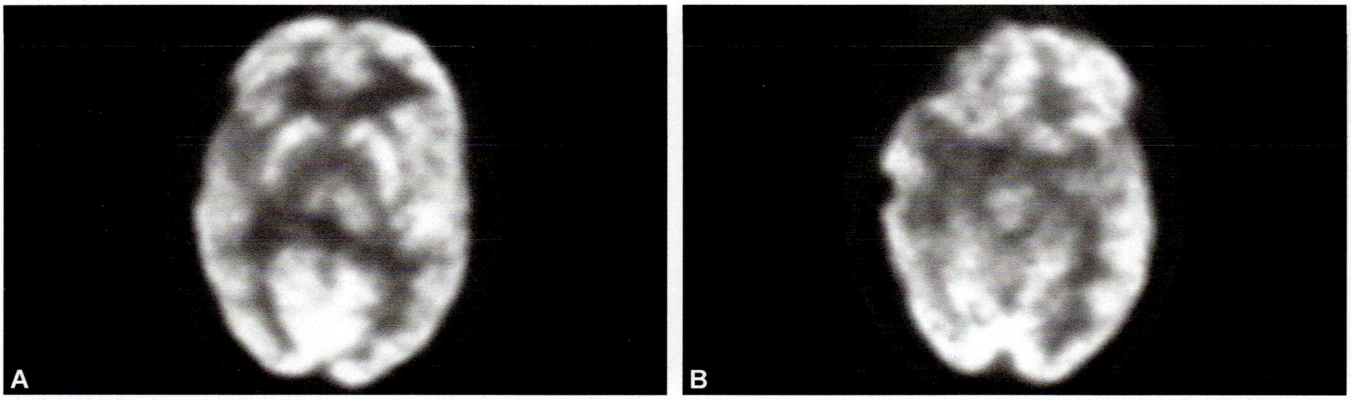

Figs. 1A and B: Both images (A and B) are adjacent slices of the brain from an FDG PET/CT study. Reduced metabolic activity is seen in the right temporal lobe on both slices, suspicious for a focus of seizure activity in the right temporal lobe.

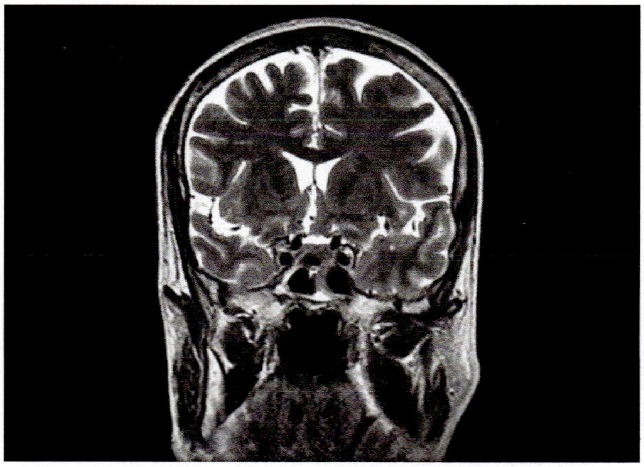

Fig. 2: A magnetic resonance imaging was also acquired for anatomic characterization. It demonstrated an atrophic right hippocampus with abnormally high T2-weighted signal compatible with medial temporal sclerosis.

REFERENCES

1. Available from http://en.wikipedia.org/wiki/Mesial_temporal_sclerosis
2. Available from http://www.ncbi.nlm.nih.gov/pmc/articles/PMC3260654/
3. Available from http://jnm.snmjournals.org/content/43/9/1167.full.pdf

CASE 5: FDG PET OF ALZHEIMER'S DISEASE

Brief History

A slow progression of memory loss.

Findings

Findings are shown in Figures 1 to 4.

Main Teaching Points

- It is well established that bilateral temporoparietal hypometabolism is the classic metabolic abnormality associated with Alzheimer's disease.[1]
- The sensitivity of FDG PET for detecting Alzheimer's disease is 93% based on a study with pathologic verification. However, the specificity was 63%.
- Clinical suspicion of Alzheimer's disease is 70% sensitive and 100% specific.

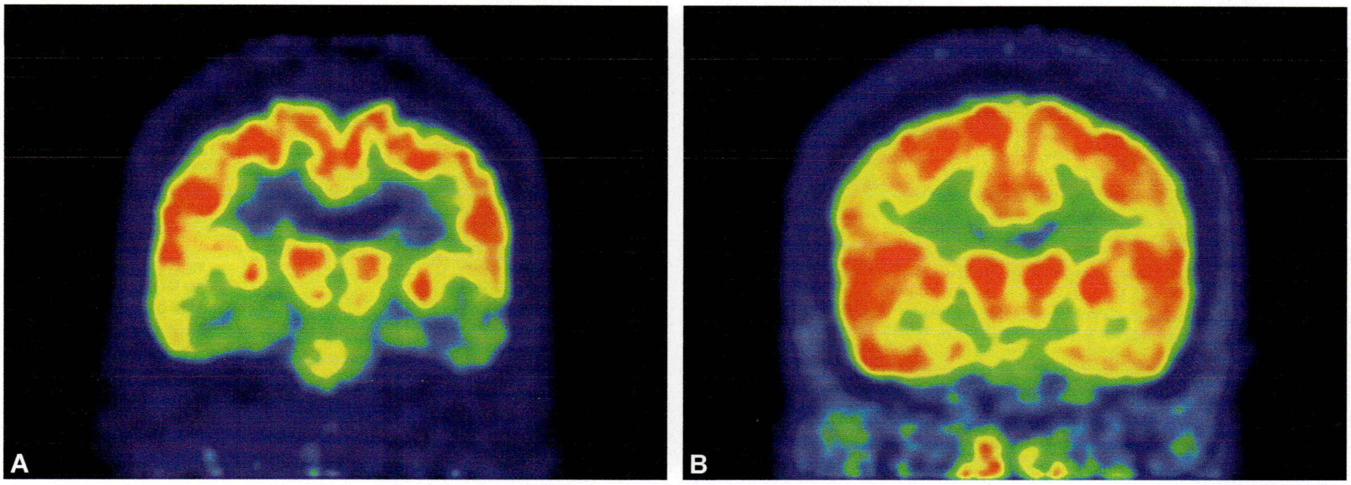

Figs. 1A and B: Significantly decreased FDG activity is seen in the bilateral temporal lobes of the first image. The second image represents a normal brain for comparison.

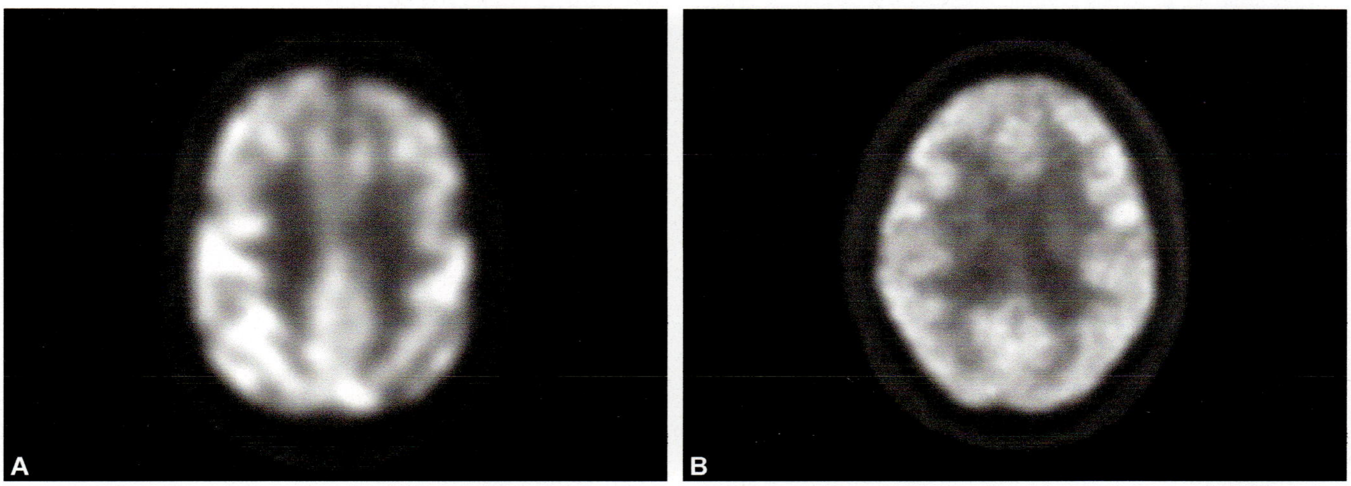

Figs. 2A and B: On the leftmost image, normal FDG activity is seen in the frontal lobes of this same patient. A normal brain is shown in the rightmost image.

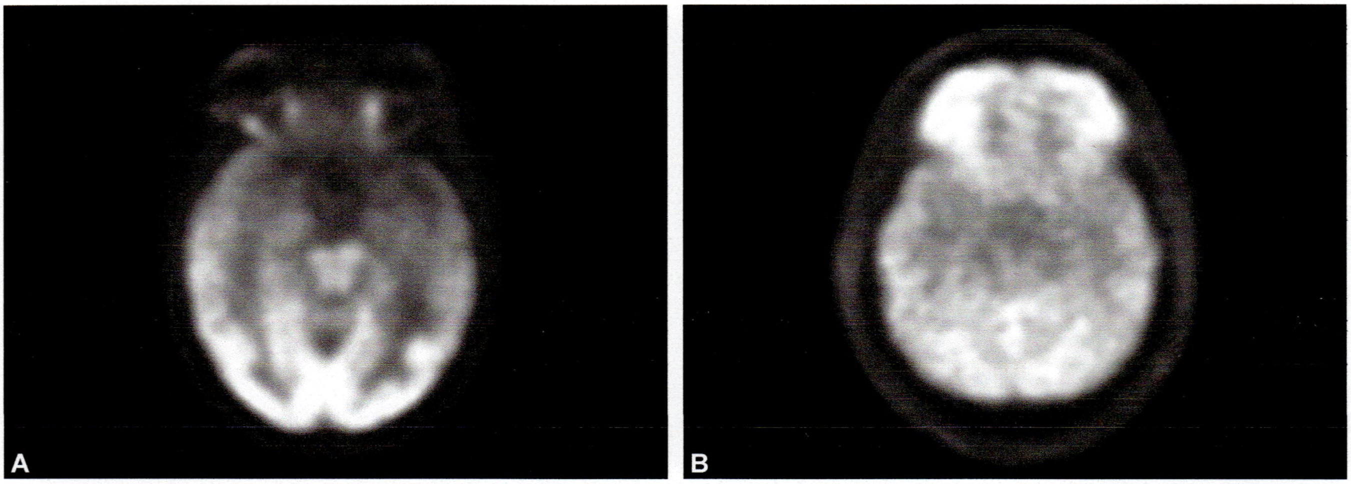

Figs. 3A and B: The abnormally decreased FDG activity is seen at the anterior and mesial aspect of the temporal lobes, a pattern most likely representative of Alzheimer's disease. In the rightmost image, the normal brain demonstrates no such decrease. Allowing for anatomic differences, the gray matter is symmetrically perfused on the rightmost image.

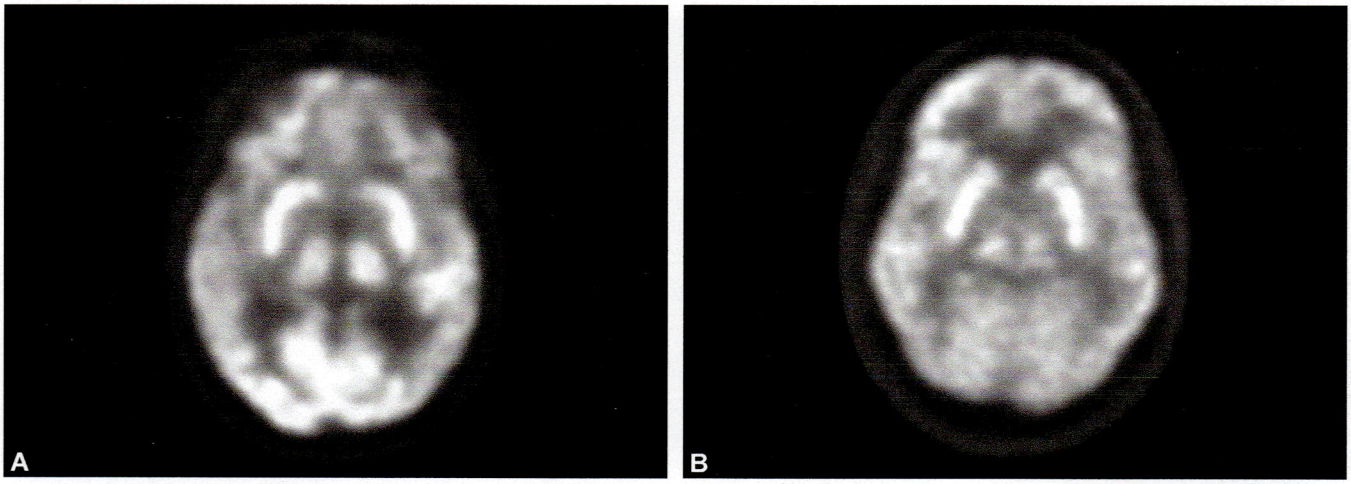

Figs. 4A and B: There is mild decreased activity in the bilateral parietal lobes, but the occipital lobes of this patient and the normal patient are similar appearing and demonstrate normal activity.

REFERENCE

1. Available from http://jnm.snmjournals.org/content/41/11/1920.short

CASE 6: PET FDG OF FRONTAL TEMPORAL DEMENTIA

Brief History

Personality changes and memory loss.

Findings

Findings are shown in Figures 1A to C.

Main Teaching Points

- The hallmarks of frontotemporal dementia (FTD) are behavior and language disturbance as opposed to symptom of Alzheimer's disease (AD) which is memory loss.
- Frontotemporal dementia lacks the cholinergic deficiency of AD and is clinically managed differently thus emphasizing the importance of differentiating the two.
- In FTD, hypometabolism is predominantly in anterior regions including the frontal lobes, anterior temporal cortex and anterior cingulate cortex.[1]
- In a study, hemispheric asymmetry of hypometabolism (more frequently lateralized to the left) was common in patients with FTD.[2]

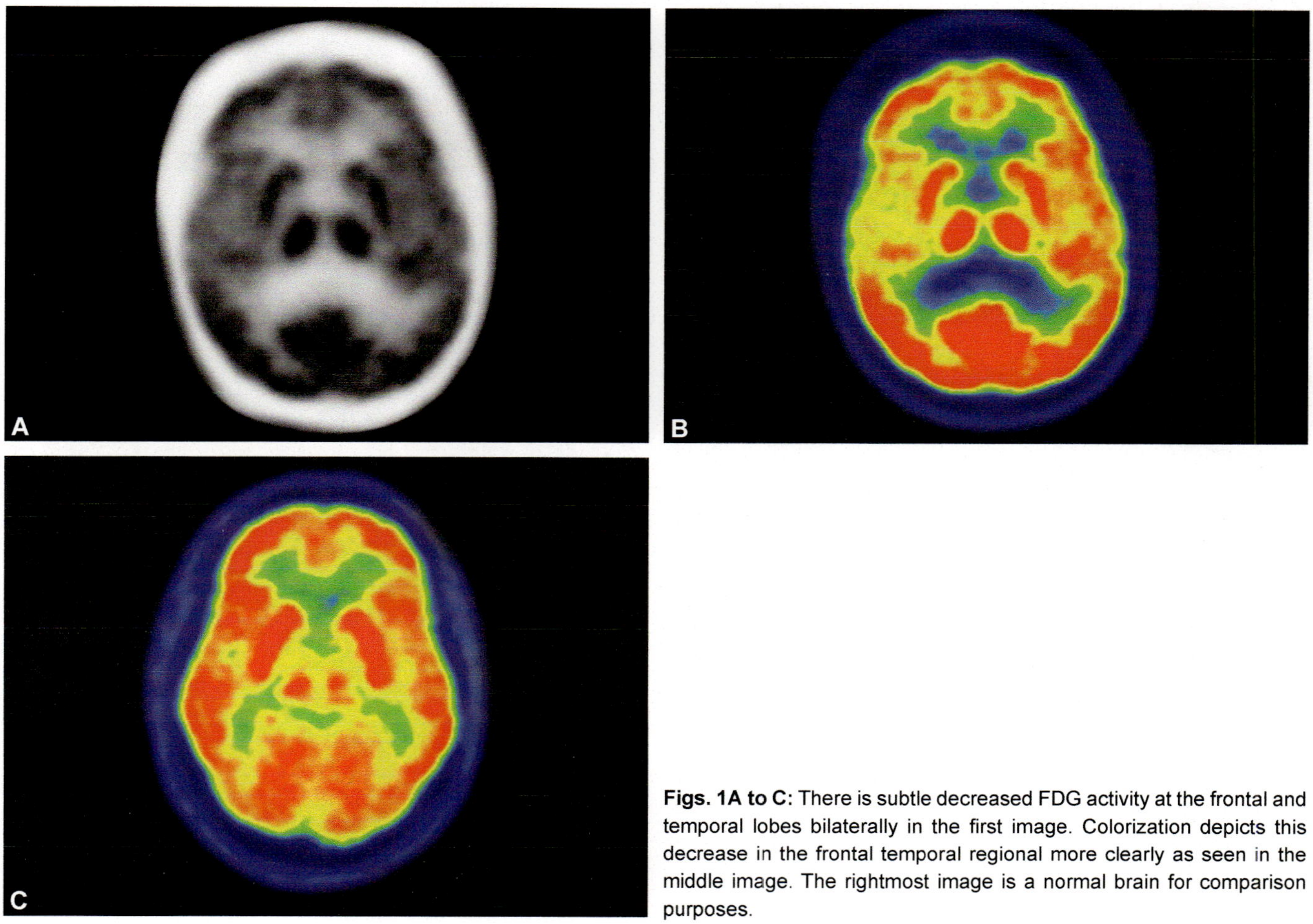

Figs. 1A to C: There is subtle decreased FDG activity at the frontal and temporal lobes bilaterally in the first image. Colorization depicts this decrease in the frontal temporal regional more clearly as seen in the middle image. The rightmost image is a normal brain for comparison purposes.

REFERENCES

1. Available from http://brain.oxfordjournals.org/content/130/10/2616.full
2. Available from http://jnm.snmjournals.org/content/46/2/233.short

CASE 7: PET FDG OF LEWY BODY DEMENTIA

Brief History

Symptoms of visual hallucinations and progressive memory loss.

Findings

Findings are shown in Figures 1A and B.

Main Teaching Points

- Dementia with Lewy bodies (DLB) show posterior brain hypometabolism classically at the parieto-occipital regions.[1]
- Lewy body dementia (LBD) is a term that includes two clinical diagnoses: dementia with Lewy bodies and Parkinson's disease dementia. LBD usually presents with fluctuating attention and concentration, visual hallucinations, and spontaneous parkinsonian motor signs.[2]
- In the majority of DLB cases, reduction in FDG uptake is seen bilaterally but unilateral reduction can be seen in 21% of cases.

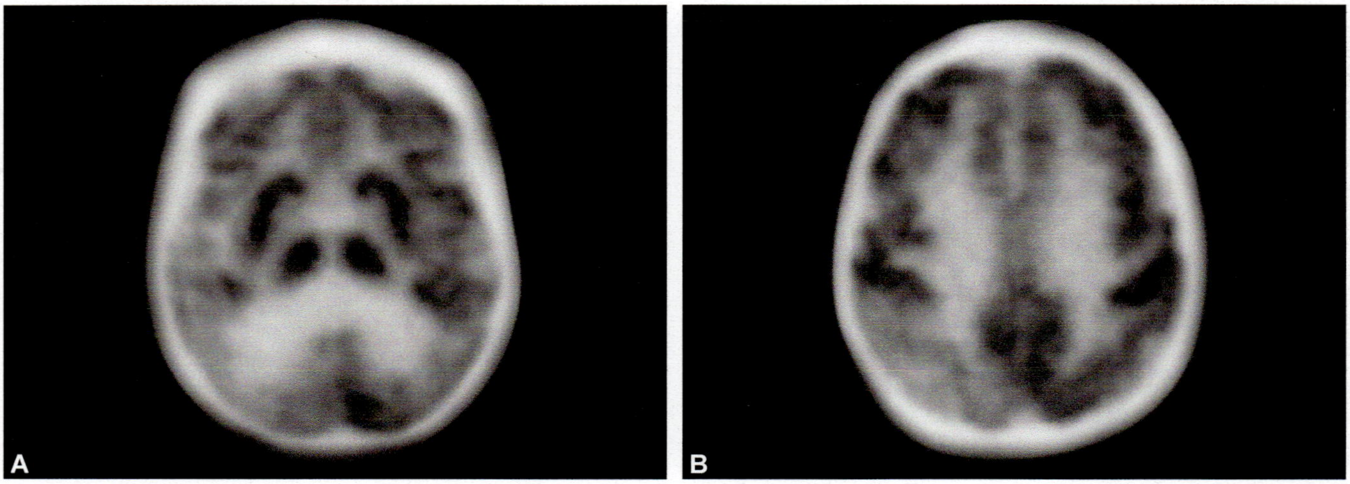

Figs. 1A and B: Two slices (A and B) from a single FDG PET study were performed on the same patient. Prominent decreased metabolic activity is seen in the entire right occipital lobe but the left occipital lobe also demonstrates mild decreased activity. Mild decreased FDG activity was also noted in the bilateral parietal lobes. Sparing of the primary sensorimotor cortex is observed between the frontal and parietal cortices.

REFERENCES

1. Available from http://jnm.snmjournals.org/content/49/3/390.full.pdf+html
2. Available from http://www.lbda.org

CASE 8: ^{18}F-AV45 PET

Brief History

Cognitive decline.

Findings

Findings are shown in Figures 1 and 2.

Main Teaching Points

- Plaques containing amyloid-β (Aβ) peptide are found in Alzheimer's disease (AD) brains and can confirm the diagnosis via autopsy. ^{18}F-AV45 or florbetapir F18 is a radiopharmaceutical for detecting this plaque formation that may precede cognitive symptoms.
- In AD patients, AV45 tend to accumulate in the gray matter of the frontal, temporal and precuneus regions.[1]
- A negative scan will demonstrate sparse or no neuritic plaques, reducing the likelihood that a patient's cognitive impairment is due to AD.
- A positive scan does not does not establish a diagnosis of AD and may be seen in other types of neurologic conditions as well as older patients with normal cognition.[2]

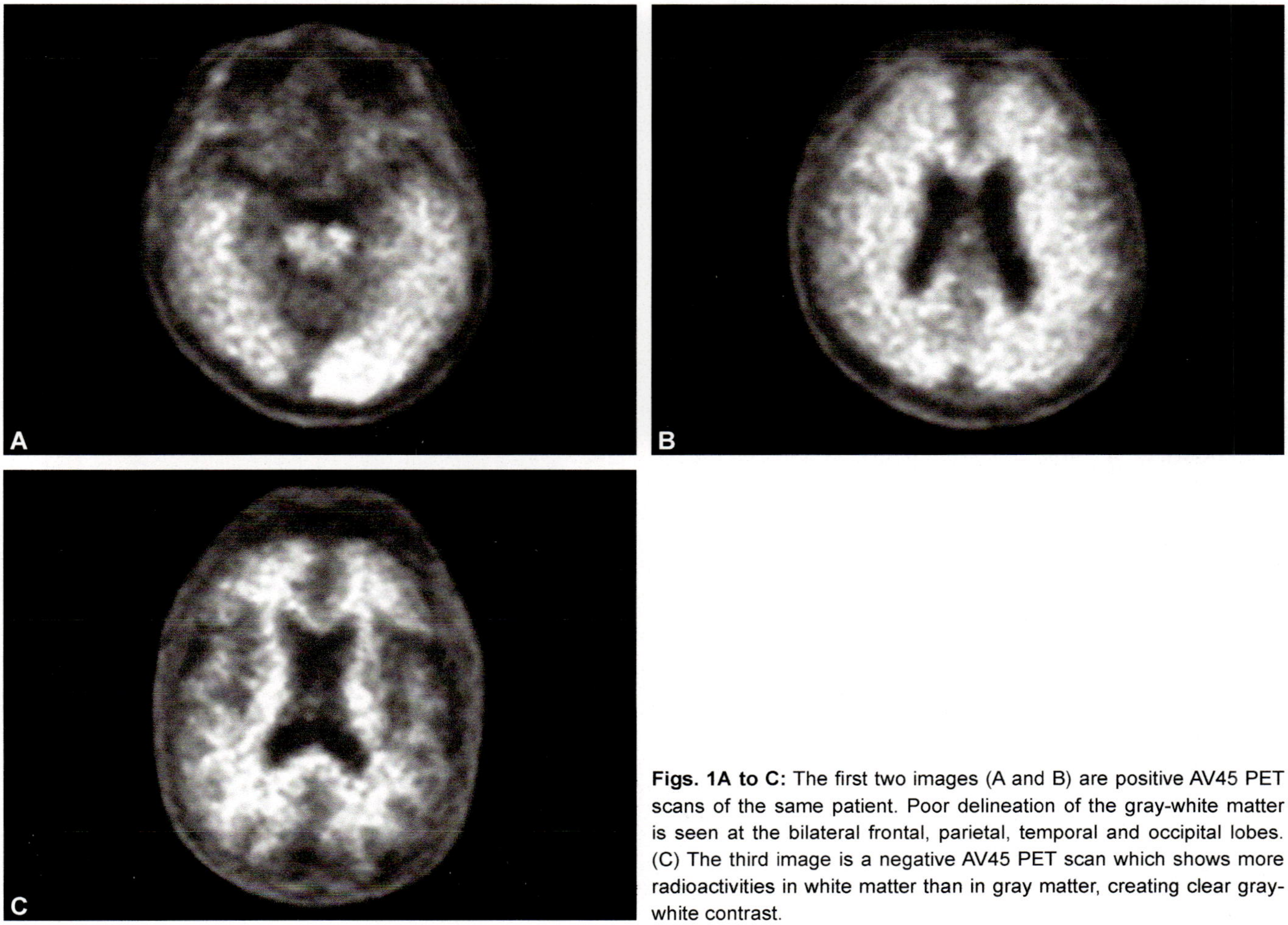

Figs. 1A to C: The first two images (A and B) are positive AV45 PET scans of the same patient. Poor delineation of the gray-white matter is seen at the bilateral frontal, parietal, temporal and occipital lobes. (C) The third image is a negative AV45 PET scan which shows more radioactivities in white matter than in gray matter, creating clear gray-white contrast.

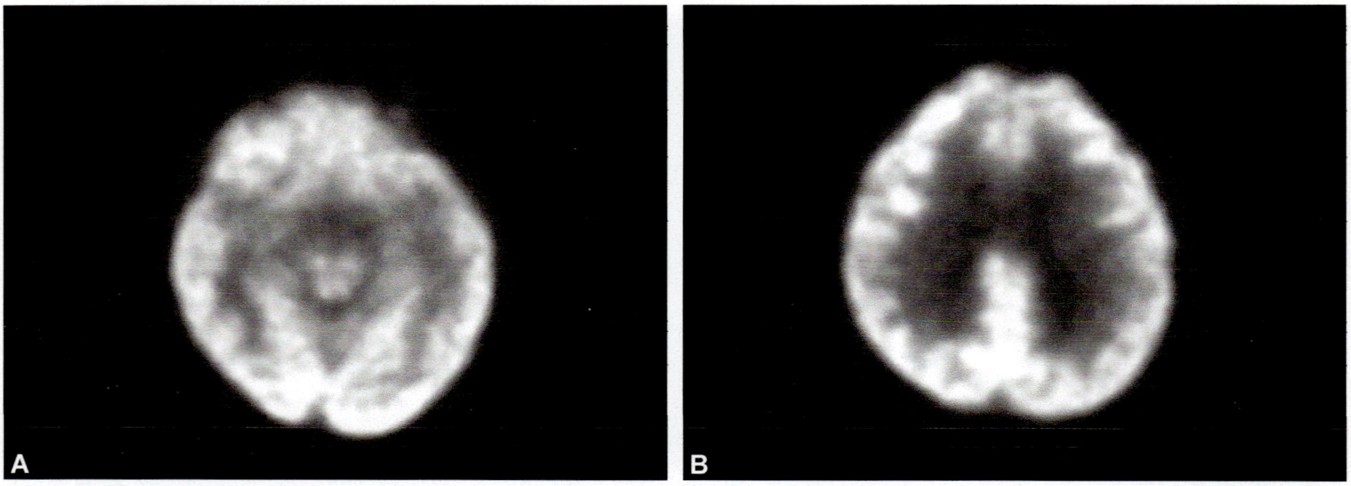

Figs. 2A and B: These are the respective image slices from a concurrent FDG PET scan. They demonstrate symmetric and normal metabolism.

REFERENCES

1. Available from http://jnm.snmjournals.org/content/51/6/913.full.pdf
2. Available from http://www.amyvid.com/Pages/index.aspx

CASE 9: FDG PET WITH MILD COGNITIVE IMPAIRMENT

Brief History

Mild cognitive impairment with a mini mental state examination of 24.

Findings

Findings are shown in Figures 1 and 2.

Main Teaching Points

- Mild cognitive impairment (MCI) is a clinical term describing reduced cognitive capacity between normal aging and dementia.
- In one study based on FDG PET, MCI patients showed primarily posterior cingulate cortex and hippocampal hypometabolism.[1]
- In another study based on MRI, gray matter loss in the medial temporal lobe characterized MCI, while gray matter loss in the parietal and cingulate cortices suggested Alzheimer's disease.[2]

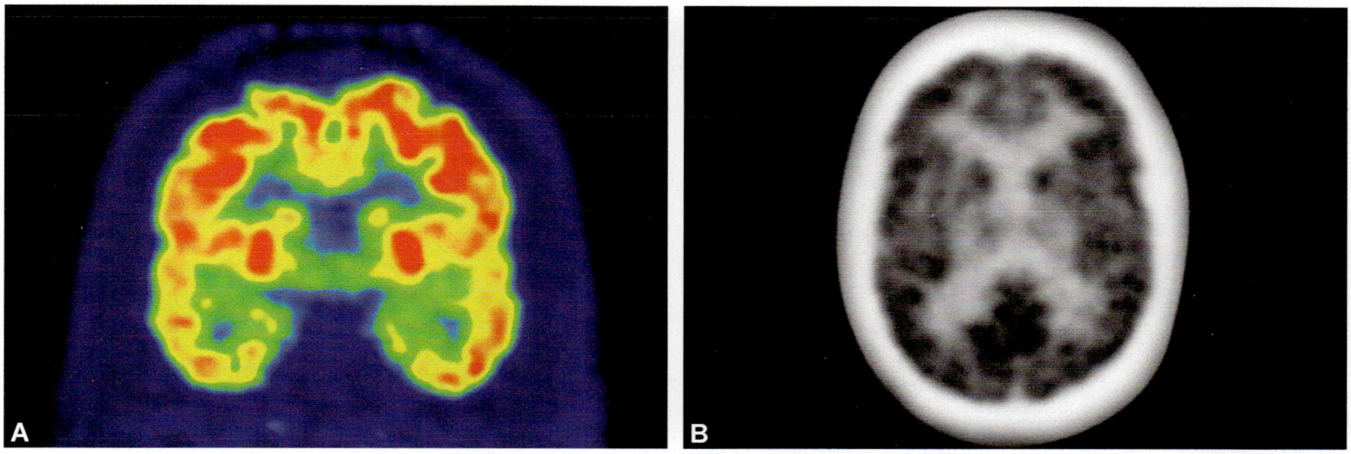

Figs. 1A and B: In this FDG PET, mild decrease in FDG metabolism is seen within the mesial temporal lobes bilaterally. This may be a sign of mild cognitive impairment but could also be an early sign of Alzheimer's dementia.

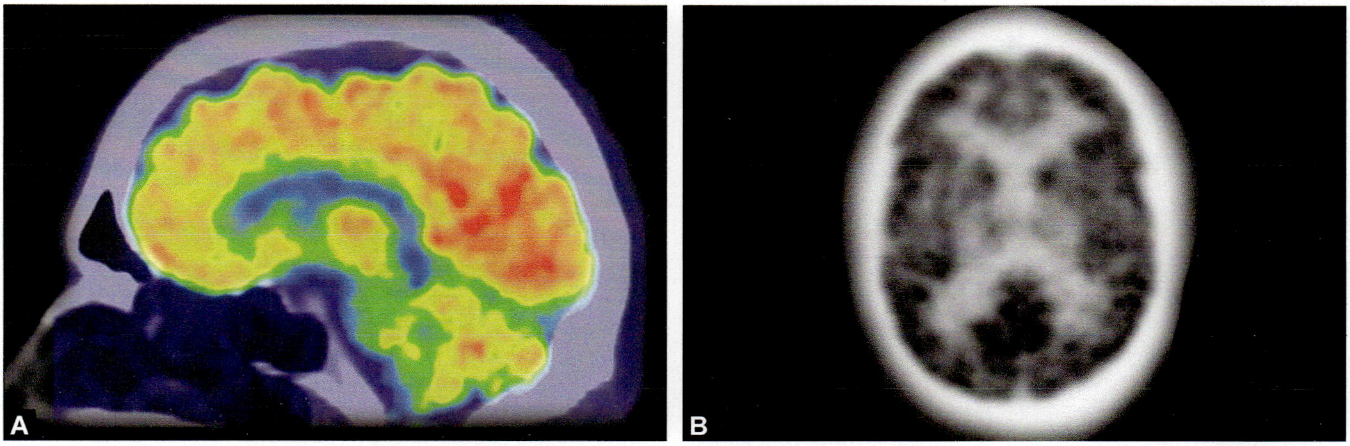

Figs. 2A and B: The other regions of the brain demonstrate preserved metabolism including the cingulate, frontal, parietal and occipital cortex.

REFERENCES

1. Available from http://jnm.snmjournals.org/content/49/3/390.full.pdf+html
2. Available from http://www.sciencedirect.com/science/article/pii/S1053811904003714

CASE 10: FDG PET/CT AND GLIOBLASTOMA MULTIFORMES

Brief History

Radiation therapy to a right temporal lobe mass 2 months ago. Needs evaluation for recurrent tumor or radiation necrosis.

Findings

Findings are shown in Figures 1 to 4.

Main Teaching Points

- In postradiation cases, focal hypometabolism is characteristic of necrosis.[1]
- Positron emission tomography was 80–90% sensitive and 22–80% specific for differentiating recurrent tumor from radiation necrosis. Some institutions report high accuracy, whereas others report that PET is not sensitive/specific enough to be used for managing brain primary brain tumors.[2,3]
- FDG PET can determine prognosis in patients by grading the gliomas.[4]

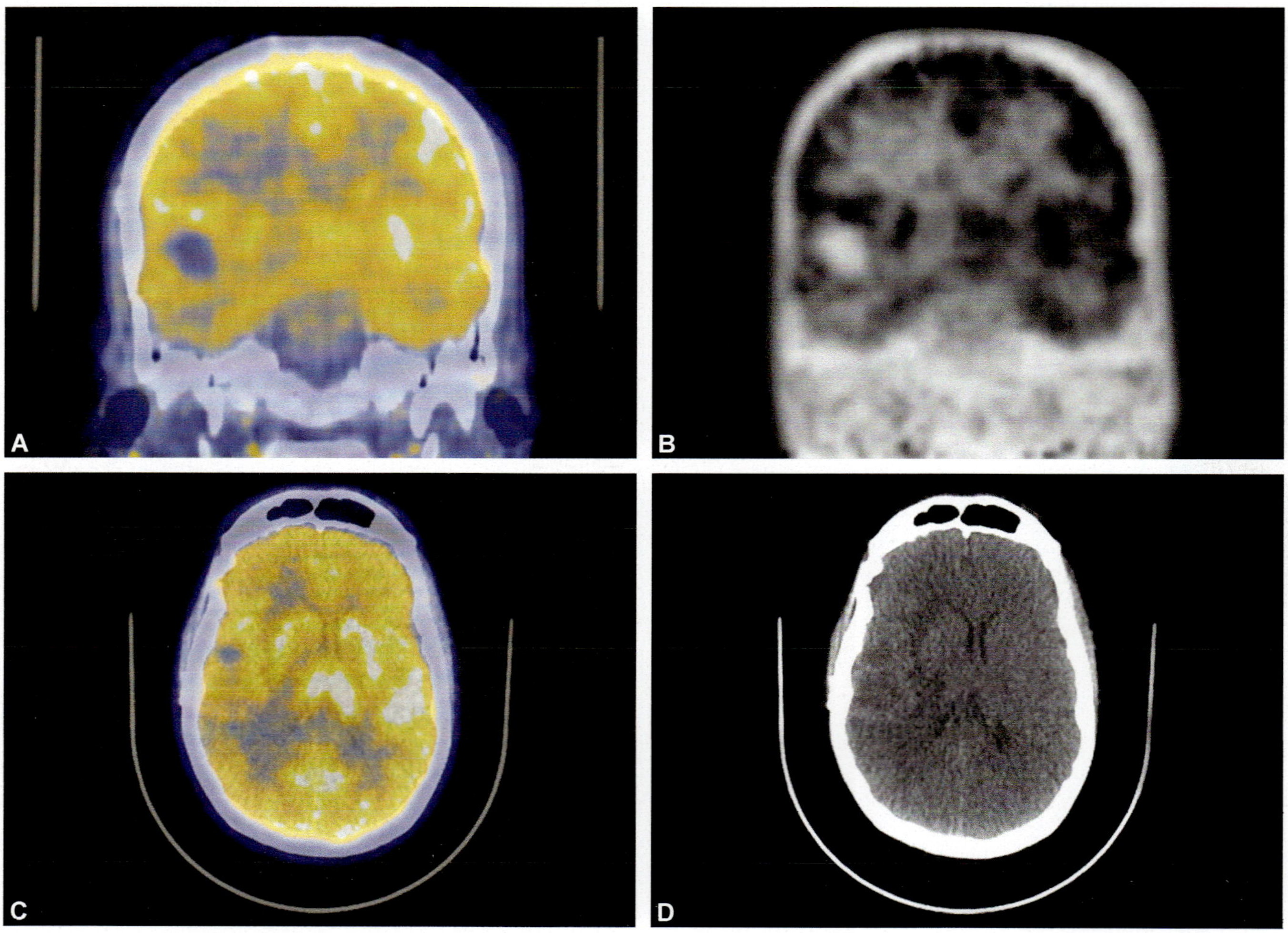

Figs. 1A to D: These images all demonstrate FDG activity at the periphery of an enhancing right temporal lobe mass with a hypometabolic center. The question is if this is active tumor or radiation necrosis, and unfortunately, this could not be determined. The time between the radiation therapy and this scan is too short and postradiation activity could still be present. A follow-up brain PET/CT in 3–4 weeks was requested.

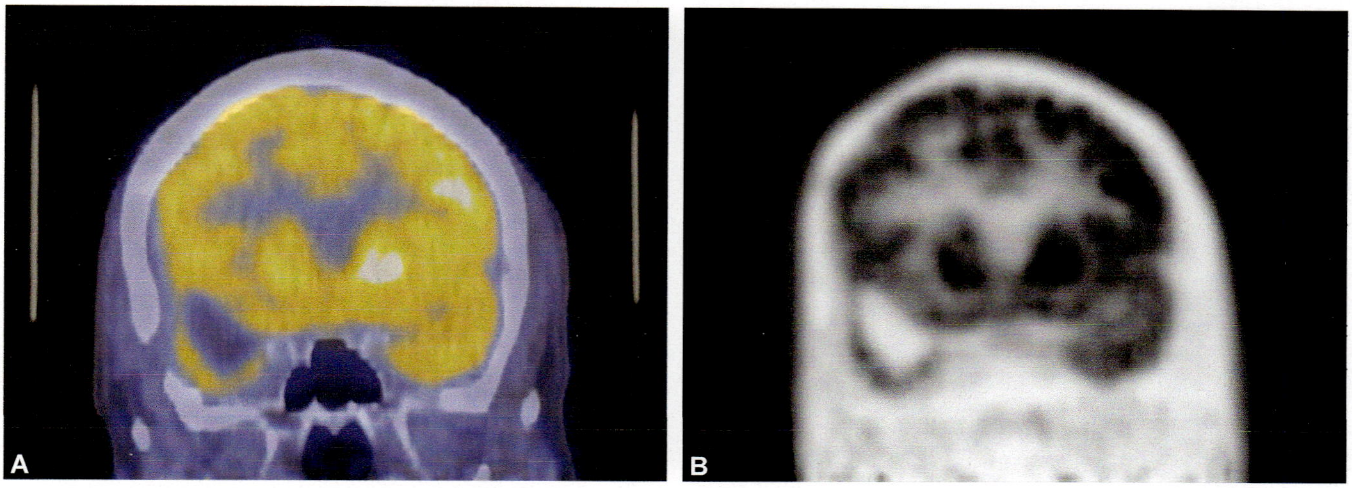

Figs. 2A and B: Subsequently, another PET/CT study was obtained and this one demonstrated postradiation changes in the right temporal lobe with decreased FDG activity. Recurrent tumor is much less likely and this could favor radiation necrosis.

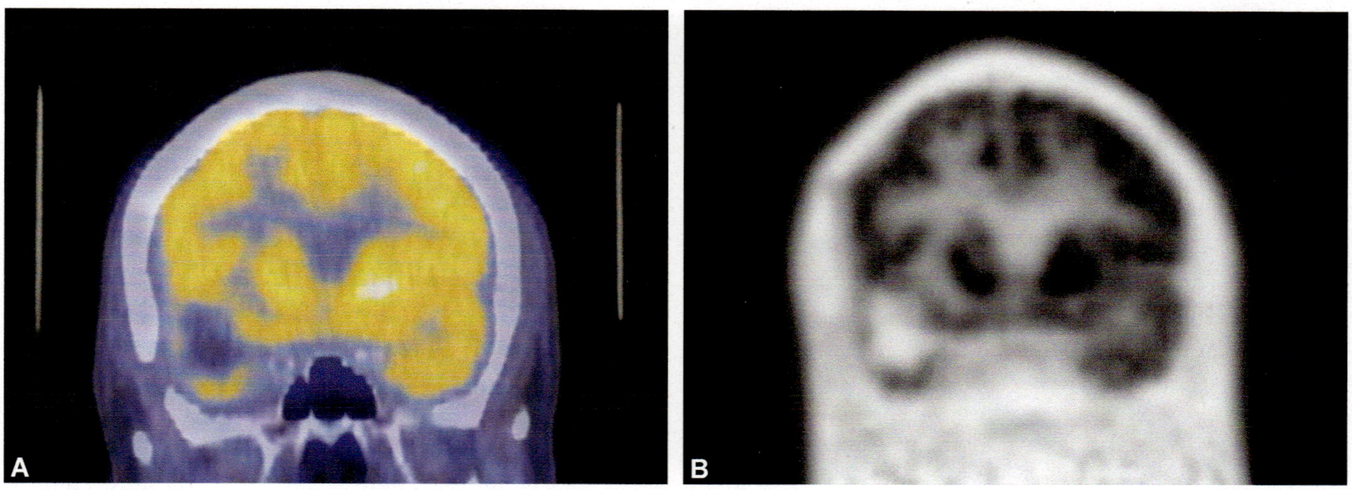

Figs. 3A and B: A third PET/CT was obtained after 1 month from the prior. The coronal view appears relatively unchanged and there is shrinkage of the hypometabolic mass, which still favors radiation necrosis.

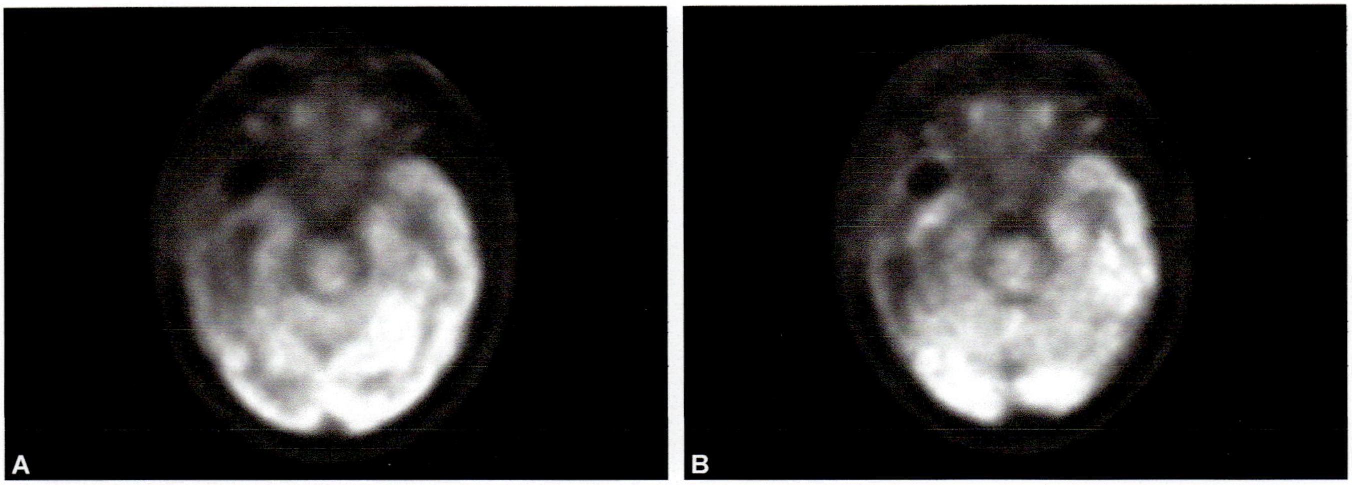

Figs. 4A and B: The fourth PET/CT was performed, and a selected slice is depicted in the second image (B). Compared to the prior [first image (A)], interval increase in metabolic activity surrounds the right temporal resection cavity, compatible with residual or recurrent disease.

REFERENCES

1. Available from http://www.ajronline.org/content/150/1/189.full.pdf+html
2. Available from http://www.ajnr.org/content/19/3/407.short
3. Available from http://onlinelibrary.wiley.com/doi/10.1002/ijc.1016/full
4. Available from http://tranow.com/assets/library/Brain_Colorectal_Lymphoma.pdf

CASE 11: FDG PET OF BRAIN METASTASIS

Brief History

Recent diagnosis of anaplastic thyroid carcinoma. PET/CT ordered for staging.

Findings

Findings are shown in Figures 1 to 3.

Main Teaching Points

- Lung cancer is the most common primary that metastasizes to the brain.[1] Other types of cancers that spread to the brain, in order of decreasing frequency, include breast, melanoma, kidney and colon cancer.
- FDG PET is only 75% sensitive and 83% specific for detecting cerebral metastases. Contrast enhanced MRI is a better tool, but has an 11% false positive rate.[2,3]
- 11C-methionine radiopharmaceutical can characterize amino acid transport in brain tumors and are considered more sensitive to recurrent tumor than FDG.[4] Unlike FDG, 11C-methionine has the advantage of low background cortical activity.[5]

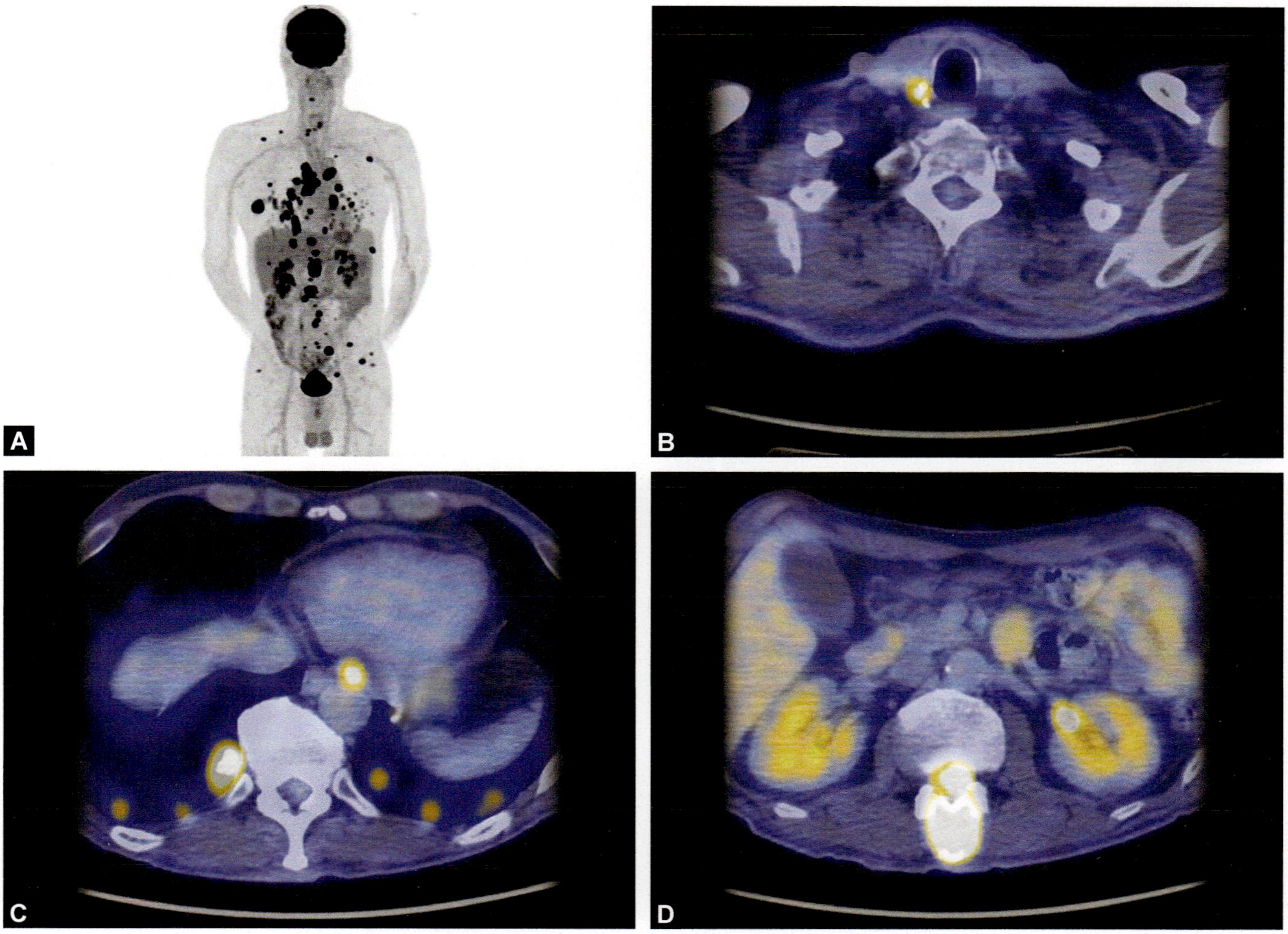

Figs. 1A to D: Widespread metastatic disease is seen above and below the diaphragm with evidence of osseous involvement.

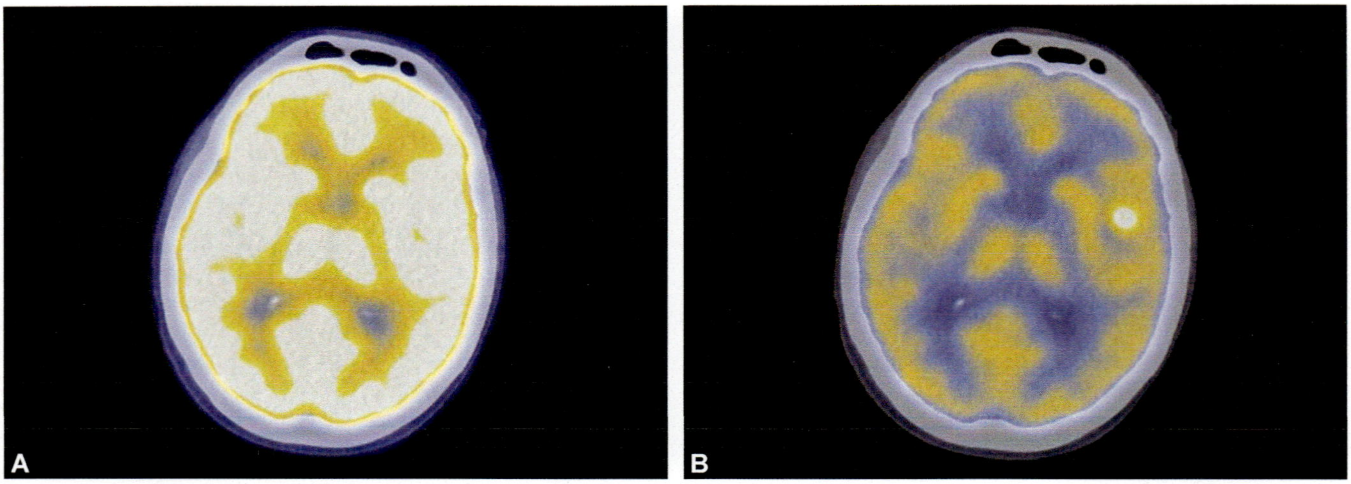

Figs. 2A and B: The first image (A) is improperly windowed. The cortex of the brain normally consumes glucose, so it has high FDG signal. After setting the window appropriately, the second image (B) reveals a hypermetabolic focus in the left temporal lobe.

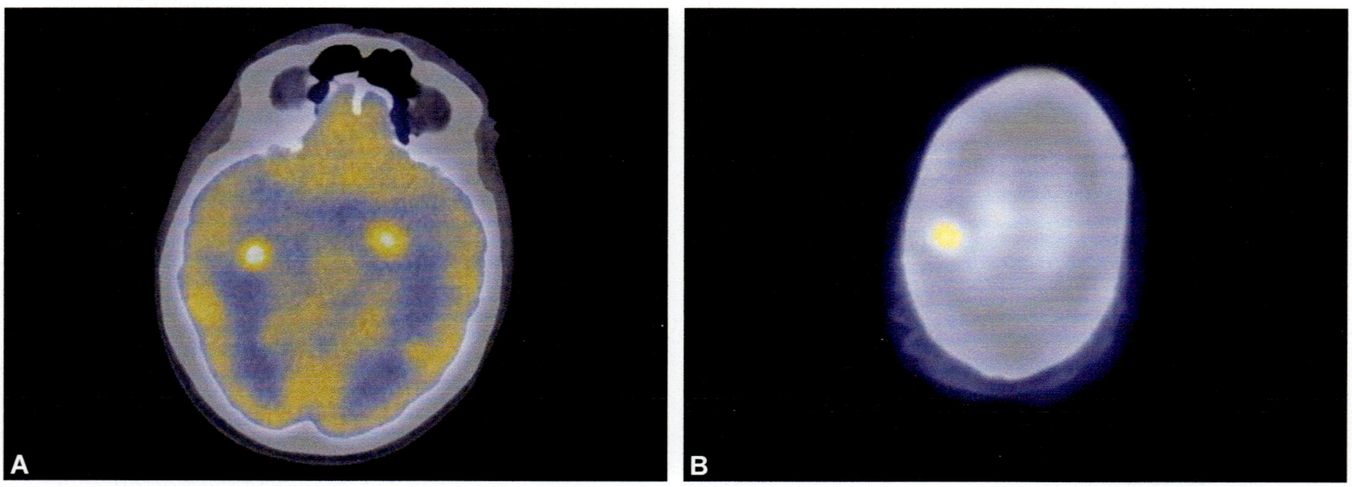

Figs. 3A and B: Several other hypermetabolic foci are seen in the brain and skull.

REFERENCES

1. Available from http://jnm.snmjournals.org/content/43/11/1432.short
2. Available from http://radiology.rsna.org/content/226/1/181.short
3. Available from http://www.ncbi.nlm.nih.gov/pmc/articles/PMC1420862/
4. Available from http://link.springer.com/article/10.1007%2Fs00259-004-1564-3?LI=true#page-1
5. Available from http://europepmc.org/abstract/MED/12687915

CASE 12: FDG PET FALSE NEGATIVE FOR GLIOBLASTOMA

Brief History

Glioblastoma status postradiation therapy.

Findings

Findings are shown in Figures 1 and 2.

Main Teaching Point

- Magnetic resonance imaging co-registration can improve the sensitivity of FDG PET from 65% to 75% for all tumor types. Specificity remains unchanged.[1]

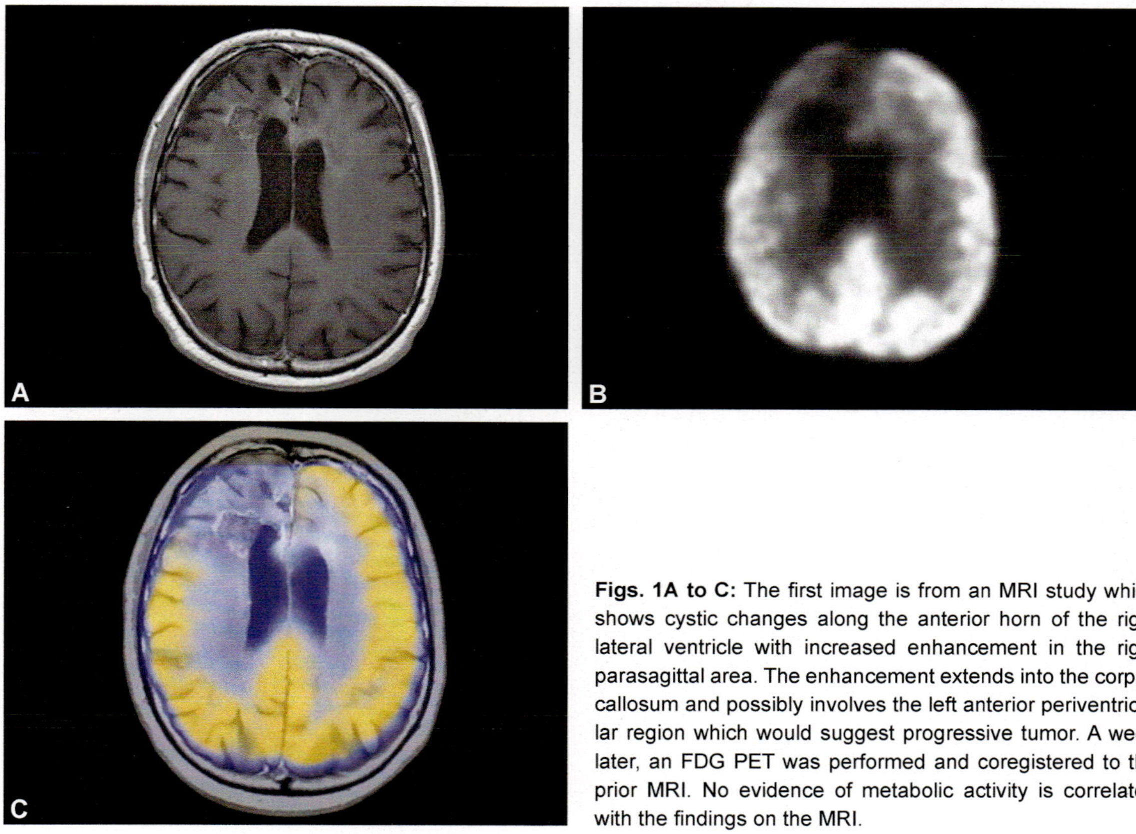

Figs. 1A to C: The first image is from an MRI study which shows cystic changes along the anterior horn of the right lateral ventricle with increased enhancement in the right parasagittal area. The enhancement extends into the corpus callosum and possibly involves the left anterior periventricular region which would suggest progressive tumor. A week later, an FDG PET was performed and coregistered to the prior MRI. No evidence of metabolic activity is correlated with the findings on the MRI.

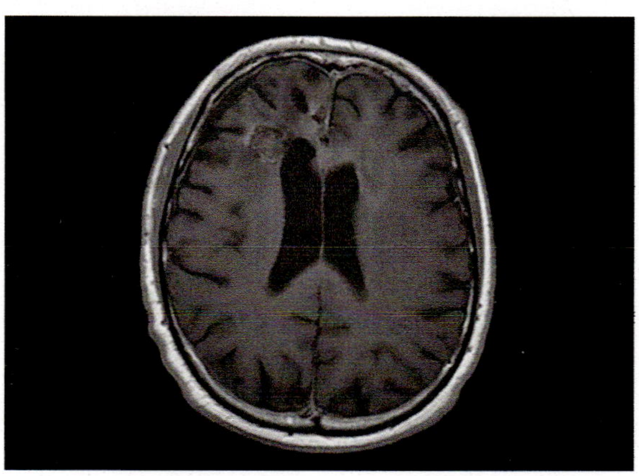

Fig. 2: A month later, MRI was repeated. No progression was seen but patient was clinically worse and eventually passed away.

REFERENCE

1. http://onlinelibrary.wiley.com/doi/10.1002/ijc.1016/full.

CASE 13: FDG PET/CT WITH BROWN FAT ACTIVITY VERSUS TUMOR

Brief History

Non-Hodgkin's lymphoma in need of restaging status post chemotherapy.

Findings

Findings are shown in Figures 1 to 4.

Main Teaching Points

- FDG PET/CT has a sensitivity of 90% and specificity of 94% for detecting metastatic lymph nodes in the neck, superior to other imaging modalities including CT or MRI.[1]
- Post-treatment images of the head and neck can be complicated and difficult to interpret because of the surgical/radiation changes. PET/CT is best suited for detecting recurrence.[2]

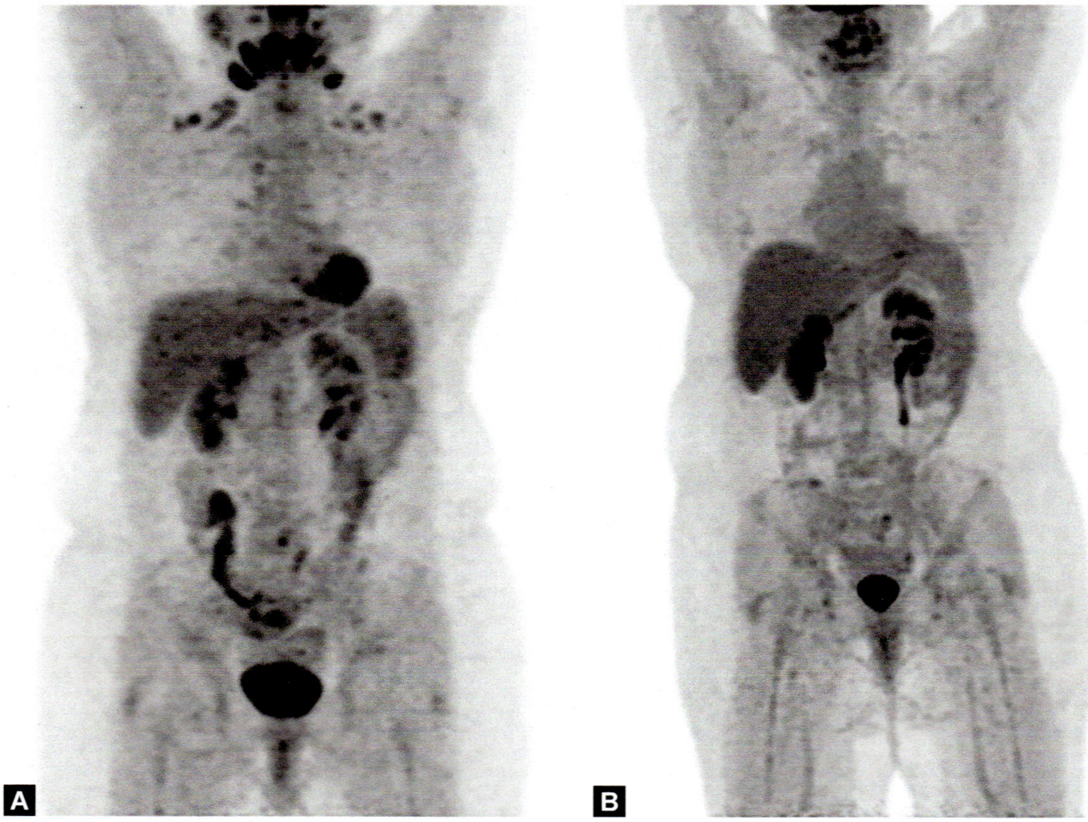

Figs. 1A and B: Hypermetabolic bilateral supraclavicular activity is seen in the first image. This pattern is consistent with brown fat activation. The second image is from a subsequent FDG PET/CT which no longer demonstrates the brown fat activation.

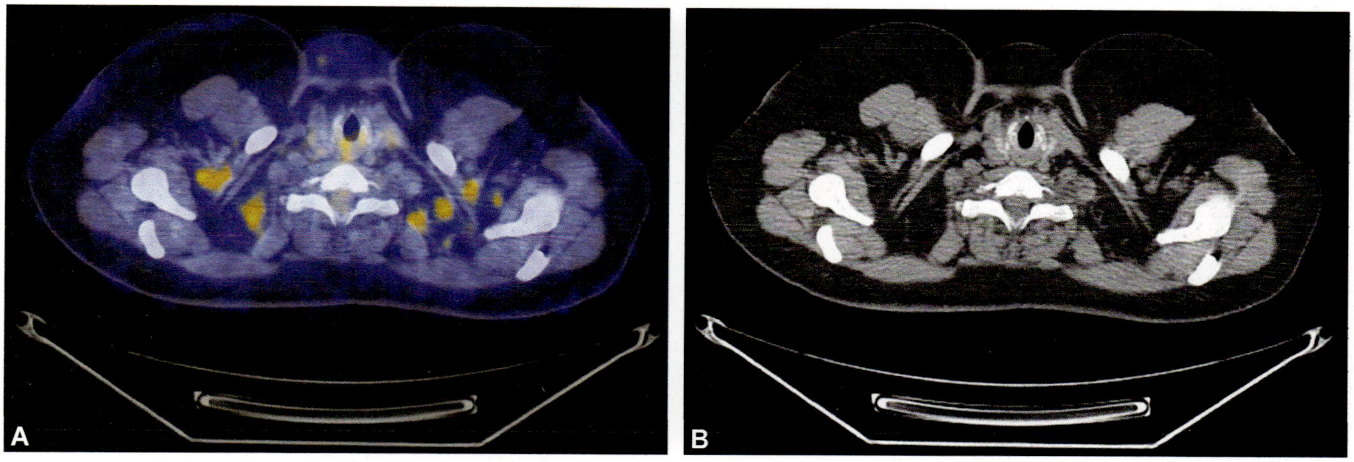

Figs. 2A and B: Brown fat activation can be confirmed by localizing the activity to the CT scan and ensuring that they do not overly any solid lesions or lymph node. All the spots observed in the first image are in fatty tissue.

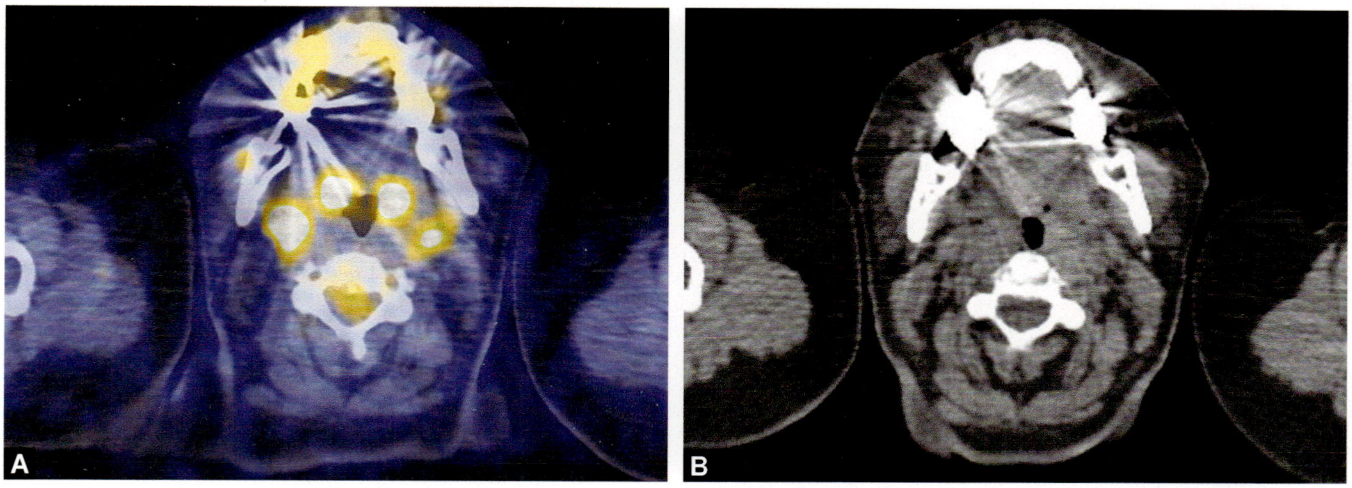

Figs. 3A and B: Bilateral jugulodigastric lymph nodes are seen. They are not brown fat activation because they are associated with solid tissue as seen on the CT slice.

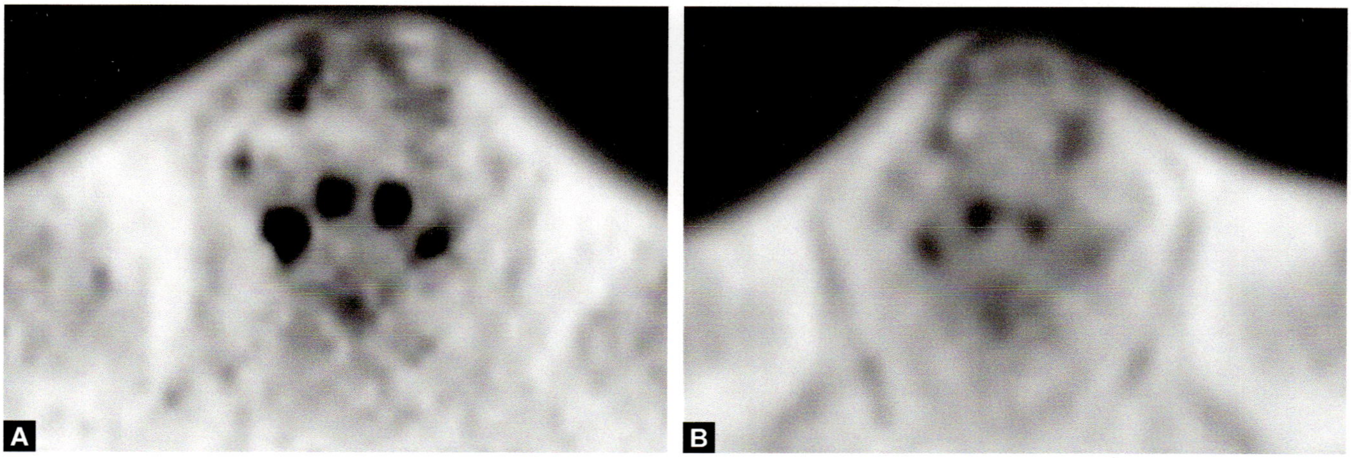

Figs. 4A and B: The two index lesions among other hypermetabolic foci within the neck have demonstrated interval decrease in size and FDG activity when compared to the prior examination [first image (A)]. This would be compatible with partial response to therapy [second image(B)].

- Brown fat activation is mainly observed in female patients with low body mass index. Correlation with CT is essential to distinguish between benign increased tracer uptake and malignant findings.[3]
- After completion of surgical/radiation therapy, a 10–12 week waiting period is recommended to minimize false-positive findings due to inflammation, edema, or distortion.[4]

REFERENCES

1. http://link.springer.com/article/10.1007%2Fs002590050293?LI=true#page-1
2. http://radiographics.rsna.org/content/32/5/1261.full.pdf+html
3. http://link.springer.com/article/10.1007%2Fs00259-006-0066-x?LI=true#page-1
4. http://radiographics.rsna.org/content/32/5/1261.full.pdf+html

Non-FDG PET/CT Cases

CASE 1A: ASSESSMENT OF NEUROENDOCRINE TUMORS (NETS)

Brief History

A 64-year-old female with biopsy proven grade 1 NET underwent ^{18}F-dihydroxyphenylalanine (DOPA) positron emission tomography/computed tomography (PET/CT) imaging for staging.

Findings

Focal increased tracer uptake is visualized on the central part of left upper lung lobe (yellow arrow).

Mild diffuse tracer uptake is seen on the pancreas with intensive tracer accumulation in kidneys, ureters and the urinary bladder (Figs. 1A and B).

Main Teaching Points

- ^{18}F-DOPA PET/CT shows promising results for the assessment of low grade (G1) NETs with Ki67-index less than or equal to 2%.
- 18F-FDG PET/CT shows superior results in the assessment of aggressive, high grade (G3) NETs with Ki67-index more than 20%.
- In the assessment of intermediate grade (G2) NETs with Ki67-Index of 3–20%, performing of both ^{18}F-DOPA and ^{18}F-FDG PET/CT may be the most suitable approach.

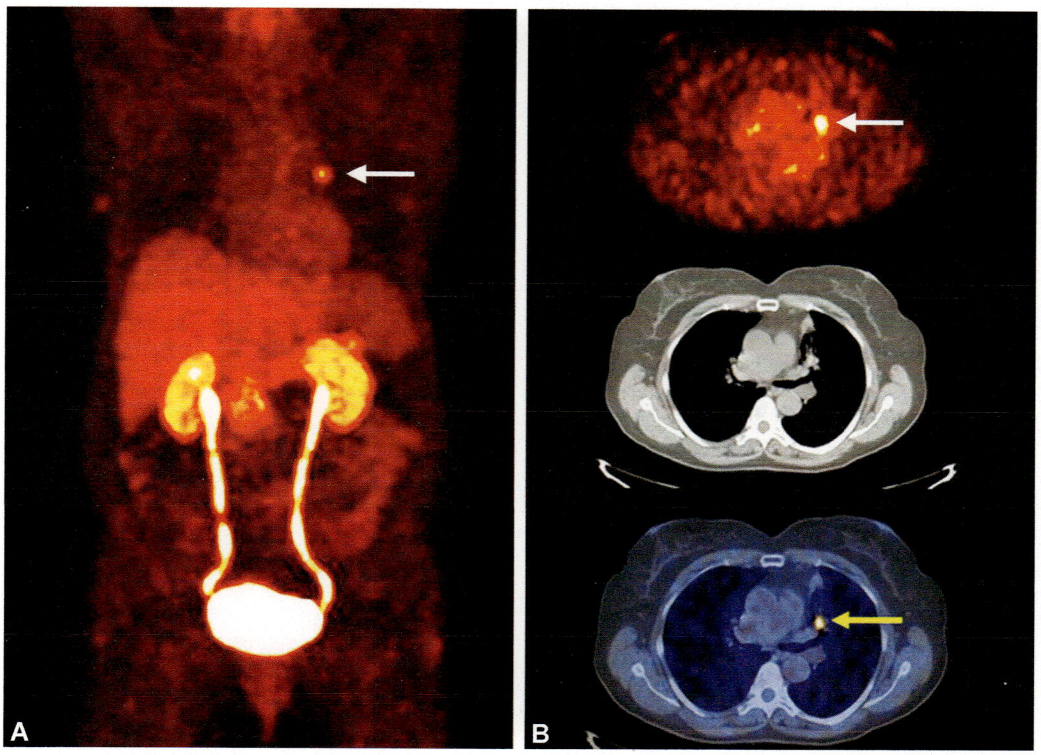

Figs. 1A and B: ^{18}F-DOPA PET/CT.

CASE 1B: ASSESSMENT OF NEUROENDOCRINE TUMORS (NETS)

Brief History

A 65-year-old female with:

- Rectal carcinoid tumor and rectal resection.
- Progression of the disease with liver metastasis in 2005 and liver resection.
- New development of the disease with well-differentiated NET in Pancreas (2008).
- Five cycle of peptide receptor radionuclide therapy (PRRT) between 2008 and 2010.

Findings

Multiple increased tracer uptakes is noticed (Fig. 1A) in the in the left supraclavicular region, hilus of the left lung, left lung (Fig. 1B), liver (Fig. 1C), abdomen and pelvis as well as skeleton (Fig. 1D), suggestive of generalized metastases.

Main Teaching Points

- 68Ga labeled somatostatin receptor (SSTR) analogs PET/CT shows promising results in the assessment of patients with low (G1) to intermediate (G2) NETs and is indicated for:
- Staging
- Restaging after therapy
- Identification of the site of cancers of unknown primary
- Selection of cases eligible for PRRT
- Recent meta-analysis (Treglia et al. Endocrine. 2012) of 16 SSTR PET/CT studies and 567 patients showed a sensitivity of 93% [95% confidence interval (CI): 91–95%] and a specificity 91% (95% CI: 82–97%) in the assessment of NETs.

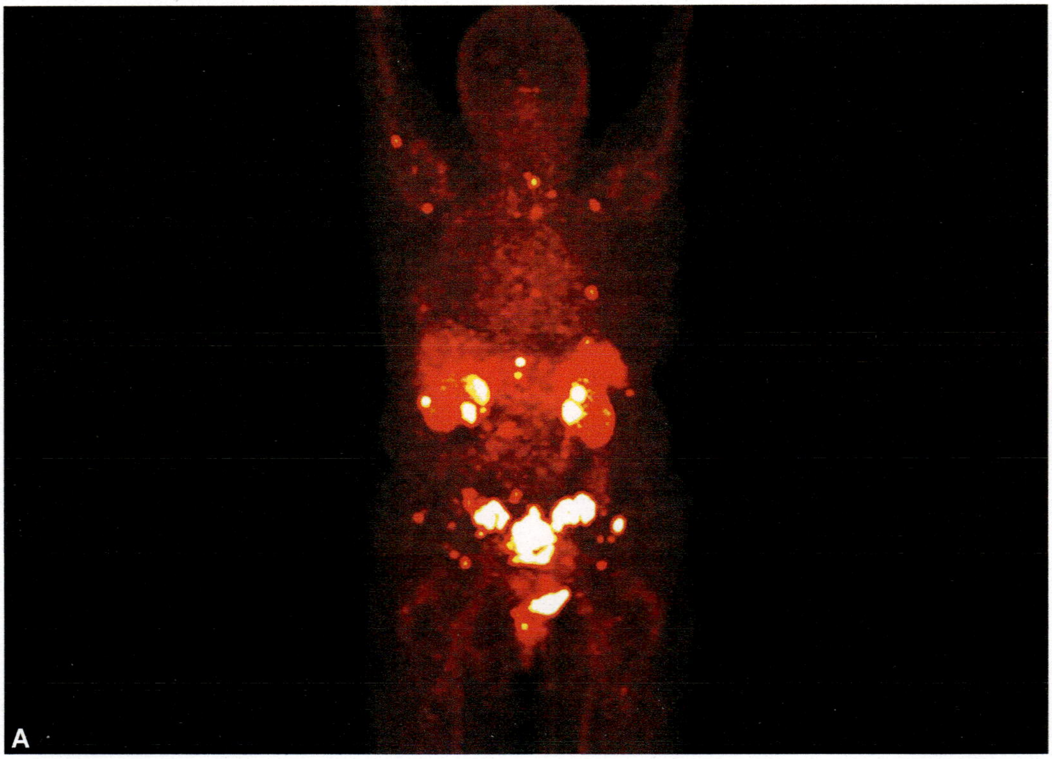

Fig. 1A

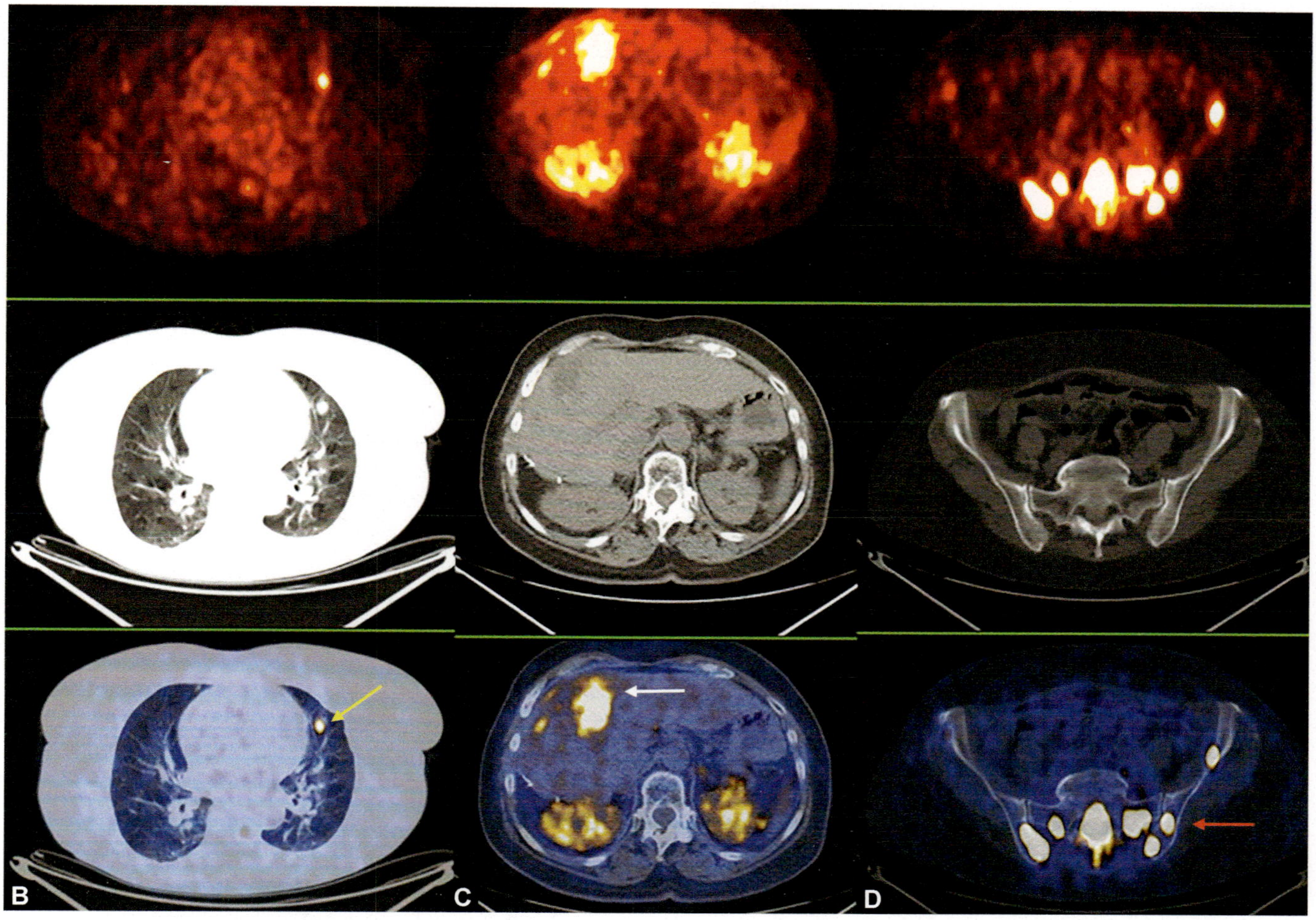

Figs. 1A to D: 68Ga DOTA-NOC PET/CT.

CASE 2: ASSESSMENT OF PROSTATE CANCER

Brief History

Preoperative staging of a 66-year-old man with biopsy proven prostate cancer with prostate specific antigen (PSA) level of 53 ng/mL, Gleson score of 8, cT3-4, G3.

Findings

Pathologic increased tracer uptake is seen in the prostate at both sides (Figs. 1A and 1B).

Multiple pathologic hypermetabolic lymph nodes are seen on the right iliac nodes groups as well as retroperitoneum at both sides (Fig. 1A and 1C).

Abnormal bony lesions are seen on spinous process of L2 (Fig. 1D), right ischium and proximal part of left femur (Fig. 1A).

Main Teaching Points

In spite of good agreement (81%) between regions with maximum choline uptake on PET/CT and sextants with maximum tumoral involvement in the histopathologic examinations, choline PET/CT cannot differentiate between malignant lesions and prostatitis.

- ^{18}F-Choline PET/CT has a limited value in the detection of lymph node metastases less than 5 mm.
- ^{18}F-Choline PET/CT can be useful especially for the evaluation of high risk prostate cancer patients to exclude distant metastases when surgical treatment is scheduled. It changed the therapeutic management of 20% of high risk patients, which suggests an appropriate clinical indication for referring prostate cancer patients to metabolic PET/CT imaging procedures (Beheshti et al, Radiology, 2010).

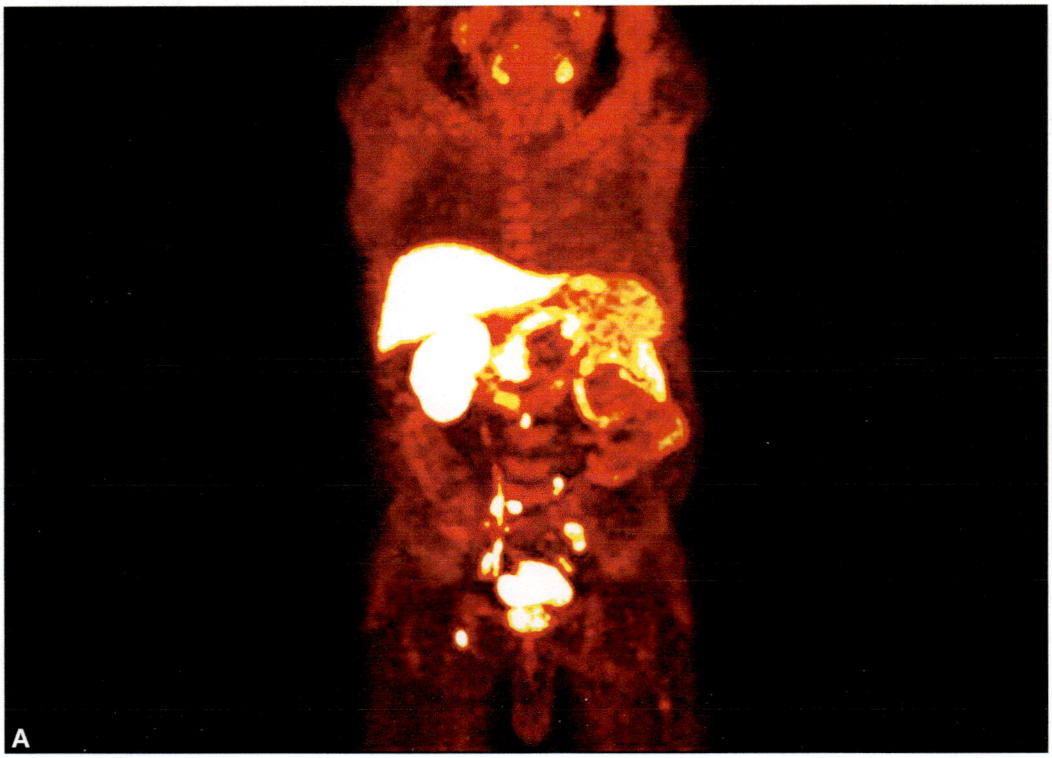

Fig. 1A

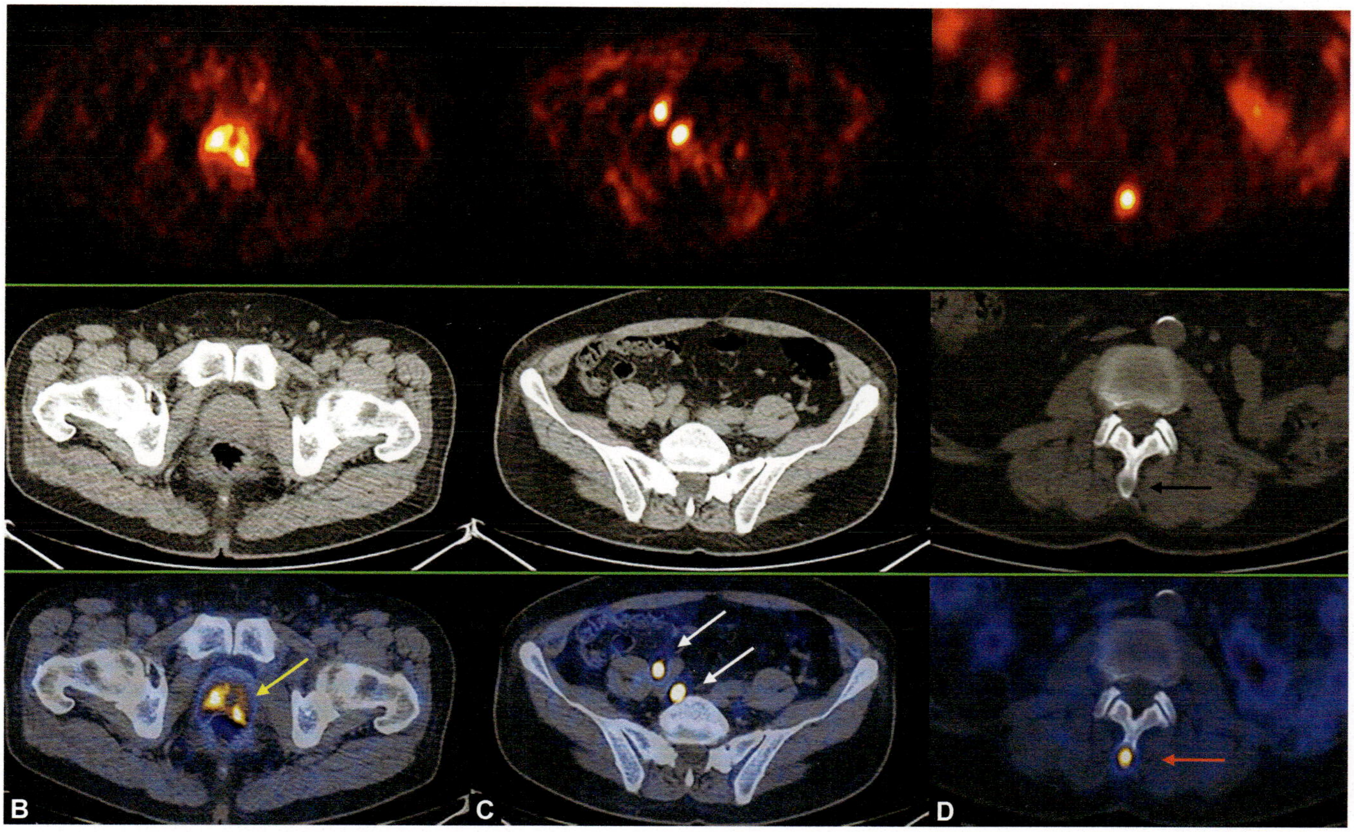

Figs. 1A to D: ^{18}F-Choline PET/CT.

CASE 3: ASSESSMENT OF BREAST CANCER

Brief History

Treatment monitoring of a 66-year-old woman with breast cancer after hormonal treatment and bisphosphonate therapy.

Findings

Pathologic increased tracer uptake is seen in the left ilium (Figs. 1A and B)—suggestive of bone metastasis.

Pathologic hyperactive bone remodeling is seen L4 with central hypoactivity presenting the healing process and sclerotic bony formation as a sign of response to treatment (Figs. 1A and C).

Abnormal bony lesion is seen on the left facet joint of T12/L1 (Fig. 1D) suggestive of degenerative bony change, clearly differentiable from malignancy due to exact localization and morphological pattern on CT (Figs. 1A and D).

Main Teaching Points

- ^{18}F-sodium fluoride (^{18}F-NaF) PET/CT is a highly sensitive imaging modality for the evaluation of bone metastases in a variety of cancers.
- Further it has been suggested that ^{18}F-NaF, while a marker of osteoblastic activity, may also be highly sensitive for detection of lytic and bone marrow metastases.
- The higher resolution of PET systems with the ability of acquiring tomographic studies and morphological correlation with CT findings has made the ^{18}F-NaF PET/CT a promising modality for the evaluation of bone metastases with higher sensitivity for lesion detection when compared with the routine conventional bone scan. It is established as the more accurate method with the ability to classify a significantly larger number of undetermined lesions as being malignant or benign [97% vs 80.5% in ^{18}F-NaF PET/CT vs Tc-99m—methylene diphosphonate (MDP) bone scan, respectively].

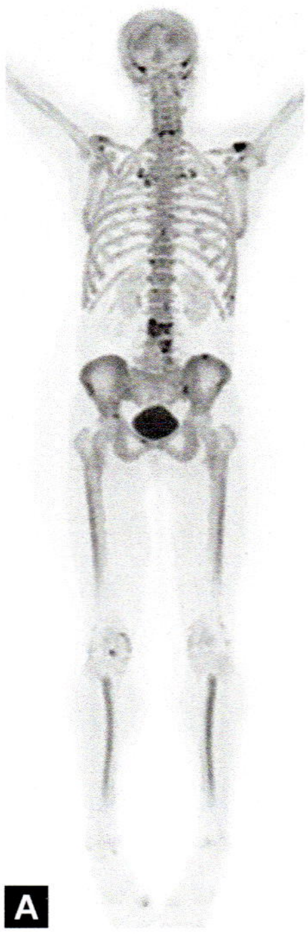

Fig. 1A

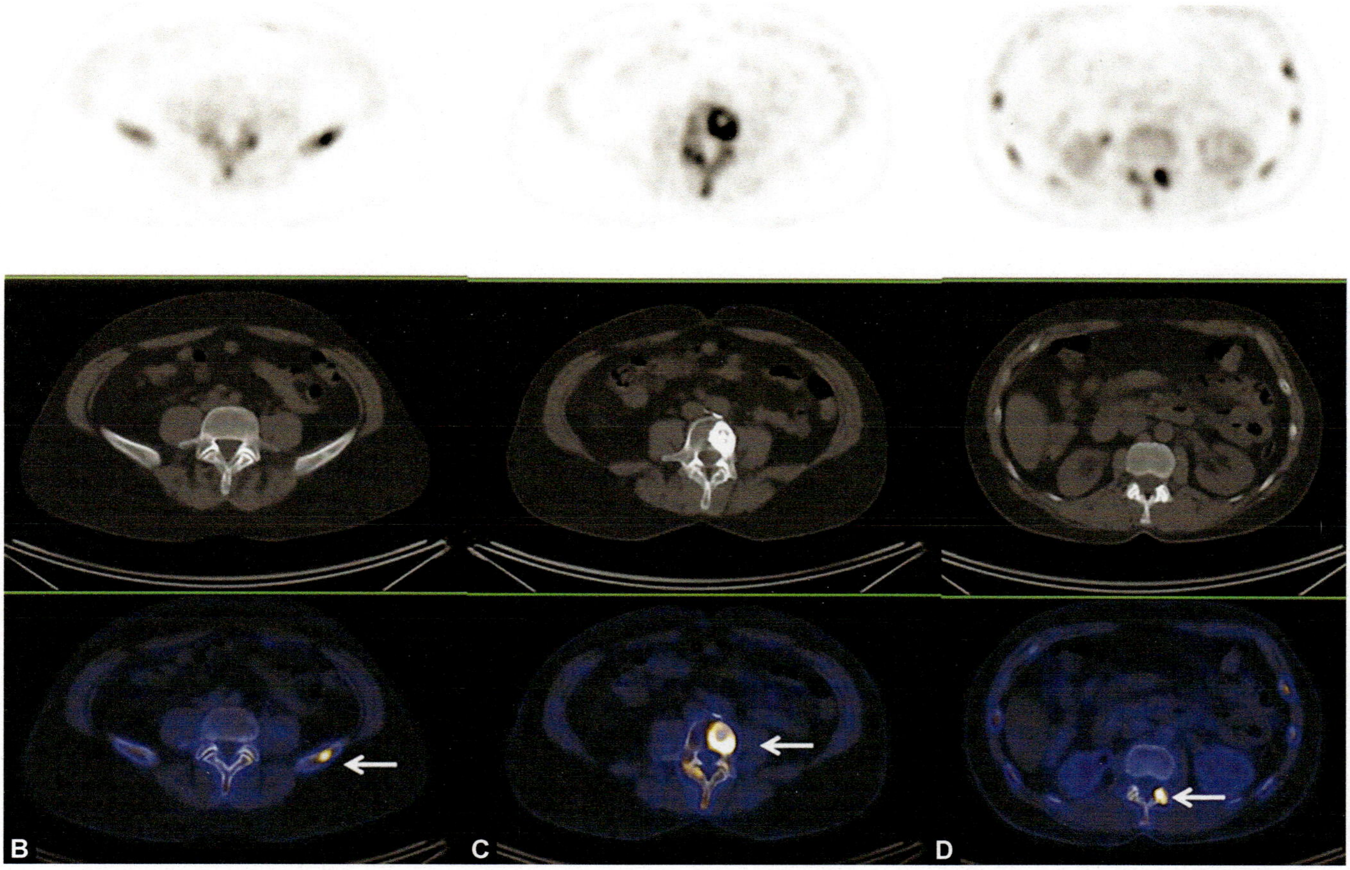

Figs. 1A to D: ^{18}F-NaF PET/CT.

CASE 4: ASSESSMENT OF RECTAL ADENOCARCINOMA RESPONSE TO THERAPY

Brief History

A 67-year-old male with rectal adenocarcinoma, clinical staging: T3, N1, M0 imaging findings before and after neoadjuvant radiochemotherapy. The patient received concomitant chemoradiation during the first 4 weeks of neoadjuvant chemotherapy with capecitabine, plus weekly oxaliplatin and standardized three-dimensional conformal neoadjuvant radiation therapy for a duration of 5 weeks (25 fractions 5 × per week) with a tumor dose of 45 Gray.

Findings

Pathologic increased tracer uptake is seen in the primary rectal tumor and in right-sided perirectal lymph node metastasis (Fig. 1).

Subsequent imaging following chemoradiation therapy demonstrates interval resolution of the hypermetabolic rectal mass and right perirectal lymph node (Fig. 2).

Main Teaching Point

- Fluorothymidine (FLT) imaging might be useful to monitor the course of patients undergoing neoadjuvant radiochemotherapy.

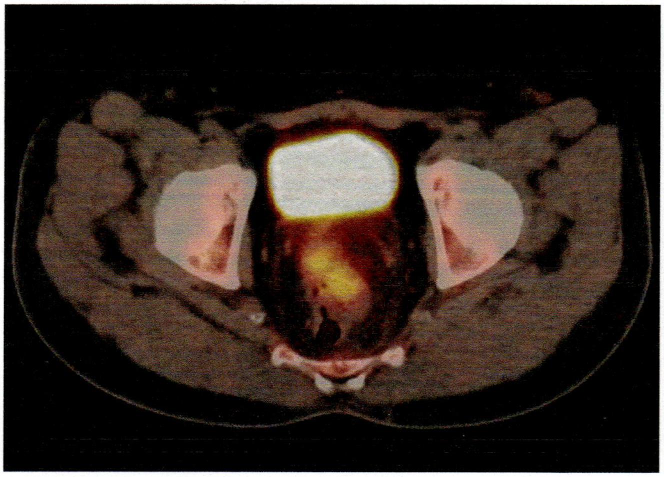

Fig. 1: ^{18}F-FLT PET/CT: increased uptake in the primary tumor (maximum diameter 60 mm, maximum SUV 10), and in right-sided perirectal lymph node metastasis.

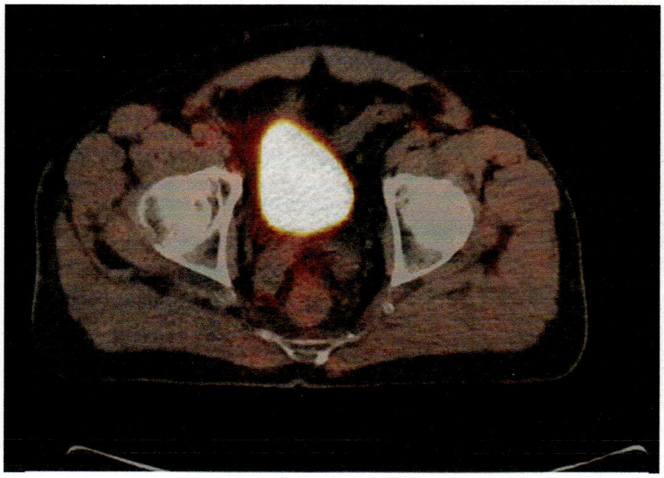

Fig. 2: ^{18}F-FLT PET/CT: absence of increased uptake in both primary tumor and lymph node metastasis. The patient was operated on and has been in clinical remission for 3 years now.

CASE 5: STAGING OF RECTAL ADENOCARCINOMA

Brief History

A 71-year-old female with rectal adenocarcinoma T3 N1 M1 imaging findings before neoadjuvant radiochemotherapy.

Findings

Pretherapy staging FLT (Figs. 1A and B) and FDG (Figs. 2A and B) images demonstrate pathologic increased tracer uptake in the primary rectal tumor and in right-sided perirectal lymph node metastasis on both sets of images. There is a focus of abnormally increased FDG activity within the left hepatic lobe (Fig. 2A). However, no FLT avid lesion is identified within the liver (Fig. 1A).

Main Teaching Point

Fluorothymidine PET/CT imaging is less accurate than FGD PET/CT imaging for staging of rectal cancer with regard to the detection of liver metastasis.

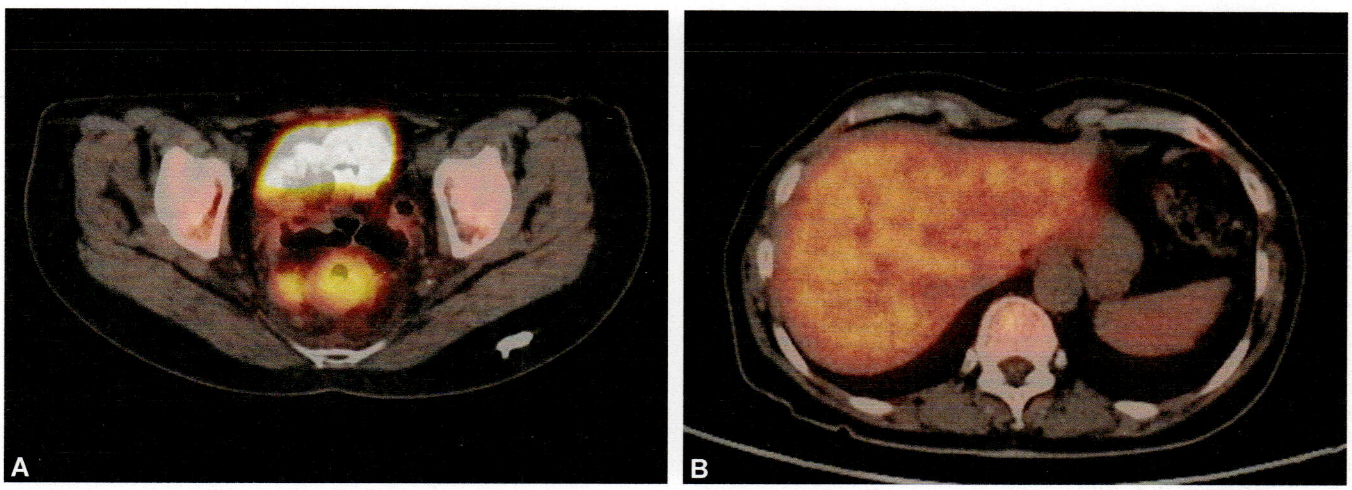

Figs. 1A and B: ^{18}F-FLT PET/CT: increased uptake in the primary tumor (maximum diameter 60 mm, maximum SUV 10), and in right-sided pararectal lymph node metastasis, while any liver metastasis was detectable.

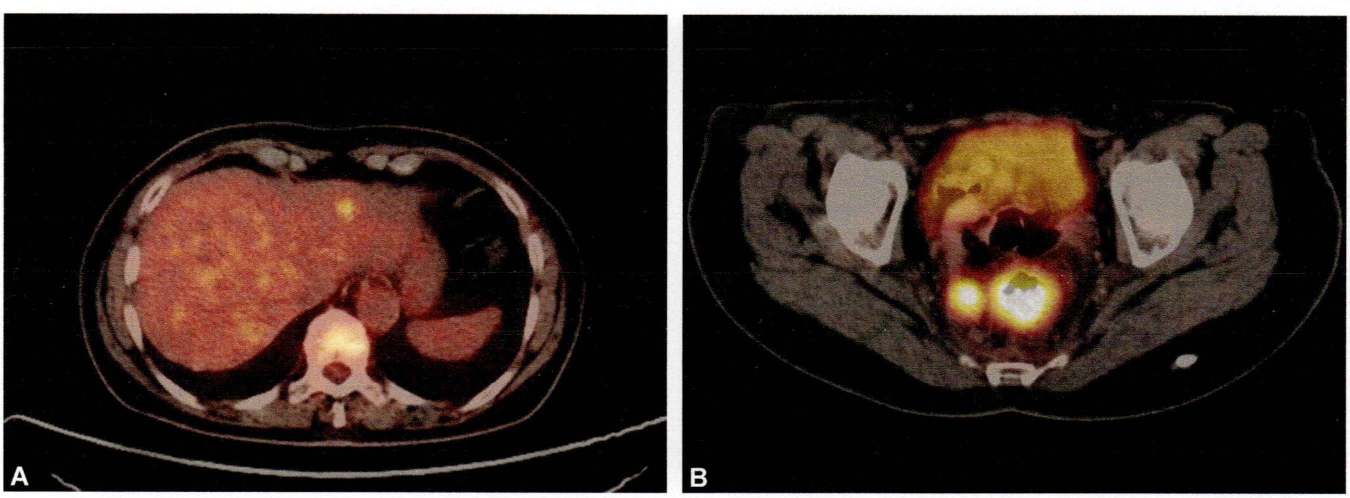

Figs. 2A and B: FDG PET/CT: pretherapeutic imaging demonstrates an increased uptake in the primary tumor and pararectal lymph nodes and in the liver.

CASE 6: ASSESSMENT OF ALZHEIMER'S DISEASE

Brief History

A 72-year-old female patient suspected of Alzheimer's disease, gradually progressing memory complaints over 2–3 years. Neuropsychology shows deficits in visuospatial functions and episodic memory. Previously treated for hypertension.

Findings

Simultaneous PET/MRI acquisition was performed 40–70 minute post injection of 432 MBq C11-PiB. There is significant cortical amyloid binding particularly in frontal and mesial parietal areas (red arrows). The Standard Uptake Value (SUV) ratios relative to cerebellar cortex is 2.5–2.7. Clinical MRI show discrete white matter lesions (yellow arrows) presumably older ischemic changes (T2w, FLAIR, Diffusion). There are no microbleedings (T2*, SWI). The hippocampal volume relative to the intracranial volume segmented using FreeSurfer is significantly reduced (Fig. 1).

Main Teaching Points

PET/MRI combined with amyloid imaging PET tracers may provide a one-stop comprehensive dementia work-up identifying:

- Positive imaging biomarker such as etiological risk factors of Alzheimer's disease or Lewy body dementia and atrophy patterns including reduced hippocampal volume
- Significant comorbidity from ischemia or microbleedings (found in 10–30% of Alzheimer patients)
- In patients with negative imaging biomarker: ruling out tumor, normal pressure hydrocephalus, subdural hematoma, AV-malformations.

The combinations of clinical presentation, increased amyloid binding, and structural and neuronal damage would categorize the biomarker probability of Alzheimer's disease as high.

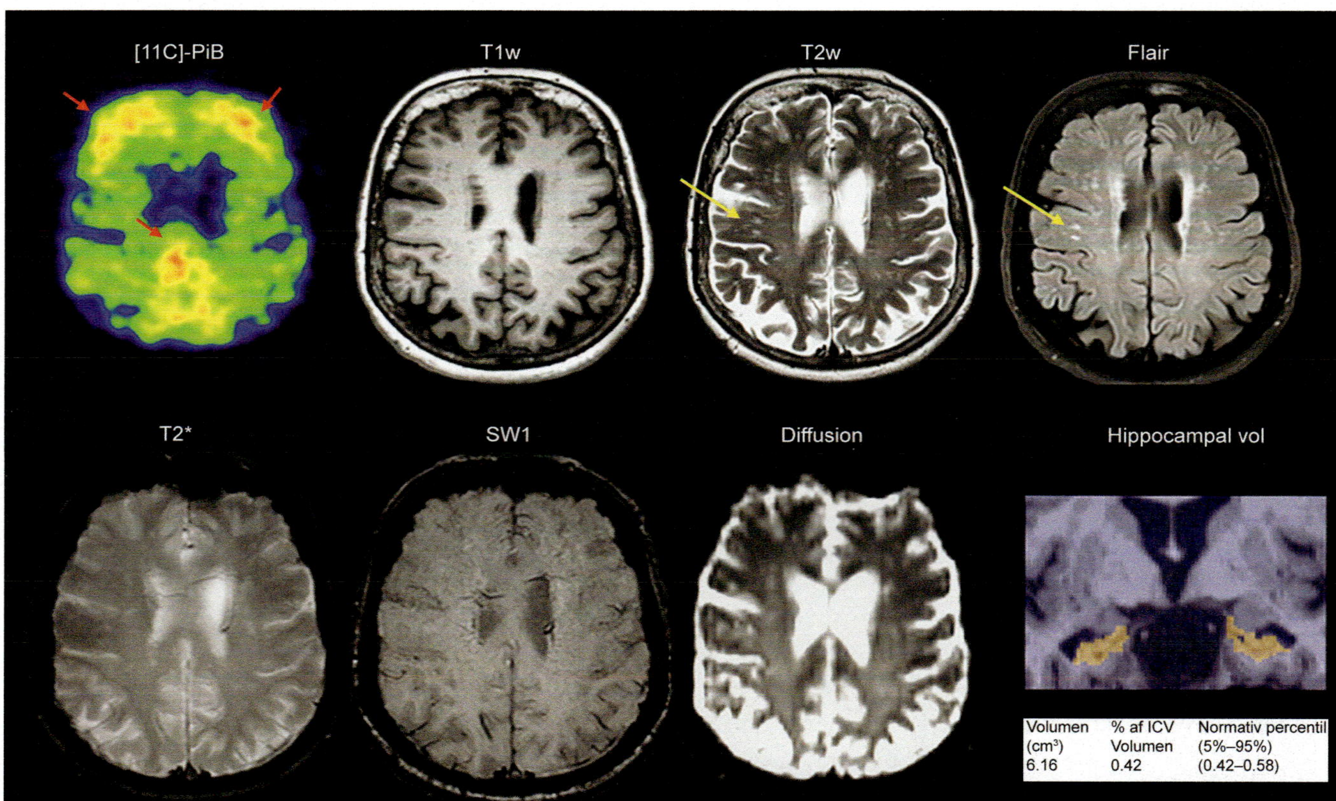

Fig. 1: 11C-Pittsburgh compound B (PiB) PET-MRI.

CASE 7: ASSESSMENT OF BONE METASTASIS

Brief History

A 51-year-old female patient diagnosed with locally advanced breast cancer 15 years ago. The patient was treated with neoadjuvant chemotherapy, surgery and postoperative radiotherapy had recurrence 10 months ago and was started on new chemotherapy. Recent clinical evaluation showed disease progression, but no bone metastasis was identified. Patient was examined with ^{18}F-sodium fluoride (^{18}F-NaF) PET/MRI.

Findings

Simultaneous PET/MRI acquisition was performed 106 minute post injection of 212 MBq F18-NaF maximum intensity projection (MIP) whole body PET image (Fig 1A) shows increased uptake in the left sixth rib, the right side of T10, the right transverse process of the T1 and the left femoral neck. Coronal PET images shows increased uptake in the left femoral neck (Fig. 2A). Corresponding MRI shows low signal intensity on T1 (Fig. 1B) and high signal intensity on STIR (Fig. 3B) consistent with bone metastasis. MRI STIR images also shows smaller but similar lesion in the right iliac bone and greater trochanteric region of a left hip (Fig 3B, red arrows), consistent with bone metastases. Corresponding PET shows faint and barely noticeable uptake (Figs. 1 to 3).

Main Teaching Point

Magnetic resonance imaging is an imaging technique that allows direct visualization of bone marrow and its components with high spatial resolution. By combining MRI with F18-NaF PET we now have a potent imaging modality with probably unbeatable sensitivity and specificity for bone and bone marrow metastasis.

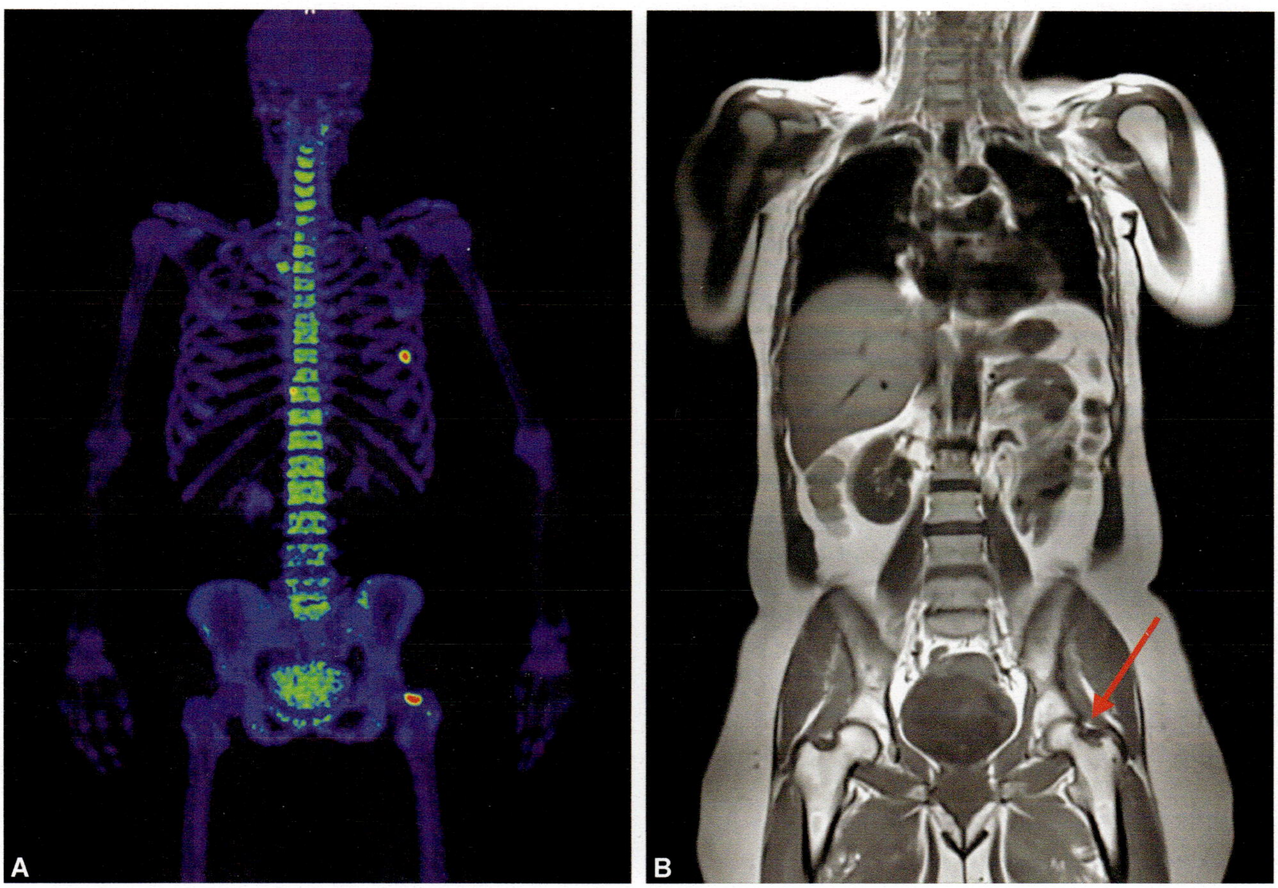

Figs. 1A and B: ^{18}F-NaF PET-MRI; (A) PET MIP; (B) MRI coronal T1 weighted.

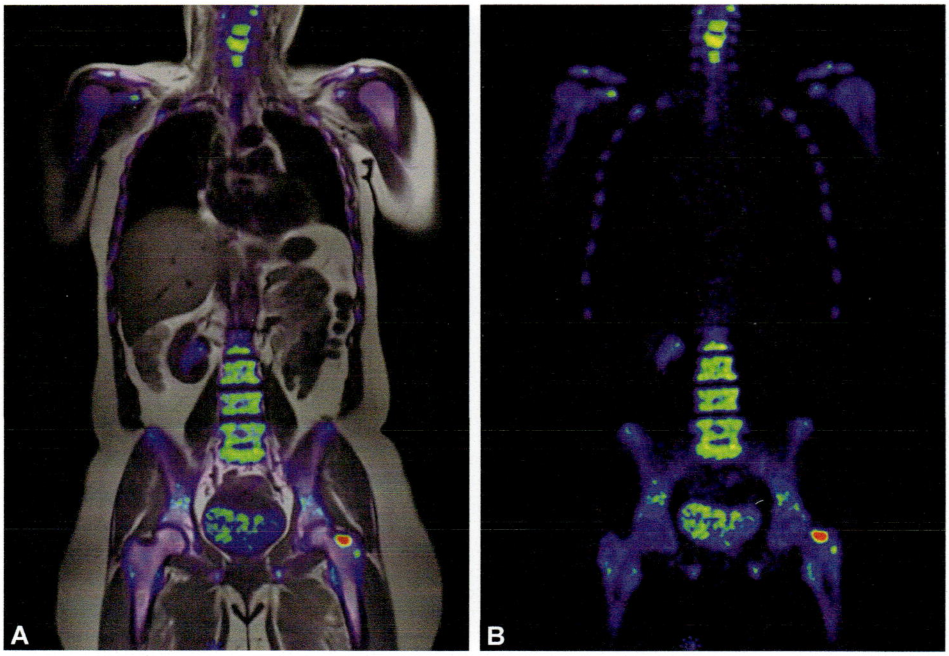

Figs. 2A and B: ^{18}F-NaF PET-MRI. (A) fused PET-MRI (T1 W). (B) PET coronal image.

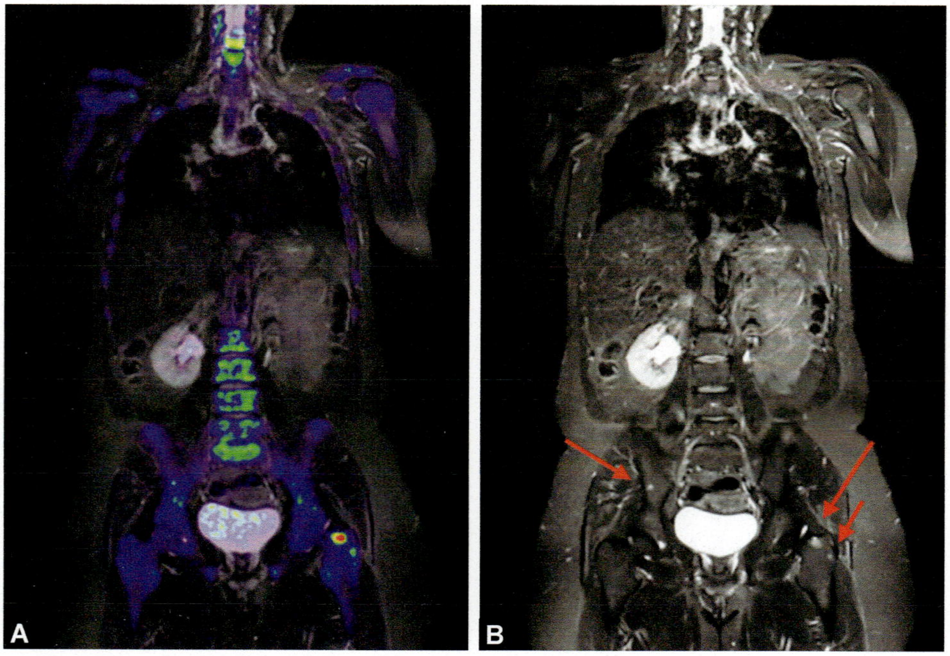

Figs. 3A and B: ^{18}F-NaF PET-MRI. (A) fused PET-MRI (coronal). (B) MRI coronal STIR.

CASE 8: ASSESSMENT OF BIOLOGIC THERAPY RESPONSE IN RHEUMATOID ARTHRITIS

Brief History

A 49-year-old female with established antinuclear antibody-positive erosive rheumatoid arthritis (RA) and osteoarthritis (OA) of the carpometacarpal (CMC) joint of the thumb. Physical examination for this patient revealed swelling and synovitis of the right wrist, and diminished range-of-motion. Radiographs and conventional contrast-enhanced MRI showed erosive changes at multiple carpal bones including the capitate, triquetrum, lunate, hamate, and scaphoid and bone marrow edema at multiple joints, consistent with RA, and CMC joint space narrowing with osteophyte formation and subchondral sclerosis, consistent with OA. The patient had failed conventional methotrexate therapy and was a candidate for receiving a tumor-necrosis-factor-alpha (TNF-α) inhibitor. The patient was imaged using the UC Davis high-resolution extremity PET/CT at 2 time points; baseline before starting TNF-α therapy and 5 weeks after initiation of TNF-α therapy.

Findings

From the baseline image, bone erosions are visualized on CT while synovitis is visualized as increased FDG uptake on PET (blue arrows). This follows the classic pattern of RA. In addition, palmar muscle FDG uptake is seen, together with increased uptake at the CMC joint indicative of OA (green arrow). "Netting" structures seen on CT are caused by attenuation from the thermoplastic hand immobilization device used (Fig. 1).

Longitudinal follow-up at the 5-week post therapy-initiation time-point showed a reduction in PET uptake associated with RA (blue arrows) while statistically insignificant change occurred in PET uptake due to OA (green arrow). The patient was determined to be a clinical responder based on a conventional rheumatologic examination that was conducted 3 months after the initiation of TNF-a inhibitor treatment (Fig. 2).

Main Teaching Point

- (1) Metabolic—hence inflammatory—activity associated of RA and OA can be detected by ^{18}F-FDG PET; (2) high-resolution PET imaging allows for radiotracer uptake at sites typically affected by RA to be measured separately from that at sites affected by OA; (3) High-resolution PET/CT may be useful for early monitoring of response to treatment; (4) OA with bone marrow edema shows increased ^{18}F-FDG uptake, and (5) thin-slice, isotropic-voxel anatomical imaging techniques have advantages for detecting erosive changes.

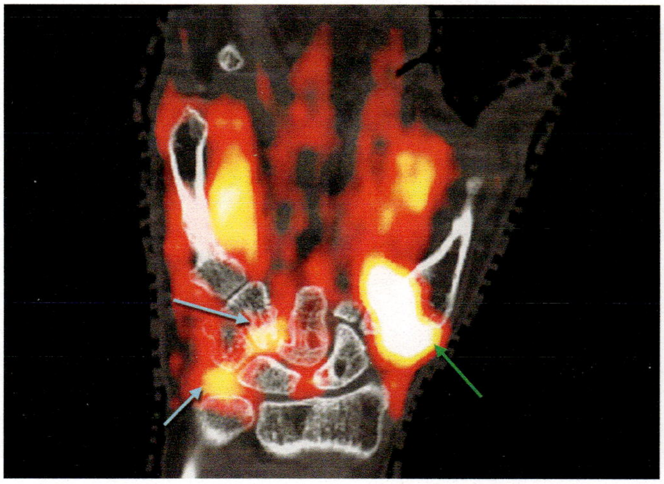

Fig. 1: ^{18}F-FDG high-resolution extremity PET/CT: Baseline high-resolution PET/CT.

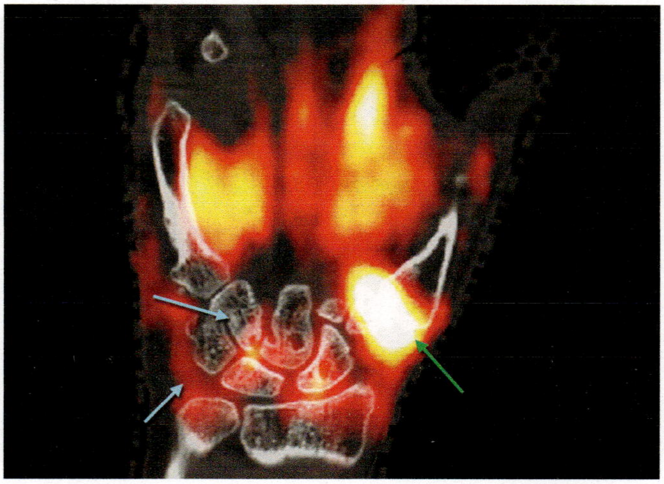

Fig. 2: ^{18}F-FDG high-resolution extremity PET/CT: Follow-up high-resolution PET/CT 5 weeks after initiation of TNF-a inhibitor therapy.

CASE 9: ASSESSMENT OF EARLY RESPONSE TO NEOADJUVANT CHEMOTHERAPY (NAC) IN BREAST CANCER

Brief History

A 46-year-old woman with a palpable mass of approximately 3 cm diameter in the right lower outer quadrant of the right breast based on physical examination, demonstrated on mammography as a lesion with architectural distortions and spiculation at the 8 o'clock position. Ultrasound-guided biopsy indicated infiltrating ductal carcinoma. The carcinoma was estrogen receptor (ER)-positive, progesterone receptor (PR)-negative and human epidermal growth factor receptor (HER2)-equivocal based on pathological analysis. The patient was a candidate for receiving NAC and eventual mastectomy, and was imaged using the UC Davis high-resolution extremity PET/CT at 3 time points; baseline before starting NAC, after 1 cycle of NAC (4 weeks from baseline) and after completion of NAC presurgery (27 weeks from baseline) but 2 days before mastectomy. The radiotracer ^{18}F-FDG was used.

Findings

From the baseline image (Fig. 1A), features consistent with results of mammography and ultrasound were visualized from PET/CT. The lesion showed an increased FDG uptake on PET (green arrows) as expected. After one cycle of NAC, a decrease of 26% compared to baseline was observed in the PET signal intensity from the lesion (Fig. 1B). At the end of NAC and 2 days before surgery, PET images indicated a decrease of 60% in signal intensity of the region of the tumor compared to baseline (Fig. 1C).

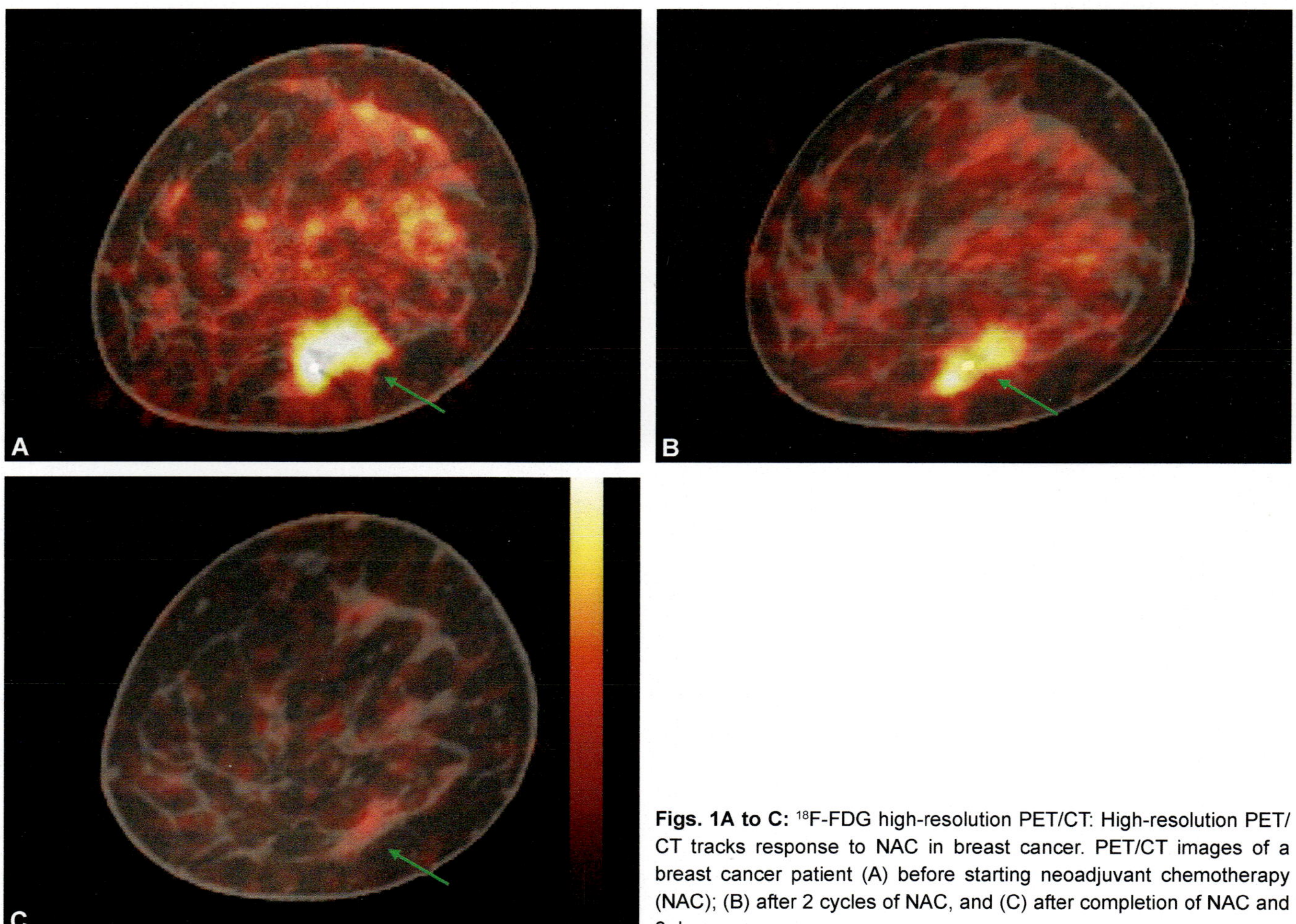

Figs. 1A to C: ^{18}F-FDG high-resolution PET/CT: High-resolution PET/CT tracks response to NAC in breast cancer. PET/CT images of a breast cancer patient (A) before starting neoadjuvant chemotherapy (NAC); (B) after 2 cycles of NAC, and (C) after completion of NAC and 2 days presurgery.

A decrease in the size of the lesion was also observed on both PET and CT. Pathological analysis of the resected breast postsurgery indicated that the patient was a partial responder to NAC. This assessment was not only consistent with the presurgery PET/CT results compared to baseline but also with those from PET/CT conducted after one cycle of NAC (Figs. 1A to C).

Main Teaching Points

- (1) Primary breast cancer lesions can be visualized by 18F-FDG PET/CT and be correlated with mammography and ultrasound; (2) high-resolution extremity PET imaging allows for radiotracer uptake for small breast lesions to be visualized; (3) high-resolution extremity PET/CT may be useful for early monitoring of response to NAC.

Index

Note: Page number followed by *f* indicates figures.

M

N

O

P

R